LAPAROSCOPY: NEW DEVELOPMENTS, PROCEDURES AND RISKS

SURGERY - PROCEDURES, COMPLICATIONS, AND RESULTS

SURGERY - PROCEDURES, COMPLICATIONS, AND RESULTS

LAPAROSCOPY: NEW DEVELOPMENTS, PROCEDURES AND RISKS

HANA TERZIĆ

EDITOR

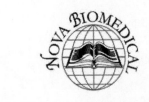

Nova Science Publishers, Inc.
New York

NOTICE TO THE READER

The Publisher has taken reasonable care in the preparation of this book, but makes no expressed or implied warranty of any kind and assumes no responsibility for any errors or omissions. No liability is assumed for incidental or consequential damages in connection with or arising out of information contained in this book. The Publisher shall not be liable for any special, consequential, or exemplary damages resulting, in whole or in part, from the readers' use of, or reliance upon, this material. Any parts of this book based on government reports are so indicated and copyright is claimed for those parts to the extent applicable to compilations of such works.

Independent verification should be sought for any data, advice or recommendations contained in this book. In addition, no responsibility is assumed by the publisher for any injury and/or damage to persons or property arising from any methods, products, instructions, ideas or otherwise contained in this publication.

This publication is designed to provide accurate and authoritative information with regard to the subject matter covered herein. It is sold with the clear understanding that the Publisher is not engaged in rendering legal or any other professional services. If legal or any other expert assistance is required, the services of a competent person should be sought. FROM A DECLARATION OF PARTICIPANTS JOINTLY ADOPTED BY A COMMITTEE OF THE AMERICAN BAR ASSOCIATION AND A COMMITTEE OF PUBLISHERS.

Additional color graphics may be available in the e-book version of this book.

Library of Congress Cataloging-in-Publication Data

Laparoscopy : new developments, procedures, and risks / editor, Hana Terzic.
      p. ; cm.
  Includes bibliographical references and index.
  ISBN 978-1-61470-747-9 (hardcover)
1. Laparoscopy. I. Terzic, Hana.
  [DNLM: 1. Laparoscopy--methods. 2. Risk Factors. WI 900]
  RG107.5.L34L37 2011
  617.5'507545--dc23
                              2011026733

Published by Nova Science Publishers, Inc. † New York

Contents

Preface

Laparoscopic surgery, also called minimally invasive surgery, is a modern surgical technique in which operations in the abdomen are performed through small incisions as compared to the larger incisions needed in laparotomy. In this book, the authors present current research from across the globe in the study of the procedures, risks and new developments in laparoscopy. Topics include laparoscopic reconstructive adnexal surgery; surgical treatment of deep endometriosis by laparoscopy; robotic assisted surgery and the challenges of laparoscopic rectal cancer surgery.

Chapter I - This chapter describes the current status of paediatric minimally invasive surgery, focusing on areas where innovation and expansion has occurred. Paediatric laparoscopy has benefited from improved instrumentation. In particular, the introduction of a range of 3mm instruments has allowed neonatal laparoscopy to advance. Gastrointestinal Surgery: The use of laparoscopy in the management of inguinal hernias in infants and children remains an area of debate. The advent of SILS and its application to appendicectomy and cholescystectomy is described. A discussion of the laparoscopic management of pyloric stenosis, duodenal atresia and web ablation is included. The value of laparoscopy in the management of Hirschsprung's disease and anorectal malformations is described. The use of single incision laparoscopic surgery (SILS) is increasing in pediatric practice: appendicectomy, cholecystectomy, pyloromyotomy and endorectal pull through have all been performed using this technique. Paediatric Urology: Access to the upper renal tracts may be obtained transperitoneally or retroperitoneally. The transabdominal route has been made more attractive by the potential of SILS. SILS nephrectromy is well described, and the author's recently performed a heminephrectomy using SILS access. Ureteric reimplantation has been refined by the transvesical approach using 3mm instruments, allowing this operation to be performed with minimal scarring. Thoracoscopy: The role of minimal access surgery in the thorax has expanded to include the resection of congenital lung lesions – employing partial and total lobectomy. Thoracoscopic repair of tracheoesophageal fistula with esophageal atresia and for H type fistula is becoming increasingly used as an alternative to open surgery. Thoracoscopy has also been employed for aortopexy. Congenital diaphragmatic hernia repairs are now commonly performed thoracoscopically; controversies exist around this area of work, particularly in relation to the high recurrence rate associated with the use of patch repair. The repair of pectus excavatum using a Nuss bar has been made safer by the introduction of thoracoscopy to guide the procedure. Oncological Surgery: Minimal access tehniques are firmly established in the diagnosis of childhood cancer, and are gradually gaining a foothold in curative resection. The evidence for these applications is reviewed. Conclusion: The frontiers of paediatric laparoscopy are expanding, with SILS further reducing the cosmetic impact of surgery in the abdomen and complex neonatal surgery being performed using a minimal access route with increasing frequency.

Chapter II - Robotic Surgery is a current procedure in endosurgery, but literature has not addressed the learning curve for the use of the robotic assisted surgery. The learning curve for robot surgical procedures varies widely. Apart from innate skill, learning curves are composed of at least two fundamentals related to the volume of cases and the incidence rate. Commonly cited reasons include lack of adequate training in residency programs because of the time devoted to abdominal, vaginal, and obstetric procedures, lack of available and adequate training opportunities outside of dedicated fellowships, lack of proctors and mentor surgeons in communities to help to further advance the skills of younger surgeons, and lack of desire to leave established surgical practices to try to develop skills requiring long learning curves to master. Currently, the training involves practice with the surgical robot in either pig or human fresh tissue in a laboratory environment in order to become familiar with the functions of the robot, the attachment of the robotic arms to the robotic trocars, and the overall functions of the robotic console. In this chapter authors reviewed current literature on learning curve in robotic assisted surgery and screened problems linked to robotic surgical skills.

Chapter III - Laparoscopy is the standard of treatment for many gynecological diseases, it is a very common procedure in gynaecology and it is widely accepted as the method of first choice for many gynaecological problems. A meta-analysis of 27 randomized controlled trials comparing laparoscopy and laparotomy for benign gynaecological procedures concluded that the risk of minor complications after gynaecological surgery is 40% lower with laparoscopy than with laparotomy, although the risk of major complications is similar. Laparoscopy has been considered a real alternative to laparotomy with numerous advantages: short hospital stay, less need of analgesia, low intraoperative blood loss and faster recovery time. Many researchers are in pursuit of new technologies and new tools of minimally invasive technologies for reducing laparoscopic complications. The industry responded to these demands with many innovations, such as new optical instruments and digital images, virtual and augmented reality, robotic assisted surgery, etc. In this chapter, authors discussed the possible utilization of novel technologies to reduce the risk of laparoscopic gynecological complications.

Chapter IV - Reconstructive gynecologic surgery is performed to treat the primary disease as well as refashion abnormal genital organs to restore anatomy and more importantly improve function. It leads to reduce potential problems and side effects from primary surgery and improve patients' quality of life. Early discharge within 24 hours after the procedure with an excellent outcome is a common sequel to reconstructive gynecologic surgery even if done via laparotomy [1]. Nevertheless, reconstructive surgery requires high level of expertise, delicate instruments, fine maneuvers, longer time, and fine energy modalities. Reconstructive gynecologic surgery is a broad term covering a lot of gynecologic subsepecielities e.g. urogynaecology [2], infertility [3], onocology [4], breast reconstruction [5] and pelvic floor dysfunction [6]. Laparoscopic approaches have been dramatically changed and in many cases replaced most of the traditional approaches. Thus, adding endoscopic approach to the principles of reconstruction is expected to achieve best results for the women's health.

Chapter V - Endometriosis is a gynecologic disorder defined by the presence of endometrial glands and stroma outside the uterus [1]. The most common site of endometriotic implants is the peritoneal cavity, but occasionally lesions have been found in the pleural cavity, liver, kidney, gluteal muscles, bladder, and even in men. The anatomical location and the inflammatory response to these injuries appear to be responsible for the signs and symptoms associated with endometriosis [2]. Macroscopically, pelvic endometriosis can be subdivided into three distinct entities [3,4]: superficial peritoneal (and ovarian) endometriosis, cystic ovarian endometriosis and deeply infiltrating endometriosis.

Chapter VI - This chapter fouses on the utilization of laparoscopic trainers and surgical virtual simulators, who provide deliberate practice, training, and assessment in a safe environment. Simulators range from simple task trainers to high-fidelity mock operating rooms, from organic to inorganic models. With the advent of laparoscopic surgery technical challenges raised, as altered depth perception, reduced tactile feedback, and the fulcrum effect. Thus surgical operations required a sophisticated level of practice, more than in open surgery. The laparoscopic box trainer was an early spark in the proliferation of depth and breadth in surgical skills training, now driven by forces including work-hour restrictions, patient safety concerns, financial cost of training, and emerging technology. Another help in surgical skills come from virtual reality, a computer simulation that enables users to perform operations on the system and shows effects in real time. Computerized simulators allow instant score reporting, feedback, and automated tutoring. Instruments' expensive cost is a major downside, but they really help young and skilled surgeons to trainee their daily work.

Chapter VII - This chapter highlights the present role of laparoscopy in colorectal cancer. There exists strong evidence supporting the use of laparoscopic approaches in the surgical treatment of colon cancer. Several randomised controlled trials comparing open and laparoscopic resection for colon cancer have confirmed the numerous short term advantages including reduced post-operative wound pain, fewer wound and pulmonary related complications, shorter hospitalization and a quicker return of bowel function without compromising the oncologic outcome and overall survival. Evidence for laparoscopic proctectomy is only now emerging from the results of ongoing trials. Laparoscopic resection for rectal cancer has not been met with the similar enthusiasm seen in colon cancer. This may be attributed to laparoscopic mesorectal excision being technically more challenging as evidenced by the high conversion rates reported in early studies. While these studies have demonstrated the similar short-term benefits seen in laparoscopic colectomy for colon cancers, trials are presently still being conducted to evaluate the long-term oncologic outcomes and survival. The COREAN trial has demonstrated similar short-term advantages whilst retaining the quality of oncological resection of laparoscopic proctectomy in mid and low rectal cancers. The outcomes of similar trials such as the ACOSOG Z6051 and the ALaCaRT will provide more concrete conclusions on the role of laparoscopic proctectomy for rectal cancer. There is emerging consensus on the various technical approaches to laparoscopic colonic mobilization, vessel ligation and creation of anastomoses, all of which aim to achieve comparable oncologic resections with the traditional open techniques. Conventional laparoscopic and hand-assisted laparoscopic techniques have been compared and evaluated extensively. Following the successful adoption of robotic technology in radical prostatectomy, robotic assisted laparoscopic colorectal surgery has seen increasing interest in an attempt to overcome the limitations of standard laparoscopy. The new technology provides a stable platform with three-dimensional visualization, endowrist range of movements with better manoeuvrability in confined spaces, and motion scaling for better precision in dissection. These advantages are most evident when performing mesorectal excision in the deeper confines of the pelvis. Early studies have shown robotic assisted total mesorectal excision to be associated with lower rates of positive resection margins and conversion. To achieve even better cosmetic outcomes, single port access surgery for colon cancer has begun to emerge with several case series reported in the literature. These procedures have been reported to be safe and feasible through a smaller incision without compromising the oncologic principles. Early surgeon-modified single incision devices have now been replaced by a number of commercially manufactured ones. Expert laparoscopists have begun to expand the role of the minimally invasive approach in non-elective situations. Recent reviews have proven the safety and feasibility of performing emergency laparoscopic surgery in well selected patients with obstructed or perforated colorectal cancers. In addition, certain conditions such as anastomotic dehiscence, adhesive small bowel obstruction and even reversal of Hartmann's procedures following prior surgery for colorectal cancer can also be treated using the laparoscopic approach. The field of laparoscopy in colorectal cancer continues to evolve and is likely to become an integral part in the management of colorectal cancer in the near future.

Chapter VIII - Splenectomy is performed for various conditions such as benign and malignant haematological diseases, secondary hypersplenism and trauma. The first laparoscopic splenectomy (LS) was reported in 1991 [1], and the advances in minimally invasive surgery have given surgeons the option to perform the LS safely in both children and adults. The current literature of comparative studies provide evidence that the laparoscopic approach to splenectomy offers advantages over open surgery in terms of reduced postoperative pain and complication rate, better cosmesis and shorter hospital stayas well as quicker recovery of gastrointestinal function [2-4] and reduced need for blood transfusion. Moreover, when quality of life was measured with the SF-36 survey, the laparoscopic approach to splenectomy was associated with better 'general health' and 'physical functioning' and lesser 'bodily pain' postoperatively compared to open surgery [5]. Although, the early experience with LS suggested that the laparoscopic approach was only safe for normal to mildly enlarged spleens, more recent evidence has shown the technique to be safe and beneficial in patients with massive and 'supramassive' (length >22cm and weight >1600g) spleen [6]. Additionally, the laparoscopic approach did not compromise the intraoperative assessment and detection of accessory spleen compared to open surgery [7]. In high volume centres, the laparoscopic approach to splenectomy was either of equal cost [2] or offered cost savings compared to open surgery [8]. As with any operative procedure, there are numerous considerations to be undertaken before performing this procedure and care should be taken when carrying it out on children and pregnant patients. Methods to search for the evasive splenunculi, pre-operatively, remain to be perfected and are yet to be vigorously tested and benefits of the radiological-guided splenic artery embolisation remains unclear. LS should be classified as the gold standard procedure and the open splenectomy should only be done if absolutely necessary.

Chapter IX - General surgery has advanced into a multitude of subspecialties over the last two decades including, but not limited to, colorectal and upper gastrointestinal (UGI). Advancements in surgical procedures in each field, specifically laparoscopic or minimally invasive surgery (MIS), have been partially responsible for this specialization. Minimally invasive surgery within each subspecialty has evolved and in many cases is advantageous or comparable to open surgery. The advantages of MIS can be demonstrated by improved recovery and subsequently shorter hospital stay following fundoplication or decreased blood loss following total mesorectal excision. As surgical procedures continue to progress in complexity, further advancements in surgical techniques are necessary to maintain safety and efficiency. Robotic-assisted surgical procedures may be the next evolution in minimally invasive surgery. With improved three-dimensional visualization and surgical instruments with seven degrees-of-freedom, robotic-assisted colorectal, UGI and biliary surgery has been shown to be safe and feasible in both comparative studies and case series. However, further studies are needed to define a clear patient benefit that justifies the increased operational impact and costs associated with robotic-assisted surgery in General Surgery.

Chapter X - Laparoscopic surgical resection has been universally accepted in the management of colon cancer since its inception in 1991 [1]. Laparoscopic surgery for colon cancer has been well proven by randomized studies to benefit patients; the procedure results in earlier recovery of bowel function, reduced blood loss, less postoperative pain, and decreased hospital stay compared with conventional open colectomy [2, 3]. Most of these studies have also shown adequate lymph node yields and tumor clearance in addition to the improved short-term outcomes in terms of reduced post operative pain, shorter hospital stay, reduced ileus and comparable long-term clinical outcomes. While the minimally invasive approach for colonic resections has become well established and accepted, its role in management of rectal cancer is evolving and remains contentious.

Chapter XI - Although still considered an experimental alternative to traditional and laparoscopic surgery, Natural Orifice Transluminal Endoscopic Surgery (NOTES) is quickly emerging as a new concept of minimally invasive surgery. The concept of NOTES advocates the lack of abdominal incisions and their related complications by combining endoscopic and laparoscopic techniques to diagnose and treat abdominal pathologies. Although still in its early days, NOTES is developing rapidly and is attracting a considerable interest from the surgical communities in all specialties. In much the same way as laparoscopy was originally developed, NOTES defies conventional surgical practices and has been the subject of understandable scepticism. The registered base of research in humans is still scarce; however, the porcine model experimental studies hold great promise. In this work, we explore the concept of NOTES from a gynaecological oncologist's perspective, highlighting its potential use in the field of gynaecological oncology and sentinel lymph nodes detection.

Chapter XII - The advantages of operative laparoscopy include small incisions, less postoperative pain, short hospital stay, earlier recovery and improved quality of life during the postoperative period. Different techniques have been described to facilitate the retrieval of excised masses without needing to enlarge the abdominal incision. Specimen extraction in laparoscopic surgery is more time consuming than open procedures and tissue removal must be performed in an expeditious manner if the cost-effectiveness of the technique is to be maintained. The authors review the various routes for the retrieval of benign specimens following laparoscopic excision and discuss associate risks and factors, which will influence the optimal choice of route. These routes include retrieval via the trocar using an endobag, morcellation, posterior colpotomy and mini-laparotomy. Natural Orifice Transluminal Endoscopy (NOTES) may be the operative and retrieval route of the future, is also briefly discussed.

Chapter XIII - The aetiological assessment of an infertile couple includes several complementary biological and morphological examinations. Initial exploration of the female genital tract requires the performance of pelvic ultrasound and hysterosalpingography. Some medical teams perform hysteroscopy on an outpatient basis prior to the initiation of any therapeutic measures. The value of systematic laparoscopy in infertility assessment is still subject to debate. After having been systematically employed in the 1970s and 1980s, laparoscopy was progressively abandoned as part of the initial infertility assessment over the following 20 years. However, systematic use of this technique has been suggested again in recent years - notably in view of the restriction of the number of in vitro fertilization (IVF) attempts to four per couple in France. The aim of the present review is to evaluate arguments against the systematic use of laparoscopy and to try to draw up recommendations for practice.

Chapter XIV - Introduction. A second operation after an unsuccessful antireflux surgery is a challenge for the esophago-gastric surgeon. A second laparoscopic access to the hiatus is usually technically demanding, as adherences of the previous operation generally complicate the identification of the anatomic structures. Inadvertent damage to abdominal or thoracic viscera is easier to perform. Besides, a functional satisfactory result is more difficult to achieve. In this setting, a thorough anatomic and functional study should be carried out for every patient to calibrate the possible benefits of a potential second operation with the risk of a revisional surgery, given that medical therapy is also available even for resistant cases. In the present work we report our last 10-year experience in the diagnostic workup and treatment of antireflux surgery failure, and we discuss the most convenient way to approach a revisional operation. Patients and method. From January 2001 to December 2010, 39 consecutive patients have been evaluated in our department for a failure of a previous antireflux operation. Patients were usually referred for a maintenance or recurrence of preoperative symptoms, and occasionally for the appearance of new symptoms after the operation. A diagnostic workup was carried out comprising a personal interview, functional tests including pHmetry and manometry, and recently high resolution manometry and impedanciometry, endoscopy, a barium swallow X-ray study and in the past two years a computed tomography (CT) with 3d reconstruction. Patients were classified according to the different mechanisms of failure into: a) fundoplication disruption, b) fundoplication slippage, c) fundoplication migration to the thorax or type I hiatal hernia, d) paraesophageal herniation, d) twisted fundoplication, e) misdiagnosis, f) mixed failure and e) another non-previously classified failure including a finally unidentified cause of failure. Results. Thirty-nine patients with failure of a first fundoplication were evaluated, 24 women and 15 men, with a mean age of 49 years at the first operation. Gastroesophageal reflux was the indication for surgery in 82% of the patients, and hiatal hernia with no evidence of reflux in the other 5. Globally, some kind of hiatal hernia was present in 22 patients, 80% of them a type I hernia; a giant hernia with an intrathoracic stomach was present in 7 patients. Seventeen patients had a histologically proven Barrett's esophagus, in 4 cases submitted previously to argon or radiofrequency ablation. Most first operations consisted on a standard calibrated Nissen laparoscopic fundoplication. The mean time for symptoms recurrence was 31 months. The first symptom of recurrence was mostly heartburn, followed by dysphagia. Thirty-four patients have been submitted to a second operation. The most frequent diagnosis was fundoplication disruption (10 cases), followed by migration of the fundoplication to the thorax (9 cases) and paraesophageal hernia (8 patients). Reoperations consisted mostly on fundoplication "redo" (21patients) and mesh hiatoplasty (17 cases). Ten patients have documented recurrence after the second operation (29%), with 6 patients being submitted to a third operation (17.6%). Conclusions. Revisional surgery of the hiatus is indicated mainly for failure to control gastroesophageal reflux or for thoracic ascension either of a part of the stomach or of the first fundoplication. Recurrence after a revisional surgery presents in one-quarter of the re-operated patients. A complete diagnostic workup and a meticulous operation are mandatory to reduce the recurrence rate, given that a third operation carries out a high risk of esophagectomy.

Chapter XV - The incidence of abdominal injury in all traumas is 1.5 to 18% and follows a pattern of continuous increase globally. Blunt abdominal injuries are usually associated with serious complications and a high mortality of 25 to 65% as a result of difficulty in prompt diagnosis and management, and are frequently associated with other types of injuries. Diagnostic peritoneal lavage, ultrasonography, abdominal radiographs, and computed tomography are commonly used for triage of patients with abdominal trauma. The listed diagnostic modalities are commonly used in hemodynamically stable patients with abdominal trauma as a means of diagnostic procedure and decision making for conservative or operative management. Some of the investigations are found to be unnecessary as the victims are hemodynamically unstable and require immediate operation. The time taken for triage using these methods sometime causes delay and leads to serious complications and even death due to inappropriate management in 17% of cases.

In: Laparoscopy: New Developments, Procedures and Risks   ISBN: 978-1-61470-747-9
Editor: Hana Terzic, pp. 1-41   © 2012 Nova Science Publishers, Inc.

Chapter I

Paediatric Laparoscopy: New Developments Procedures and Risks

Simon C. Blackburn and Anies A. Mahomed
Royal Alexandra Childrens' Hospital, Brighton, UK.

Abstract

This chapter describes the current status of paediatric minimally invasive surgery, focusing on areas where innovation and expansion has occurred. Paediatric laparoscopy has benefited from improved instrumentation. In particular, the introduction of a range of 3mm instruments has allowed neonatal laparoscopy to advance.

Gastrointestinal Surgery: The use of laparoscopy in the management of inguinal hernias in infants and children remains an area of debate. The advent of SILS and its application to appendicectomy and cholescystectomy is described. A discussion of the laparoscopic management of pyloric stenosis, duodenal atresia and web ablation is included. The value of laparoscopy in the management of Hirschsprung's disease and anorectal malformations is described. The use of single incision laparoscopic surgery (SILS) is increasing in pediatric practice: appendicectomy, cholecystectomy, pyloromyotomy and endorectal pull through have all been performed using this technique.

Paediatric Urology: Access to the upper renal tracts may be obtained transperitoneally or retroperitoneally. The transabdominal route has been made more attractive by the potential of SILS. SILS nephrectromy is well described, and the author's recently performed a heminephrectomy using SILS access.

Ureteric reimplantation has been refined by the transvesical approach using 3mm instruments, allowing this operation to be performed with minimal scarring.

Thoracoscopy: The role of minimal access surgery in the thorax has expanded to include the resection of congenital lung lesions – employing partial and total lobectomy.

Thoracoscopic repair of tracheoesophageal fistula with esophageal atresia and for H type fistula is becoming increasingly used as an alternative to open surgery. Thoracoscopy has also been employed for aortopexy.

Congenital diaphragmatic hernia repairs are now commonly performed thoracoscopically; controversies exist around this area of work, particularly in relation to the high recurrence rate associated with the use of patch repair.

The repair of pectus excavatum using a Nuss bar has been made safer by the introduction of thoracoscopy to guide the procedure.

Oncological Surgery: Minimal access tehniques are firmly established in the diagnosis of childhood cancer, and are gradually gaining a foothold in curative resection. The evidence for these applications is reviewed.

Conclusion: The frontiers of paediatric laparoscopy are expanding, with SILS further reducing the cosmetic impact of surgery in the abdomen and complex neonatal surgery being performed using a minimal access route with increasing frequency.

Introduction

Minimal access techniques are evolving rapidly in paediatric surgery. Technology has facilitated the application of laparoscopy and thoracoscopy to small infants, via the availability of 3mm instruments and improved optics, making complex procedures possible even using a 5mm laparoscope.

The advent of single incision laparoscopic surgery (SILS) has the potential to shift the paradigm once again, further minimising the size of the incision required to perform complex surgery in children.

This chapter describes the advances in minimal access surgery in children: gastrointestinal surgery, urology, thoracoscopy and oncology will be considered, and the role of SILS described.

Gastrointestinal Surgery

Introduction

The use of minimal access surgery has changed the landscape of abdominal surgery in children; most major abdominal procedures can now be performed using minimal access techniques. This section will address the laparoscopic approach to inguinal hernia, pyloric stenosis, duodenal atresia and duodenal web, Hirschsprung's disease and anorectal malformations. The role of single incision laparoscopic surgery (SILS) in paediatric practice will then be discussed.

Inguinal Hernia

The repair of inguinal hernias is one of the most commonly performed procedures in paediatric surgery. The technique of open inguinal herniotomy is firmly established and has a very low complication rate in expert hands. To justify changing this technique, therefore, minimal access surgery must demonstrate a similarly low rate of complications and an improvement in outcomes.

The potential advantages of laparoscopy are improved cosmesis and the identification of a contralateral patent processus vaginalis, eliminating the risk of a metachronous contralateral hernia, which has an incidence of 6.4 to 7.2% overall [1] [2].

Proponents of minimal access surgery argue that this risk can be eliminated by laparoscopy, without the need for potentially destructive dissection of the contralateral groin.

Technique

A large number of minimal access techniques for pediatric inguinal hernia repair have been described [3]. The simplest modification is the examination of the contralateral deep ring at an open repair, which can be achieved by passing a laparoscope, typically 70°-120°, through the opened hernia sac into the abdomen. This technique has been shown to identify contralateral patency in 13% of patients [4].

Hernia repair can be accomplished laparoscopically without the need for a groin incision. This can be achieved transperitoneally or extraperitoneally [3][5]. In transperitoneal repair, the suture is used to close the deep ring in a purse string or Z type configuration. This closure can be reinforced by using a peritoneal flap to cover the deep ring, or by suturing the medial or lateral umbilical ligaments over the repair [6]. This repair is technically demanding, particularly when the operation is performed in neonates, as it requires tying a secure intracorporeal knot in a small working space.

In female patients, where damage to the testicular vessels and vas deferens is not a concern, the hernia sac can simply be inverted into the abdomen and controlled with an endoloop[7].

The extraperitoneal technique involves passing a hook loaded with suture around the deep ring, ensuring the avoidance of the vas deferens and testicular vessels by using a laparoscope placed at the umbilicus. The suture is then tied extracorporeally, closing the deep ring. This technique has the advantage of being less technically demanding.

Outcomes

Chan et al performed a randomised single blind study, comparing intracorporeal laparoscopic repair with open surgery, in 2005[8]. Forty two patients underwent open repair and 41 patients underwent laparoscopic repair. In the open series, 12.5% of patients had a metachronous hernia. There was a 33% rate of contralateral patency at laparoscopy. The laparoscopic approach was associated with less pain, faster recovery and improved cosmesis.

Koivusalo et al performed a randomised study on 89 patients, randomising 42 patients to laparoscopic repair [9]. This study was weighted to assess the time taken for patients to return to normal activity. Patients undergoing laparoscopic repair had an increased need for analgesia and longer operations (33 v 15 minutes). 2 patients undergoing laparoscopic repair and 1 undergoing open repair had a recurrence. Time to normal activity was similar.

Shier et all performed a large study in three centres, reporting 666 children with 933 hernia defects [10]. The mean operative time was 16 minutes for unilateral hernias and 23 minutes for bilateral hernias. There was 3.1% recurrence rate. Contralateral patency of the processus vaginalis was identified in 23% of boys and 15% of girls.

A recent paper by Chen et al compared two intracorporeal techniques: simple suture of the internal ring and suture of the internal ring with reinforcement using the medial or lateral umbilical ligament, with 214 patients in each group [6]. This study demonstrated a decrease from 4.8% recurrence to 0% recurrence with this change in technique.

The laparoscopic approach to inguinal hernias is most demanding in infants. Esposito et al recently described a series of transperitoneal repairs in 50 children under 1 year of age. One recurrence occurred in this series [11]. Turial et al reported a series of 147 infants in 2010, with a 2% recurrence rate. 4% of patients in this series required a subsequent orchidopexy [12].

The laparoscopic approach to inguinal hernia repair in children offers several advantages over the open approach. Superior cosmesis is certainly possible, although many would argue that the small groin incision associated with open hernia repair is not unsightly. The laparoscopic approach offers good visualisation of the bowel in an incarcerated hernia, reducing the possibility of reduction of necrotic bowel without it being identified. The management of recurrences is also more simple, they can either be approached in an open manner through an undisturbed groin, or the hernia repair can simply be repeated laparoscopically. The laparoscopic approach can also be used to identify femoral hernias, which are poorly diagnosed at open operation and have a high recurrence rate [13].

There are, however, concerns that the recurrence rate for laparoscopic hernia is higher than the less than 1% rate for standard open hernia repair in children [14], although the laparoscopic repair competes well with the higher recurrence rate associated with open repairs in neonates, typically 11-15% [15] [16]. Additionally, the high rate of surgery for a contralateral patent processus vaginalis, typically around 30% [4] [8] [10], is substantially higher than the 7% rate of metachronous hernia [1], leading some to argue that the laparoscopic approach exposes many children to unnecessary contralateral surgery, with the accompanying risk of damage to the vas deferens and testicular vessels.

Pyloric Stenosis

Pyloric stenosis is one of the most commonly treated surgical conditions of infancy. The operation of pyloromyotomy was described by Ramstedt in 1912 [17]. This operation has stood the test of time, but the operative approach to exposing the pylorus in order to perform the myotomy has evolved. The original midline laparotomy was replaced by a right upper quadrant transverse incision, which has been superseded in most centres by a cosmetically superior incision through the umbilicus [18]. More recently the laparoscopic approach has once again shifted the paradigm. Although the difference in cosmetic result is arguably small, surveys have indicated a strong parental preference for the reduced scarring associated with laparoscopic pyloromyotomy [19].

Technique

The most commonly used technique is that described by Najmaldin and Tan [20]. A 5mm port is placed at the umbilicus and a pneumoperitoneum established, to a maximum insufflation pressure of 10mmHg. Three millimeter working instruments are then introduced directly through the abdominal wall. Either the stomach or the duodenum is held with a laparoscopic grasper, and a myotomy is performed either with an endotome or hook diathermy. One the muscle has been incised, the pyloromyotomy is spread using a second laparoscopic grasper. A specialist laparoscopic spreader is available for this purpose (Karl Storz). Once the myotomy is completed, air is insufflated and the mucosa inspected to ensure no perforation has occurred. The instruments are then removed and the incisions closed.

Outcomes

Laparoscopic pyloromyotomy is one of the few treatments in paediatric surgery that has been subjected to rigorously conducted randomised controlled trials.

In an early meta-analysis Hall et all raised concerns that the rate of complication after laparoscopic pyloromyotomy might be higher than that associated with an open operation [21]. Their analysis of 8 studies demonstrated a higher rate of mucosal perforation and incomplete myotomy in patients undergoing laparoscopic pyloromyotomy.

These concerns were mirrored in a single centre prospective randomised trial, in which 183 infants were subjected to either an open or laparoscopic pyloromyotomy [22]. This study demonstrated that infants undergoing laparoscopic pyloromyotomy had a longer operation and a higher incidence of incomplete myotomy (3 v 0).

These conclusions have, however, been refuted by two other studies. The first is a single centre, prospective, randomised study of 200 infants, which showed no difference in operating time between the two techniques [23]. Length of stay and time to full feeds were the same in both groups. The patients undergoing laparoscopic pyloromyotomy had less pain and emesis.

The second is a 6 centre double blind randomised controlled trial in which 180 infants were recruited [24]. Parents and staff were blinded to the procedure performed by the use of standardised dressings. A standardised feeding protocol was used to compare patients. This study demonstrated no increase in complication rate with laparoscopic pyloromyotomy, and showed that infants undergoing laparoscopic pyloromyotomy gained full feeds significantly sooner, and went home significantly earlier, than those undergoing open surgery.

There is, therefore, good evidence to show that the laparoscopic approach to pyloromyotomy is as safe as, and in some respects superior to, the open approach.

Duodenal Atresia

The repair of duodenal atresia involves a technically challenging anastomosis between a dilated proximal segment, and a collapsed segment distal to the atresia. This operation has, however, been described laparoscopically.

Technique

A 4mm port is placed at the umbilicus with a 3mm port in the right lower quadrant and a 5mm port in the left upper quadrant [25]. The surgeon stands at the patient's feet. The duodenum is exposed by mobilising the ascending colon medially and the atresia is identified. Once a duodenotomy has been made proximal and distal to the atresia, the anastomosis is completed in a "diamond" fashion. This can be accomplished using either a running or interrupted suture with vicryl or PDS [26] [27]. Intracorporeal knots are used. The anastomosis can be facilitated by bringing the apical stitch out through the abdominal wall

[27]. Other authors have described the use of "U clips", originally designed for vascular anastomoses, to perform the anastomosis [26] [28].

Repair of a duodenal web may also be accomplished laparoscopically, using a 3 port technique [30](Figures 1 and 2).

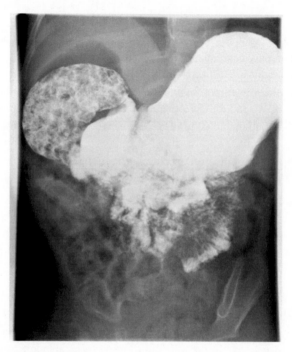

Figure 1. Upper GI contrast study in a two-year-old patient, demonstrating proximal duodenomegaly with food retention secondary to a web in the second part.

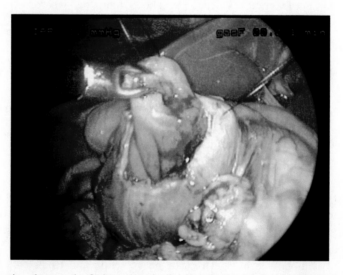

Figure 2. Intraoperative photograph of a laparoscopic division of a duodenal web via a duodenotomy.

A duodenotomy is performed between stay sutures and the web everted through it. The web may then be held in position by means of a stay suture. Once the ampulla of Vater has been identified, the web is excised. The duodenotomy is then closed in the same line as it is opened, using intracorporeal sutures.

Outcomes

Kay et al recently reported a series of 19 cases of congenital duodenal obstruction, in whom laparoscopic repair was completed successfully in 17 [27]. These infants underwent surgery at a mean age of 5 days. There were no anastomotic leaks or missed distal obstructions, secondary to further atresias, in this series. The infants reached full feeds at an average of 12 days.

This positive report was mirrored by a series in which U clips were used, where patients undergoing laparoscopic repair of duodenal atresia were shown to be faster in regaining full feeds and to require shorter periods of hospitalisation [28].

Anorectal Anomaly

The repair of high anorectal anomalies has traditionally required the use of an open laparotomy and a perineal dissection. Lower anomalies can be repaired via a posterior sagittal anorectoplatsty (PSARP), which requires dissection via the perineum to divide the fistula almost invariably associated with this anomaly. Minimal access surgery has been used to reduce the morbidity associated with an abdominal incision, and to minimise the perineal dissection required.

Technique

The technique of laparoscopic assisted anorectal pull through (LAARP) was described by Georgeson [30]. The abdomen is insufflated using a Veres needle placed to the right of the umbilicus, and a 4mm trocar placed at this site. Two addition trocars are then placed 2cm superior to the umbilicus and 2cm to its left. A 5mm trocar is placed in the left hypogastrium.

The peritoneal reflection is dissected and the distal mesorectum divided. The associated fistula between the rectum and the urinary tract is then identified. This may simply be divided [31] or controlled with a suture or linear stapler [32]. It has been suggested that submuscosal dissection commencing approximately 1 inch proximal to the fistula site may prevent the formation of a diverticulum at the fistula site [33].

As the dissection proceeds the pubococcygeus muscle is identified. At this point electrostimulation is used externally at the perineum to map the position of the external anal sphincter. A track is then created using a Veres needle passed from the perineum to the pelvis. A radially expanding trocar is then employed to dilate this track and the rectal fistula pulled through to the perineum, before an anorectal anastomosis is performed.

The advantage of this technique is that a high anorectal anomaly can be managed with minimal perineal dissection, without division of the levator complex from below. The visualisation achieved with the laparoscope also allows very precise mapping of the pelvic musculature. Creating a track with a Veres needle allows precise placement before it is dilated.

Outcomes

The literature on laparoscopic assisted correction of anorectal anomalies was recently subjected to systematic review [34]. This was limited by its retrospective nature and the heterogeneous nature of the results reported. A total of 124 patients were reported of whom 77.4% were male. 88.7% of patients had a colostomy at the time of definitive surgery, the remainder had a primary pull through. This review concluded that there is an urgent need for randomised studies to compare the LAARP to more established techniques.

Several non-randomised studies have compared outcomes from LAARP to PSARP. Lin et al compared anorectal manometry in 9 patients who had undergone LAARP with 13 who had undergone PSAARP, demonstrating more favourable anorectal manometry in the LAARP group [35]. An MRI study comparing LAARP and PSARP has shown better anatomical reconstruction when LAARP is used, although the functional consequences of this are not clear [36]. Other studies have suggested that continence following LAARP is as good as [37], or better than [38] PSARP.

This area of practice would benefit from a properly constructed randomised controlled trial, although this would take some time to demonstrate a difference as the outcomes in terms of long term continence would take some years to become apparent.

Hirschsprung's Disease

The management of Hirschsprung's disease necessitates removal of the aganglionic segment of bowel, followed by an anastomosis of ganglionic colon to the aganglionic rectum. Minimal access surgery has made a contribution to the evolution of the endorectal pull through (Soave) operation, the Duhamel and Swenson pull through, and the former two will be described.

Laparoscopic Assisted Endorectal Pull Through

This technique requires a similar setup to that described for the LAARP. Once access to the abdominal cavity has been gained, the colon is assessed and seromuscular biopsies taken above the transition zone. These biopsies are then sent for histology, and no further dissection is performed until it is established that the site for proposed pull through is ganglionic.

Once this step is complete, the mesentery of the aganglionic segment is divided with the monopolar hook or a harmonic scalpel, maintaining dissection close to the bowel wall to avoid the risk of injury to nearby structures. Once this dissection reaches the level of the pelvic floor the operation is completed via the perineum. A submucosal plane is created transanally, the anus first having been everted with stay sutures. This allows the resection specimen to be removed through the anus. Once the level of resection has been reached the bowel is divided. A posterior internal anal spinchterotomy is then performed.

Adequate position of the pull through is then confirmed with laparoscopy.

The advantages of this technique, apart from those associated with avoiding a laparotomy, are that the visualisation of the bowel and operative result are excellent, seromuscular biopsies can be taken intraoperatively without the need for an open incision and that the mesocolon can be divided intraabdominally, making the transanal portion of the operation much easier [39].

Outcomes

Georgeson reported an early series of 80 patients in 1999 [40]. Eighty patients underwent laparoscopic assisted endorectal pull through, of whom 86% had a transition zone in the sigmoid colon or rectum. The mean operative time was 147 minutes. Full feeds were achieved at a mean of 28 hours post operatively. There were 2 anastomotic leaks, and 2 conversions to open surgery. Six patients suffered with enterocolitis post operatively, 6 had chronic diarrhoea and 1 patient had recurrent constipation.

This encouraging early series has been followed by more recent comparative studies. Cragie et al compared 20 laparoscopic assisted endorectal pull throughs to 22 open operations, showing similar operative times and length of stay [41]. Fujiwara et al assessed continence 7 years after pull through and showed a tendency towards better continence following laparoscopic assisted surgery, although this was not statistically significant [42]. 54% of patients in this series had moderate to severe incontinence, compared to 23% of those undergoing laparoscopic surgery. Mattioli et al mirrored these findings, demonstrating similar complication rates and continence rates in patients undergoing laparoscopic repair [43].

Laparoscopic Assisted Duhamel Pull Through

Bax et al described the technique of lap assisted Duhamel pull through in 1995 [44]. A primary port is placed and ports are added halfway between the ziphoid and umbilicus, and pararectally at the level of the umbilicus. Extramucosal biopsies are taken to confirm the proposed level of pull through is ganglionic. Dissection is continued to the pelvic floor and the rectum is divided with an endo GIA stapler (Figure 3). An incision is made in the posterior rectum transanally and the bowel pulled through. A transanal anastomosis is completed between the ganglionic colon and native rectum. The spur superior to the site of the anastomosis is then obliterated using a stapler passed from below.

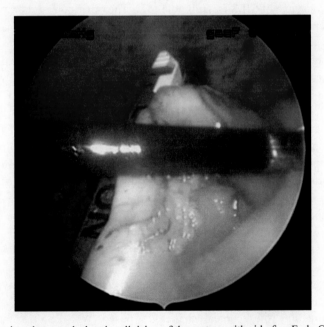

Figure 3. Intra-operative photograph showing division of the rectum with aid of an Endo GIA stapler.

Outcomes

Travassos et al compared 62 open to 55 laparoscopic assisted Duhamel pull throughs in 2007 [45]. They demonstrated a shorter hospital stay and time to full feeds, with no difference in complication rate. These authors did however caution that this operation is technically demanding, with accounts for the longer operating time observed in this series.

SILS

Muensterer et al recently described a SILS approach to laparoscopic assisted endorectal pull through, describing its use in 6 patients [46]. 2 4mm trocars are placed in the periumbilical fascia through the same umbilical skin incision. A grasper is placed through a simple stab incision. Levelling biopsies are taken using a similar technique to that described for open surgery. The colonic dissection is then achieved using electrocautery.

SILS

Single incision laparoscopic surgery (SILS) has become established in recent paediatric practice. In the hands of experienced minimal access surgeons SILS has the advantage of limiting the number of visible incisions, potentially decreasing trauma to the abdominal wall and also has the potential to lead to shortened hospital stay and faster recovery [47]. Another potential advantage of SILS is that it utilises a skills set which surgeons performing paediatric laparoscopy already possess. This is in contrast to NOTES, which requires an entirely different set of skills.

There are potential disadvantages, however. Some authors argue that scars from smaller laparoscopic instruments, particularly 3mm instruments in babies, heal almost invisibly and so the cosmetic advantage of SILS is negligible [47]. The other potential drawback of SILS is that the more extensive dissection required to gain access to the abdominal cavity may lead to increased post operative pain.

A variety of techniques have been described to access the abdomen in children. The same proprietary devices as are used in adult practice can be applied to paediatric patients. The Covidien SILS port (Covidien, Dublin Ireland), Advanced Surgical Concepts Triport (Advanced Surgical Concepts, Bray, Ireland) and the Uni-X device (Pnavel Systems, Brooklyn, NY) have all been used in children [49]. The disadvantage of these devices in smaller children and infants is that they require a minimum incision of 20mm to be inserted, which is not a length of scar which can be hidden in a small umbilicus [46]. One potential solution to this problem is to dissect the fascia around an umbilical incision and then place separate ports through the abdominal wall at different sites, thus facilitating the placement of the laparoscope and instruments without the need for a specialised insertion device [46] [47] [50] [51].

There are a variety of instruments being developed to increase the triangulation that can be achieved with a SILS approach. The Realhand (Novare Surgical Systems, Cupertino, CA) system is one example. It is, however, possible to perform SILS surgery using standard laparoscopic instruments [50] [52].

There are a number of technical challenges posed by SILS, particularly when the technique is "downsized" to the paediatric abdomen. The small size of the paediatric umbilicus has already been mentioned. There are currently no proprietary access devices small enough to be used in a small umbilicus. Foam based devices, such as the SILS port (Covidien, Dublin, Ireland) can be trimmed to fit through a smaller facial defect [49]. If separate incisions in the fascia are made, then the closure of an open umbilical ring may increase the fascia available to place additional trocars [49]. Trocar crowding, and instrument clashing are, once again, more of a challenge when confronted in a smaller working space. A 45° endoscope, varying instrument grips, different instrument lengths and an in-line camera and light cord can help to overcome these problems.

One of the major limitations of SILS in current practice is the difficulty in tying intracorporeal knots posed by the lack of triangulation. This can be overcome by the use of extracorporeal knots and knot pusher, but this difficulty is likely to limit the application of SILS in complex reconstructive operations until technology develops sufficiently to facilitate this.

The have been an increasing number of reports of SILS procedures in the paediatric population in recent years. Dutta reported a series of 20 procedures in 2009, including splenectomy, cholecystomy and appendicectomy. Realhand instruments (Novasurgical, Cupertino, California) where employed in this series, together with a 2.5 cm umbilical incision, similar results were achieved to conventional laparoscopic cases [53]. In the same year Rothenberg described the use of an umbilical laparoscope to perform cholecystectomy, appendicectomy and adhesiolysis with the addition of a single additional 3mm port [50].

In a large series published in 2010 Hansen at all describe an accumulated series of 224 patients undergoing SILS procedures. This series includes 130 appendectomies, 32 pyloromyotomies, 32 cholecystectomies, 11 inguinal hernias, 6 fundoplications and 4 SILS assisted endorectal pull through procedures [49].

Some consideration will know be given to individual SILS procedures.

SILS Appendicectomy

Technique

Abdominal access is gained via an umbilical incision, typically in a "yin-yan" configuration. Access to the abdomen can be gained either by use of a SILS port [54] or by dissecting the periumbilical fascia and placing instruments through fascial stab incisions [51]. The appendix is then identified and mobilised using hook diathermy. The mesoappendix is taken down with diathermy or a stapler and the appendix divided with a stapling device. The appendix is removed using a retrieval bag.

Outcomes

Chandler et al performed a retrospective comparison of 50 single port appendicectomies with 46 open controls in 2010 [54]. Perforated appendices were excluded from analysis. This study demonstrated a comparable length of stay, but a longer operative time for the SILS procedures (33.8 v 26.8 minutes). Muensterer et al report a series of 75 patients managed with SILS appendicectomy; 50 of these patients had acute appendicitis, 16 perforated appendicitis and 9 were undergoing interval appendicectomy. The mean operating time in this series was 40 minutes, which is faster than the same authors' laparoscopic experience. 20% of patients in this study required an additional trochar for safe completion of the procedure [51]. Oltman reviewed 39 patients who had appendicectomy, 19 of whom had had a SILS approach [55]. There were 2 conversions to conventional laparoscopy in the SILS group. Longer operative times were again observed.

SILS Cholecystectomy

Technique
Abdominal access is gained via the umbilicus. The dissection is aided by placing a transabdominal suture through the fundus of the gallbladder, which allows Callot's triangle to be visualised without the use of a further laparoscopic port [53] [56]. This procedure has been achieved using standard laparoscopic instruments [56], although articulated graspers are thought to be helpful by some authors [53]. The gallbladder is removed through the umbilical incision with or without the aid of a retrieval bag.

Outcomes
Emani et al recently published a series of 25 pediatric cholecystectomies performed by SILS [56]. 2 patients required an additional port to accomplish the procedure. The SILS approach was associated with a longer operative time than the open procedure. Length of stay was similar.

SILS Pyloromyotomy
The SILS approach to pyloromyotomy has been described [50][57]. Muensterer recently reported a series of 15 cases in which 2 mucosal perforations occurred [50]. This technique is in its infancy and is associated with a higher complication rate than the laparoscopic approach. The cosmetic benefit of a larger umbilical incision in exchange for saving two 3mm abdominal scars, which heal almost invisibly in most infants, is also questionable [49].

SILS Splenectomy
Splenectomy using SILS has been described [53]. The gastrosplenic ligament is divided with a thermaseal device. The splenic hilum can then be divided using a roticulating stapler. The spleen is placed in an endobag and morcilated before being removed through the umbilical incision.

Minimally Invasive Paediatric Urology

Introduction

The use of minimally invasive techniques is firmly established in paediatric urology, both in the use of cystoscopic intervention and in the use of laparoscopy to access the upper renal tracts. This section will consider the relative merits of the retroperitoneal and transperitoneal routes to access the kidney, before briefly considering nephrectomy and heminephrectomy. Laparoscopic pyeloplasty and transvesical ureteric reimplantation will then be described.

Retroperitoneoscopic and Transperitoneal Access

The technique of retroperitoneoscopic access to the kidney using a balloon was first described by Gaur [58]. This technique involves entering the retroperitoneal space via a small lumbar incision. The space is then expanded using the balloon, which can be constructed using a surgical rubber glove and a catheter, and inflated by means of a syringe connected to a 3 way tap. Gaur described the application of this technique to a diverse range of procedures in adults, including renal biopsy, lymph node biopsy, pyeloplasty, varicocelectomy and adrenal exposure. This technique has become widely used in paediatric urology. The advantage of this approach is that it allows access to the upper renal tracts without breaching the peritoneum and, therefore, allows direct access to the kidney. In the context of heminephrectomy, less dissection of the hilum of the moiety to be preserved is required [59]. There is also a decreased risk of damage to the abdominal organs [60] [61] [62], less ileus and shoulder pain as well as fewer adhesions [63]. If a haematoma or urinoma forms as a consequence of surgery, then this is confined to the retroperitoneum, rather than entering the peritoneal cavity [60] [61].

The paediatric application of retroperitoneoscopy is not limited to the upper renal tracts. By developing the retroperitoneal space, access to other retroperitoneal structures is possible, including the para-aortic nodes [64].

The major limitation of the retroperitoneoscopic approach is the limited working space available. This is a particular problem when suturing is required, for example in the context of laparoscopic pyeloplasty. The kidney is also located cephalad to the trocars, leading to potential difficulty in accessing the upper pole of the kidney [65].

By contrast, the transperitoneal route allows a capacious working space, at the expense of disturbing the peritoneal cavity and the need to dissect the colon to access the kidney. In the presence of significant adhesions, especially in the presence of a previous severe pyelonephritis, the transperitoneal approach has significant advantages over the open approach [63]. Although postoperative adhesion formation is a potential concern, this is not necessarily a significant problem [66] [67].

Kim et al performed a systematic review comparing 401 retroperitoneal nephrectomies with 488 transperitoneal procedures. The mean operative time was shorter in the retroperitoneal group (129 v 154 minutes). Both groups of patients had the same length of stay. Two vascular injuries occurred in the retroperitoneal group. The authors concluded that both approaches were reasonable, and that surgeon preference should govern the operative approach taken [68].

Castellan et al reviewed their experience of 48 laparoscopic heminephrectomies performed using the trasnperitotoneal and retroperitoneal approach. They noted that complications were related to the age of the patient rather than to the operative approach [69].

The operative approach to the kidney, therefore, should be governed by the surgeon's knowledge of both techniques, and the ability to apply them to the clinical case in hand. There is no evidence that either approach is superior.

Nephrectomy and Heminephrectomy

The first paediatric laparoscopic nephrectomy was reported by Koyle et al in 1993 [70]. This was shortly followed by the first report of laparoscopic heminephrectomy in a child [71]. Whilst uptake of laparoscopic or retroperitoneoscopic nephrectomy in paediatric practice has been rapid, application of these techniques to heminephrectomy has been slower [72]. This is, perhaps, because of the lower frequency of this operation, the younger patient population and the potential for more serious complications: including urinoma, haematoma and ischaemia of the remaining renal parenchyma [60]. There are, however, potential advantages from the laparoscopic technique, particularly the precise division of the kidney offered by magnification from the laparoscope [73]. Laparoscopy also facilitates dissection of the vascular pedicle without mobilisation of the kidney, thus potentially decreasing the risk of ischaemia to the remaining renal tissue [59].

Traxel et al recently reviewed 5 comparative studies of open versus laparoscopic partial nephrectomy in children [59] [65] [74] [75] [76] [77]. They comment on an increased operating time with laparoscopic surgery, although a trend was observed towards a decrease with increasing experience. Length of stay was shorter in all studies and the majority demonstrated a decrease in analgesic requirement. Of particular note is that some patients undergoing open surgery required a second incision to remove the distal ureter [75].

Laparoscopic Pyeloplasty

Pyeloplasty is a one of the most commonly performed procedures in paediatric urology. The technique of open pyeloplasty has a high success rate. The laparoscopic approach to pyeloplasty has the potential to offer advantages in terms of improved cosmesis and reduced operative trauma, but is competing with a well-established open procedure in which the success rate is high and the incision small.

Technique

Transperitoneal laparoscopic pyeloplasty offers the advantage of a large working space. The procedure may be preceded by a cystoscopy and retrograde pyelogram, a J-J stent may also be placed at this point. Some authors leave the ureteric guide wire in place to facilitate dissection of the ureter later in the procedure [78].

Laparoscopic access is gained to the abdomen via a 5mm port placed at the umbilicus. Two working ports are then placed in the mid epigastrium and in the ipsilateral midclavicular line. The colon can be mobilised to gain access to the kidney [78]. Alternatively, it is possible to access the pelvico-ureteric junction (PUJ) by making a window in the colonic mesentery [80]. The PUJ is mobilised and the ureter divided. An intracorporeal ureterouretostomy is then performed using 5-0 or 6-0 absorbable suture. The placement of a stay suture in the renal pelvis can facilitate the anastomosis.

The retroperitoneoscopic approach utilises the Guar balloon technique [58]. Access to the kidney can be achieved via a posterior or flank incision. The flank incision has the advantage of offering a standard incision in the event of conversion being necessary, at the expense of a higher risk of causing an inadvertent pneumoperitoneum [80]. A 10mm primary trocar is placed and 2 or more 5mm ports are added. An intracorporeal anastomosis can then be achieved.

Outcomes

Penn et al recently published early results of a randomised series comparing open and laparoscopic pyeloplasty [79]. Twenty patients who underwent laparoscopic pyeloplasty had a slightly longer operative time than 19 who underwent open pyeloplasty (151 minutes v 130 minutes). There was a trend to shorter hospital stay in the laparoscopic group (29.3 v 36.3 hours). Neither of these differences approached statistical significance [79].

In a descriptive study, Tan reported his experience with 18 patients from 3 months to 15 years in age; good results were achieved with a mean operative time of 89 minutes [81]. Ravish et al reviewed a series of 29 patients undergoing pyeloplasty, of whom 15 underwent a laparoscopic operation [82]. The mean operative time in the laparoscopic group was longer (215 v 159 minutes).

In a retrospective analysis of a multi-institutional database Tanaka reviewed the results of 324 laparoscopic pyeloplasties and compared them to the results of 4937 open procedures [83]. Because of the large number of patients in this study the authors were able to stratify them by age, and showed that the greatest benefit offered by laparoscopy, in terms of length of stay and analgesic requirement, was to patients over 10 years.

In a more recent series, Sweeney et al report a series of 112 patients who underwent laparoscopic pyeloplasty. This was successful in 97%, with 3% of patients requiring further procedures. Mean operative time was 254 minutes [78].

Laparoscopic pyeloplasty, therefore, offers modest benefit in terms of length of stay and analgesic requirement, which may be most beneficial to older children. This is at the expense of a longer operating time and a technically challenging intracorporeal anastomosis.

Transvesical Ureteric Reimplantation

The endoscopic treatment of vesico-ureteric reflux by subureteric injection of Deflux has reduced the need for ureteric reimplantation, achieving success rates of 70-90%. This technique does, however, sometimes fail and is less effective at treating higher grades of reflux [84]. Where surgery is required to correct vesico-ureteric reflux the use of minimal access surgery has the potential to decrease morbidity.

Various minimal access approaches to ureteric reimplantation have been described. Laparoscopic extravescial reimplantation has been achieved using the Lich-Gregoir technique. This technique has the limitation of requiring retrovesical dissection and a significant proportion of children subsequently develop voiding dysfunction [85], although there is some evidence that this can be ameliorated by adopting a nerve sparing technique [86].

Minimal access intravesical surgery has the potential to minimise the impact of extravesical dissection, whilst avoiding the morbidity associated with an open cystostomy. The techniques of trigonoplasty and ureteric advancement have been achieved transvesically [87] [88]. More recently, the technique of intravesical cross trigonal ureteric reimplantation has made minimal access surgery applicable to the Cohen reimplantation.

Technique

The technique of intravesical cross trigonal ureteric reimplantation was originally described by Yeung [89]. The patient is placed supine with the legs apart such that the ureteric orifice can be accessed during the procedure. The laparoscopic stack is placed at the patient's feet and the surgeon stands at the head. A cystoscope is passed into the bladder, which is then distended with saline. Under cystoscopic guidance, a traction suture is placed through the abdominal wall and the dome of the bladder. A 5mm port is then inserted into the bladder under cystoscopic vision. The bladder is drained using a urethral catheter and insufflated to a pressure of 10-12mmHg. Further working ports are then inserted. The catheter balloon is inflated and used to occlude the internal urethral meatus such that no gas leak occurs. Two further working ports are inserted and a stent is placed in the ureter to assist with its mobilisation. The stent is secured with a suture. The operation then proceeds according to Cohen's technique: the ureter is circumscribed and mobilised with scissors and a diathermy hook, and a submuscosal tunnel created. The ureter is then drawn through the tunnel and anastomosed to the bladder mucosa using 5-0 or 6-0 suture. Yeung et al describe this operation without the routine use of a ureteric stent in the majority of patients [89].

The advantage of this technique is the very clear intravesical vision that can be achieve by replacing urine with air. The view is not clouded by blood, as bleeding pools at the base of the bladder rather than being diluted in fluid. In addition, retrovesical dissection is completely avoided.

Outcomes

Yeung reported a series of 16 patients who underwent transvesical reimplantation between 10 months and 13 years of age [89]. All procedures except 1 were completed successfully. The mean operating time was 136 minutes. There was suprapubic and scrotal emphysema in two patients. Successful resolution of VUR was achieved in 96%.

Kawuchi et al described 30 patients in whom this technique was employed, 15 of whom were children. This procedure was successful in 96% of patients [90]. In an earlier series Kuitkov described this technique in 32 patients, with an operative time of 2.8 hours [89]. Failures were more common in patients of 2 years or younger. The authors noted a high complication rate in bladders with a volume of less than 130ml. Ureteric strictures were encountered in 6.3% of patients.

Although the technique is still developing, transvesical cross trigonal ureteric reimplantation has the potential to offer a good outcome to patients requiring surgical correction of VUR, without the morbidity associated with an open incision.

SILS

Single incision laparoscopic surgery (SILS) has the potential to offer further advantages over a three port laparoscopic approach, especially in terms of cosmesis and reduced postoperative pain. SILS has gained popularity in adult practice over recent years and has started to be employed in paediatric urology, having been applied to varicocelectomy, nephrectomy, pyeloplasty and nephroureterectomy [92]. Jeon et al recently described a single port lower pole heminephrectomy for a patient with a 3.5cm lower pole metanephric adenoma

[93]. In our institution we have recently performed a heminephrouretectomy for a duplex kidney using a SILS technique (Figure 4). SILS has also been used to perform pyeloplasty. Tugcu et al recently reported a series in which transperitoneal access was used to perform laparoscopic pyeloplasty in 11 patients [94].

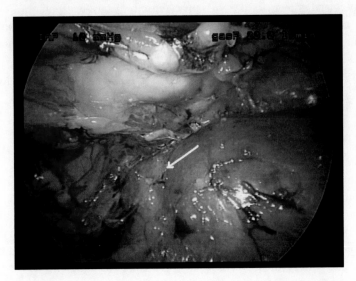

Figure 4. Exposure of left duplex kidney using SILS approach. Arrow indicates line of demarcation of upper from lower pole.

Conclusions

Paediatric urology continues to gain immensely from the application of minimal access techniques. The optimum operative approach to the kidney is dependent on surgeon preference and the procedure being performed, with both retroperitoneal and transperitoneal access having advantages and disadvantages. Pyeloplasty is increasingly being performed using minimal access techniques, offering modest benefits over open surgery at the expense of increased operating time. Transvesical surgery offers alternative access to the bladder, without the need for traumatic retrovesical dissection.

Thoracoscopy

Introduction

The first use of thoracoscopy was described in 1912 by Jacobeus in a patient with pulmonary tuberculosis. He went on to describe a personal series of 100 patients [95]. The use of thoracoscopy in the paediatric population was described in the 1970s by Rodgers et al, who used thoracoscopy to perform lung biopsies, diagnostic inspection of the pleural cavity and limited decortication of empyema [96].

As the technology associated with minimally invasive surgery has improved, major intrathoracic procedures are now possible using the thoracoscopic approach, including the repair of tracheo-esophageal fistula with esophageal atresia (OA/TEF), repair of congenital diaphragmatic hernia (CDH) and pulmonary lobectomy. Thoracoscopy has also been used to enhance the safety and efficacy of the Nuss procedure for pectus excavatum.

The major advantage offered by the thoracoscopic approach is the reduction in morbidity associated with a thoracotomy, which includes winging of the scapula, asymmetry of the chest wall and scoliosis [97].

Anaesthetic Considerations

There are several considerations when anaesthetising patients for thoracoscopic procedures. The main concern is to allow adequate working space for the procedure to take place, usually by achieving collapse of the ipsilateral lung. A variety of ventilation strategies can be utilised to facilitate this [98]. One possibility is the use of a double lumen endotracheal tube. This approach is, however, limited by smallest size of double lumen tubes available, most usually 28 Fr [98]. The other approaches are selective intubation of the mainstem bronchus using a smaller endotracheal tube, which may need to be facilitated by the use of bronchoscopy, particularly on the left side. Finally, a bronchial blocker may be used to achieve occlusion of the ipsilateral bronchus.

Where lung collapse cannot be completely achieved by these methods, the use of carbon dioxide insufflations of the thoracic cavity may facilitate it [98]. There has been some recent concern about the effect of this $CO2$ pneumothorax in neonates. A recent study demonstrated that approximately 30% of the exhaled $CO2$ in neonates undergoing thoracoscopic repair of TEF/OA and CDH was derived from the CO_2 pneumothorax rather than being a product of metabolism. This was accompanied by a drop in cerebral oxygen saturations, which persisted after surgery [99].

Thoracoscopic Repair of Esophageal Atresia with Tracheo-Esophageal Fistula

History

The first thoracoscopic oesophageal atresia repair was performed in 1999 at the meeting of the International Pediatric Surgical Endoscopy Group in Berlin [100]. This was followed in 2000 by the first successful repair of a tracheo-esophageal fistula and associated atresia [101]. Thoracoscopic repair of EA/TEF is now performed worldwide.

Technique

The patient is endotracheally intubated and placed prone at 45 degrees, with the right side uppermost. The lung is then collapsed by means of a CO_2 pneumothorax. Usually, one camera port and two working ports are employed. In order to identify the important structures for this procedure, the azygos vein may need to be controlled. This can be achieved by use of clips, monopolar diathermy or ligation [102] [103]. Control of the azygos vein may also be achieved using alternative energy sources such as the Plasmakinetic [102] or Ligasure devices.

The next stage in the operation is to gain control of the trachea-esophageal fistula and divide it. This may be achieved by suture ligation or clips. Once the fistula has been controlled then the upper oesophageal pouch is dissected and opened before an anastomosis is performed using 4 or 5-0 absorbable PDS or vicryl [102] [103] [104]. Most surgeons employ a silastic trans-anastomotic tube, placed through the anastomosis, to allow feeds to be commenced soon after surgery and to facilitate the anastomosis being performed [103].

Once the anastomosis is completed, a chest drain is placed and the port sites closed.

Experience to Date

The largest single series of TEF/EA repairs to date was published by Holcomb et al in 2005. This multi-institutional analysis reported 104 patients from 6 centres around the world. This paper reported an 11.5% early leak rate, with 31.7% of patients requiring oesophageal dilatation. There was a 4.8% rate of conversion to open surgery with an average of a 129 minute operating time [103].

Al et al reported a comparative series in 2007, in which 23 neonates undergoing EA/TEF repair were compared to controls who had undergone conventional open repair. This study demonstrated shorter operative times when open repair was compared to laparoscopic repair (149 v 179 minutes). The rate of anastomotic leakage was comparable (17.4% v 13%) [104].

Van der Zee reported a series of 51 neonates with EA/TEF treated thoracoscopically, with a mean operating time of 178 minutes. 2 patients in the series were converted to a thoracotomy, 18% of patients had a leak and 45% of patients developed a stenosis requiring dilatation [105].

The thoracoscopic approach has also been shown to be of use in treatment of the rarer 'H'-type trachea-esophageal fistula [106](Figure 5). Repair of this anomaly is traditionally undertaken through the neck, with the accompanying risk of damaging the recurrent laryngeal nerve, or through a thoracotomy. Thoracoscopy offers a method of correcting this anomaly whilst avoiding the morbidity of either of these approaches.

Advantages

Given that the procedure can be accomplished with comparable complication rates to open thoracotomy, the major advantage is the avoidance of the long term morbidity associated with a thoracotomy, which was 32% at three years in one study [92]. Some authors experienced at performing thoracoscopic repair believe that the use of thoracoscopy also facilitates better visualisation of the anatomy than can be achieved with a conventional thoracotomy [103].

Disadvantages

One disadvantage of the thoracoscopic technique is that it converts an extrapleural operation to a transpleural operation, making the consequences of an anastomotic leak potentially more severe. This has yet to be reflected in an increased complication rate in published studies, however. It has also been suggested that the data regarding the long term sequelae of thoracotomy in neonates refer to older techniques which have been superseded by less destructive approaches to thoracotomy, which might carry a lesser risk of causing long term morbidity. There is however, little data to support this assertion.

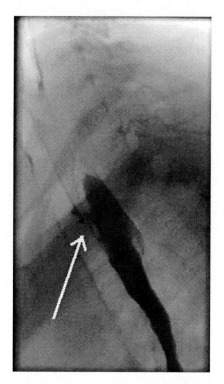

Figure 5. Upper GI contrast study, showing an H-type tracheo-esophageal fistula (arrowed).

One theoretical advantage of the thoracoscopic technique for EA/TEF repair is that the degree of esophageal dysmotility seen after the procedure, which so plagues these babies as they start feeding, might be reduced because of the more limited dissection required. This is not supported by a recent study, which demonstrated no difference is oesophageal motility when open and thoracoscopic approaches were compared [107].

Aortopexy

Aortopexy is a surgical treatment for tracheomalacia, in which the aorta is apposed to the sternum to prevent collapse of the trachea during expiration. This operation is traditionally performed via a median sternotomy, but is increasingly being performed using minimal access techniques. The first thoracoscopic aortopexy was reported by DeCou in a 13 year old girl with Down's syndrome and tracheomalacia [108].

Technique

The patient is placed supine and the mediastinum is approached from the left. Access is achieved via two working ports and a camera placed in the left chest wall, with the camera looking superiorly [109]. The left lobe of the thymus gland is then mobilised and then moved away or resected. In order to appose the aorta to the posterior aspect of the sternum, the chest wall is depressed, and 3-0 ethibond sutures placed through the sternum. An endoclose device may be used to facilitate this [109]. Bronchoscopy at the end of the procedure confirms that the aortopexy has opened the trachea sufficiently.

Van der Zee et al report 6 children requiring aortopexy from a series of 51 neonates undergoing thoracoscopic repair. Of these, 2 patients required a second procedure to achieve an adequate result [105]. In the international series of patients who had thoracoscopic EA/TEF repairs, 7 patients required an aortopexy, of which 6 were successfully accomplished thoracoscopically [103].

Congenital Diaphragmatic Hernia

Congenital diaphragmatic hernia most commonly occurs at the posterolateral margin of the diaphragm, this is known as a Bochdalek defect. This defect is found more frequently on the left than the right. The less common Morgagni hernia occurs in the anterior part of the diaphragm, just posterior to the xiphisternum.

Morgagni Hernia

The anterior, Morgagni, defect is often diagnosed incidentally later in life, and causes little respiratory embarrassment during the neonatal period. There is an emerging consensus that these defects are amenable to laparoscopic repair [110] [111] [112] [113].

Technique

An initial port is placed at the umbilicus, and further working ports are added to allow triangulation and access to the upper abdomen. The hernia is reduced and the defect repaired. Closure of the defect may be achieved by sutures placed through the anterior abdominal wall and diaphragm, with extracorporeal knots being placed through small incisions in the anterior abdominal wall.

Closure of a larger defect that may be facilitated by the insertion of a prosthetic patch [111].

Bochdalek Hernia

Posterolateral congenital diaphragmatic hernia is associated with a high mortality. The overall mortality of 50% has now improved, with recent series reporting an overall survival of 80% [114].

Most surgeons choose to perform open repair of Bochdalek hernias through a left subcostal laparotomy.

The literature surrounding minimal access repair of Bochdalek hernias is difficult to interpret, as many series report patients who are diagnosed both during the neonatal period and later in life. The management of neonatally diagnosed Bochdalek hernias is dominated by the physiological disturbance caused by the associated pulmonary hypoplasia and pulmonary hypertension, which accounts for the majority of deaths in this group. Patients diagnosed later in life, however, have much less marked physiological disturbance and, as such, have outcomes which are much more favourable, regardless of the surgical technique employed.

Thoracoscopic Repair

The majority of Bochdalek CDH repairs which are performed using minimal access surgery are performed thoracoscopically. This has the advantage of avoiding reducing the hernia contents, which often include the spleen, towards the laparoscope, and thus achieves superior visualisation of the defect.

Technique

The patient is placed in the lateral position with the side of the defect uppermost. The surgeon stands towards the head of the patient, standing at the patient's front. The initial port, used for the camera, is placed just below the scapula. Two working ports are added, one in the 5th intercostal space and another between the endoscope and the spine [111]. A pneumothorax is then induced, with a pressure between 4 and 10mmHg, depending on the size of the patient. The pneumothorax alone may be sufficient to reduce the hernia contents into the abdomen. Gentle instrumental manipulation is often required for reduction, in addition.

The defect is then repaired using non-absorbable sutures. These may be tied intra or extra corporeally. The sutures can be buttressed with Teflon pledgets [116]. A prosthetic patch may be added if the defect cannot be closed without tension.

Outcomes

Despite early concerns about the use of thoracoscopy [117], there have been an increasing number of successful thoracoscopic CDH repairs reported in the literature [115] [116] [117] [118] [119] [120] [121]. Nguyen and Le [118] reported a series of 45 successful thoracoscopic CDH repairs in 2006, of which 19 were in newborns. In 2007, Becmeur et al [115] reported a series of 17 patients, including 6 neonates, reporting 1 recurrence in the neonatal series and 1 conversion. In 2008, Shah et al [121] reported a series of 17 diaphragmatic hernias repaired successfully using thoracoscopy in neonates and infants; they reported only 2 neonatal recurrences (11%). Guner et al [119] recently reported a series of 15 neonatal thoracoscopic CDH repairs for 4 years. Five of their patients required a patch, and there were 3 recurrences (20%). In a comparative study, Cho et al [120] demonstrated a higher recurrence rate in their thoracoscopic group compared to open Bochdalek repairs. In a recent series of right-sided thoracoscopic CDH repairs, Liem et al [122] reported one conversion and one recurrence.

The high recurrence rate associated with thoracoscopic Bochdalek CDH repair has led some authors to suggest that patient selection might be required to confine minimal access surgery to those babies in whom success is likely. Yang et al proposed that smaller defects, less likely to require patch closure, could be identified by an intrabdominal stomach (the tip of the NG tube lying below the diaphragm) and by a peak inspiratory pressure of less than 24mmHg [118]. Gourlay et al reported a series in which thoracoscopic repair was associated with earlier return to full feeds and reduced narcotic use [123]. They postulated that successful repair was most likely in patients with limited respiratory compromise, who are most likely to have the functional reserve needed to overcome respiratory acidosis. In their series, thoracoscopic patients matched to similar open controls had comparable outcomes.

Lansdale et al performed a meta-analysis of three studies comparing open and thoracoscopic Bochdalek hernia repair, in a total of 143 patients [124]. Although this analysis is limited by the retrospective use of the studies compared, the mortality was similar. This study did, however, demonstrate a higher recurrence rate associated with thoracoscopic repair (risk ratio 3.3). Operative times were also longer in the thoracoscopic group, with a weighted mean difference of 50 minutes.

Disadvantages

The literature seems to suggest a higher recurrence rate is associated with thoracoscopic repair of Bochdalek CDH repair. There is a possibility that selecting the most appropriate patients for minimal access surgery might help to overcome this [118][125]. Further prospective studies are required to further delineate this.

Another well founded concern is that the thoracoscopic technique may lead to further compromise of respiratory function in neonates who have limited functional reserve because of the pulmonary hypoplasia associated with this condition [124]. The pneumothorax may cause physical compression of the contralateral lung, with absorption of CO_2 from the pneumothorax further worsening acidosis and depressing cerebral oxygen saturation [99] [126]. The increased requirement for ventilation leads to a need for increased minute volumes and airway pressures, leading to an increase in barotrauma.

Pulmonary Lobectomy

Indications

Pulmonary lobectomy in the paediatric population is most commonly performed for benign congenital lesions. Malignancy is encountered much less frequently than in adult practice. Pulmonary lobectomy may be performed for intralobar sequestration, congenital cystic adenomatous malformation (CCAM) (Figure 6), congenital lobar emphysema, severe bronchiectasis and, rarely, for malignant lesions [98] [128]. As mentioned in the introduction to this section, the use of thoracoscopy to allow visualisation and lung biopsy is very well established [96].

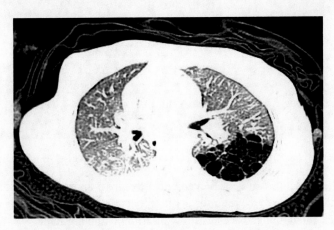

Figure 6. CT scan demonstrating CCAM involving the lower lobe of left lung.

Technique

In order to facilitate adequate working space the ipsilateral lung must first be collapsed. This can be achieved by any of the means described above: a double lumen ET tube, bronchial blocker or selective intubation.

The patient is placed in the lateral decubitus position and a primary trocar is inserted. A pneumothorax is instituted and the position of the fissure identified. For lower lobectomies, placement of a 5mm port in the anterior axillary line of the 7th or 8th interspace is recommended [98]. Dissection along the line of this fissure will reveal the major structures to be encountered, a second port is then placed in the 4th or 5th interspace to aid dissection. For upper lobectomy, the port placement may be higher in the chest to allow access to the superior pulmonary vessels [98].

In benign cystic lesions, working space can be facilitated by rupture of the cyst to increase the working space within the thorax [128].

Following a survey of the chest to confirm the anatomy, dissection continues, mobilising the lobe of the lung to be resected. In lower lobectomies this requires division of the inferior pulmonary ligament. Dissection then proceeds along the fissure, and control of the lobar vessels is achieved. An incomplete fissure may require division before the relevant anatomy can be displayed. Vascular control is achieved most easily by use of the Ligasure device, which facilitates sealing of the vessels at two locations without division, offering superior control over the vessels, which can then be divided between the seals (Figure 7).

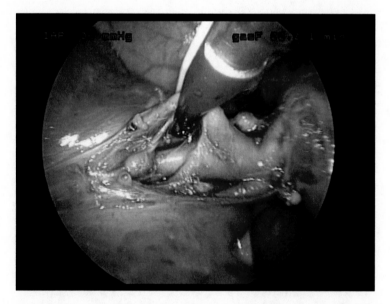

Figure 7. Intra-operative photograph demonstrating control of a bronchial vessel using the ligasure device.

Control of the bronchus can be achieved either by sharp division and suture, or by use of an Endo GIA stapler. This device requires a 12mm port for insertion, limiting its use to older children with wide enough interspaces to allow insertion without trauma.

The specimen is then retrieved with minimal extension of one of the port sites. A specimen bag can be employed and is advised in the presence of infection [98].

Outcome

In an early series reporting thoracoscopic resection of CCAMS, Albanese et al demonstrated the feasibility of thoracoscopic resection of CCAMs in 14 patients, with a mean operating time of 110 minutes [127].

Rothenberg reported a personal series of 93 pulmonary lobectomies in 2007 [98]. Of these, 89 were completed endoscopically. Four conversions were required. Only 2 patients had post operative complications: 1 developed a pneumothorax and another, a post operative pneumonia. The operating time varied from 35-210 minutes, and the length of stay from 1-5 days.

Vu et al published a comparative series in 2007, in which 24 patients undergoing open resection of CCAMs were compared to 12 patients undergoing thoracoscopic resection [129]. The mean operating time in the thoracoscopic group was 60 minutes longer. 33% of patients in this series were converted to an open operation, of whom all had pre-operative history of pneumonia.

Correction of Pectus Excavatum

Pectus excavatum is a common chest wall deformity, with in incidence of 1 in 700 births [130]. The main indication for repair is aesthetic, although the surgery may also be undertaken for patients who have pulmonary or cardiac dysfunction or who have limitations to physical activity.

The placement of a retrosternal bar to correct pectus excavatum was described by Nuss [131]. This procedure was initially performed blindly, leading to several serious complications, including cardiac perforation.

Thoracoscopic control has added safety to this procedure, with some authors describing the right sided thoracoscopy [132] [133]. This technique can be further refined by performing thoracoscopy bilaterally [134]. The placement of a trocar inferior to the port of entry for the bar permits visualisation of the track being created to the mediastinum [132]. The use of a 70 degree thoracoscope can facilitate the construction of a mediastinal tunnel [130]. The technique has even been modified to facilitate the placement of a bar completely extrapleurally [135].

Minimally Invasive Oncological Surgery

Introduction

The use of minimally invasive surgery (MIS) in the management of childhood cancer has been a feature of paediatric surgery for some years. In 1979, Rodgers and Talbert described a series of 65 thoracoscopic procedures in children, of which 8 were biopsies of lung masses, and 7 biopsies of mediastinal tumours [96]. Evidence for the use of minimal access techniques in paediatric oncology has been limited and exemplified by the failure of two randomised studies, looking at laparoscopic and thoracoscopic procedures, which were initiated in 1996 by the Childrens' Cancer Group (CCG) and the Paediatric Oncology Group

(POG). These studies were abandoned because of an inability to recruit patients [136]. Evidence for the use of MIS in paediatric cancer is, therefore, limited to the synthesis of data from single institutions, the majority of which is retrospectively collected [137].

MIS has been used in children for diagnostic and therapeutic treatment of the primary lesion. These techniques also have a role in the biopsy and treatment of metastatic disease as well as being applicable to other areas of oncology; for example diagnostic inspection of the abdomen, the placement of peritoneal catheters and the insertion of feeding gastrostomies in patients undergoing chemotherapy [137].

The role of MIS was established in two large studies published at the end of the last century. In 1995, Holcomb et al described a retrospective series of 88 procedures performed by members of the CCG [138]. This series included 63 thoracoscopic and 25 laparoscopic procedures, the majority of which were diagnostic. Saenz et al also described a large series of 93 MIS procedures, the majority of which were also diagnostic [139].

MIS has subsequently been used to diagnosis and treat a wide variety of malignant diseases including neuroblastoma [140], Wilms tumour [141] [142] hepatoblastoma and hepatocellular carcinoma [143], ovarian teratoma [143], rhabdomyosarcoma [66] and lymphoma [137] [143]. This section will consider the advantages and disadvantages of MIS, before outlining the evidence for the role of MIS in thoracic and abdominal malignancy.

Advantages

Minimal access techniques have the potential to decrease the morbidity of oncological diagnosis and treatment. The avoidance of a large incision may decrease the risk of wound infection, minimise fluid shifts, decrease the rate of incisional hernias and lead to a reduced hospital stay [137][143]. In the chest, as has previously been discussed; the avoidance of an open thoracotomy has the potential to avoid the associated long-term musculoskeletal morbidity [97]. In the context of oncological surgery, faster recovery also has the potential to allow chemotherapy to be started or resumed earlier.

Limitations

There are limitations to the use of MIS, however. One of the major disadvantages is the loss of ability to palpate tissue, which may lead to small lesions being missed, such as with metastatic lesions in the lung [144]. The use of MIS techniques for resection is also associated with higher conversion rates than in other applications [143]. The long-term outcomes from minimally invasive techniques have yet to be established, and there are suggestions of an increased rate of complications, for example bowel perforation, bleeding and port site seeding [145]. In addition the technical difficulty associated with these complex operations limits application to centres with suitably experienced surgeons and supporting staff.

Thoracoscopy for Malignancy

Diagnostic

As described in the introduction to this section, thoracoscopy has been used in the diagnosis of intrathoracic malignancy since the 1970s. Cribbs summarised the literature to date in a review published in 2007, which described 474 procedures, of which 167 were incisional biopsies [137]. Of these 163 were successful, leading to an overall success rate of 97.6% [138] [139] [140] [143] [145] [146] [147] [148] [149] [150] [151] [152] [153].

Metzelder et al published a series of prospectively collected data from their institution in the same year [144]. The figures from this review are included in that by Cribbs [137], but they are interesting in that they describe the surgical management of malignancy over a five-year period and indicate the proportion of patients who were subjected to conventional and minimal access surgery. This series describes 34 thoracic biopsies of which 14 were attempted thoracoscopically, with one conversion.

Thoracoscopy is, therefore, firmly established as a technique for the biopsy of thoracic and mediastinal lesions.

Resection Using Thoracoscopy

Resection of intrathoracic lesions using thoracoscopic techniques is less well established. Port site recurrence is a potential concern, but is not well documented in the literature. Only one port site metastasis was reported in 410 adults undergoing thoracoscopic resection [154], and only one case has been reported in a child [155].

Mediastinal Tumours

Mediastinal lesions may be amenable to resection using thoracoscopy. In 2001, Partrick and Rothenberg described the resection of 33 undiagnosed mediastinal masses, of which the majority were foregut duplications [147]. Twenty-three of the lesions encountered were malignant. All procedures in this series were completed thoracoscopically, with the exception of one conversion because of extensive disease from a sarcoma.

The technique described involved placement of the patients in a supine position with a 10 degree anterior tilt on the affected side if the lesion was in the anterior mediastinum, and in the prone position with a posterior tilt if it was in the posterior mediastinum. Single lung ventilation was achieved and a pneumothorax induced using a Veres needle. The addition of 3 to 4 additional working ports facilitated the dissection. The authors' comment on the utility of energy sources, particularly the Ligasure device, in maintaining meticulous haemostasis. The tumour may then be removed in a specimen bag.

In addition to the 11 patients discussed in the Partrick series, the resection of neurogenic mediastinal tumours (NMTs) has been reported by other authors. Petty et al described the resection of 17 NMTs with similar success rates to open surgery and a shorter hospital stay [152], and Nio describe successful removal of a further 6 lesions [151].

Lung Lesions

The majority of lung lesions encountered in paediatric oncological practice are metastases from malignant disease at an alternative site, most commonly Wilms tumour [137]. The excision biopsy of these lesions can be safely achieved thoracoscopically as described above. The further management of the majority of patients is the intensification of chemotherapy, which is facilitated by the faster recovery associated with a minimal access approach.

Particular care, must, however be applied to osteosarcoma. Yim described 11 wedge resections in 7 patients with pulmonary metastases from osteosarcoma [144]. They noted good recovery from surgery in all patients, but 3 of seven had further metastases 3-6 months after the procedure. These authors concluded this had happened as a consequence of incomplete resection. Castagnetti et al had similar issues, reporting conversion in 8 of 10 children because of inconsistency between operative findings and the preoperative CT scan [156]. In 3 of these converted patients more nodules were evident than were found at thoracoscopy. These authors concluded that tactile feedback is essential in these patients and that thoracotomy should be performed if more than one pulmonary nodule is suspected.

There are limited reports of lobectomy for pulmonary malignancy. Two of the patients in Rothenberg's series of thoracoscopic lobectomies had malignant lesions [128].

Abdominal Lesions

Diagnostic

Cribbs et al summarise the biopsy of abdominal masses in the literature until 2007 [137]. They describe 165 biopsies reported up to this date with only 2 insufficient specimens, giving the technique a 98.8% positive yield [137] [138] [140] [143] [150] [153] [157] [158]. In the Metzelder series, 77 lesions were encountered in the abdomen or retroperitoneum, of which 41 were biopsied using laparoscopy, with a 15% rate of conversion and 98% accuracy overall [143].

Resection

Curative resection is described for several intra-abdominal tumours. Of 129 abdominal tumours in Metzelder et al's series, 24 were attempted laparoscopically, with a 30.2% rate of conversion [143].

Adrenal Gland

Up to 2007, 87 cases of minimal access resection of adrenal lesions had been described [137]. Of these 9 patients had been converted to an open operation, with the most common indication being intravascular extension of the tumour (10.3%) [159-168]. Five retroperitoneal resections had been described with 2 conversions, giving a 40% conversion rate overall [152] [169]. Figures 8 and 9 illustrate a stage 1 adrenal neuroblastoma resected laparoscopically and delivered with the aid of a pouch.

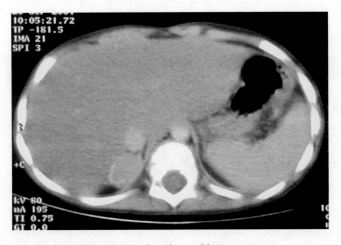

Figure 8. CT scan demonstrating a right stage 1 adrenal neuroblastoma.

Wilms Tumour

Laparoscopic nephrectomy for Wilms tumour has been avoided in some centres because of a theoretical increase in the risk of tumour rupture [143], which leads to the upstaging of the tumour and a greater burden of oncological treatment for the patient.

Duarte initially reported resection of Wilms tumours in 8 patients with good results, with only 1 child requiring further chemotherapy [141] [142]. All of these patients were managed according to the Society of Paediatric Oncology (SIOP) protocol and, therefore, had had neoadjuvant chemotherapy. Varlet described a further 5 cases in which a transperitoneal laparoscopic approach was used to successfully resect Wilms tumours [170].

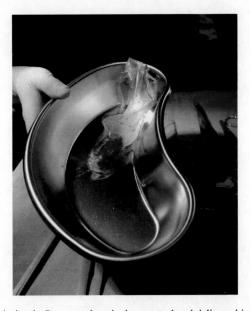

Figure 9. Photograph of the lesion in 7, comprehensively resected and delivered intact in a specimen bag.

A similar technique was employed in both studies. The colon was mobilised from the tumour and the renal hilum exposed. The vessels supplying the kidney were then controlled with a ligasure and the tumour removed through a separate abdominal incision, having been placed in a bag for removal.

Laparoscopic resection of Wilms tumour is therefore possible in selected patients. Varlet et al suggest this technique should be limited to small tumours not crossing the midline after preoperative chemotherapy and with no extension into the vena cava [170]. Duarte et al suggested that laparoscopic resection should be limited to patients where the maximum diameter of the tumour is <10% of the patient's height [141].

Neuroblastoma

Iwanaka et al reported their experience with laparoscopic management of neuroblastoma. They compared 4 laparoscopic excisions with 14 open excisions of early neuroblastoma, and 6 laparoscopic biopsies and 9 open biopsies of advanced neuroblastoma. Similar operative time and blood loss were reported, with shorter length of stay and time to full feeds in patients undergoing laparoscopic surgery [140].

Conclusions

The minimal access approach to paediatric malignancy has been a part of thoracoscopic and laparoscopic surgery in children since its introduction. Minimal access techniques are moving from a well established position in diagnostic procedures to an increasing role in therapeutic resection. The lack of randomised studies in this area is a concern, and adherence to sound oncological principles is important when undertaking such procedures.

Conclusion

This chapter has described the current status of the advances within paediatric minimal access surgery. The future is likely to involve further evolution of these techniques as technology moves forward; in particular the role of SILS and perhaps NOTES is likely to expand. This will increase the benefit of reduced surgical trauma to our patients.

References

[1]   Ron O, Eaton S, Pierro A. Systematic review of the risk of developing a metachronous contralateral inguinal hernia in children. *The British Journal of Surgery* 2007;94:804-11.
[2]   Nataraja RM, Mahomed AA. Metachronous contralateral pediatric inguinal hernia. *Open Access Surgery* 2010;2010:387-90.
[3]   Saranga Bharathi R, Arora M, Baskaran V. Minimal access surgery of pediatric inguinal hernias: a review. *Surgical Endoscopy*. 2008;22:1751-62.

[4] Niyogi A, Tahim AS, Sherwood WJ, De Caluwe D, Madden NP, Abel RM, et al. A comparative study examining open inguinal herniotomy with and without hernioscopy to laparoscopic inguinal hernia repair in a pediatric population. *Pediatric Surgery International* 2010;26:387-92.

[5] Liebert MA. IPEG Guidelines for Inguinal Hernia and Hydrocele. *Journal of Laparoendoscopic and Advanced Surgical Techniques Part A.* 2010;20:x-xiv.

[6] Chen K, Xiang G, Wang H, Xiao F. Towards a Near-Zero Recurrence Rate in Laparoscopic Inguinal Hernia Repair for Pediatric Patients. *Journal of laparoendoscopic and advanced surgical techniques* 2011; 21:445-8.

[7] Lipskar AM, Soffer SZ, Glick RD, Rosen NG, Levitt M a, Hong AR. Laparoscopic inguinal hernia inversion and ligation in female children: a review of 173 consecutive cases at a single institution. *Journal of Pediatric Surgery.* 2010 Jun ;45(6):1370-4.

[8] Chan KL, Hui WC, Tam PKH. Prospective randomized single-center, single-blind comparison of laparoscopic vs open repair of pediatric inguinal hernia. *Surgical Endoscopy.* 2005 Jul ;19(7):927-32.

[9] Koivusalo AI, Korpela R, Wirtavuori K, Piiparinen S, Rintala RJ, Pakarinen MP. A single-blinded, randomized comparison of laparoscopic versus open hernia repair in children. *Pediatrics.* 2009 Jan ;123(1):332-7.

[10] Schier F. Laparoscopic inguinal herniorrhaphy in children: A three-center experience with 933 repairs. *Journal of Pediatric Surgery.* 2002 Mar ;37(3):395-397.

[11] Esposito C, Montinaro L, Alicchio F et al. Laparoscopic treatment of inguinal hernia in the first year of life. *Journal of Laparoendoscopic and Advanced Surgical techniques* 2010; 50(5): 315-318.

[12] Turial S, Enders J, Krause K, Schier F. Laparoscopic inguinal herniorrhaphy in babies weighing 5 kg or less. *Surgical Endoscopy* 2011;25:72-8.

[13] De Caluwé D, Chertin B, Puri P. Childhood femoral hernia: a commonly misdiagnosed condition. *Pediatric surgery international* 2003;19:608-9.

[14] Morecroft J, Stringer M, Higgins M, Holmes S, Capps S. Follow-up after inguinal herniotomy or surgery for hydrocele in boys. *British Journal of Surgery* 1993;80:1613–1614.

[15] Grosfeld JL. Inguinal hernia in children: factors affecting recurrence in 62 cases. *Journal of Pediatric Surgery* 1991;26:283.

[16] Steinau G, Treutner KH, Feeken G, Schumpelick V. Recurrent inguinal hernias in infants and children. *World Journal of Surgery* 1995;19:303-6.

[17] Ramstedt C. Zur operation der angeborenen pylorus stenose. *Med. Klin* 1912;26:1191–1192.

[18] Mahomed AA, Panchalingum L, Nikolopoulos Y. The squeeze technique to assist transumbilical delivery of pyloric tumor. *Journal of Pediatric Surgery* 2006;41:1492-4.

[19] Haricharan RN, Aprahamian CJ, Morgan TL, Harmon CM, Georgeson KE, Barnhart DC. Smaller scars--what is the big deal: a survey of the perceived value of laparoscopic pyloromyotomy. *Journal of Pediatric Surgery* 2008;43:92-6.

[20] Najmaldin A, Tan HL. Early experience with laparoscopic pyloromyotomy for infantile hypertrophic pyloric stenosis. *Journal of Pediatric Surgery* 1995;30:37-8.

[21] Hall NJ, Van Der Zee J, Tan HL, Pierro A. Meta-analysis of Laparoscopic Versus Open Pyloromyotomy. *Annals of Surgery* 2004;240:774-778.

[22] Leclair M-D, Plattner V, Mirallie E, Lejus C, Nguyen J-M, Podevin G, et al. Laparoscopic pyloromyotomy for hypertrophic pyloric stenosis: a prospective, randomized controlled trial. *Journal of Pediatric Surgery* 2007;42:692-8.

[23] St Peter SD, Holcomb GW, Calkins CM, Murphy JP, Andrews WS, Sharp RJ, et al. Open versus laparoscopic pyloromyotomy for pyloric stenosis: a prospective, randomized trial. *Annals of Surgery* 2006;244:363-70.

[24] Hall N, Pacilli M, Eaton S, Reblock K, Gaines B, Pastor a, et al. Recovery after open versus laparoscopic pyloromyotomy for pyloric stenosis: a double-blind multicentre randomised controlled trial. *The Lancet* 2009;373:390-398.

[25] Rothenberg S. Laparoscopic duodenoduodenostomy for duodenal obstruction in infants and children. *Journal of Pediatric Surgery* 2002;37:1088-1089.

[26] Spilde TL, St Peter SD, Keckler SJ, Holcomb GW, Snyder CL, Ostlie DJ. Open vs laparoscopic repair of congenital duodenal obstructions: a concurrent series. *Journal of Pediatric Surgery* 2008;43:1002-5.

[27] Kay S, Yoder S, Rothenberg S. Laparoscopic duodenoduodenostomy in the neonate. *Journal of Pediatric Surgery* 2009;44:906-8.

[28] Valusek P a, Spilde TL, Tsao K, St Peter SD, Holcomb GW, Ostlie DJ. Laparoscopic duodenal atresia repair using surgical U-clips: a novel technique. *Surgical Endoscopy* 2007;21:1023-4.

[29] Mahomed A, D'hondt B, Khan K, Butt A. Technical Aspects of the Laparoscopic Management of a Late Presenting Duodenal Web. *Journal of Laparoendoscopic and Advanced Surgical Techniques* 2009;19(s1):s175-s177.

[30] Georgeson KE, Inge TH, Albanese CT. Laparoscopically assisted anorectal pull-through for high imperforate anus-a new technique. *Journal of Pediatric Surgery* 2000 ;35(6):927–931.

[31] Rollins MD, Downey EC, Meyers RL, Scaife ER. Division of the fistula in laparoscopic-assisted repair of anorectal malformations-are clips or ties necessary? *Journal of Pediatric Surgery* 2009;44:298-301.

[32] Podevin G, Petit T, Mure PY, Gelas T, Demarche M, Allal H, et al. Minimally Invasive Surgery for Anorectal Malformation in Boys: A Multicenter Study. *Journal of Laparoendoscopic and Advanced Surgical Techniques* 2009;19(s1):s233-s235.

[33] Srimurthy KR, Ramesh S, Shankar G, Narenda BM. Technical modifications of laparoscopically assisted anorectal pull-through for anorectal malformations. *Journal of Laparoendoscopic and Advanced Surgical Techniques. Part A.* 2008;18:340-3.

[34] Al-Hozaim O, Al-Maary J, Al Qahtani A, Zamakhshary M. Laparoscopic-assisted anorectal pull-through for anorectal malformations: a systematic review and the need for standardization of outcome reporting. *Journal of Pediatric Surgery* 2010 ;45:1500-4.

[35] Lin CL, Wong KKY, Lan LCL, Chen CC, Tam PKH. Earlier appearance and higher incidence of the rectoanal relaxation reflex in patients with imperforate anus repaired with laparoscopically assisted anorectoplasty. *Surgical Endoscopy* 2003;17:1646-9.

[36] Wong K, Khong P, Lin S, Lam W. Post-operative magnetic resonance evaluation of children after laparoscopic anorectoplasty for imperforate anus. *International Journal of Colorectal Disease* 2005;20:33-7.

[37] Kudou S, Iwanaka T, Kawashima H, Uchida H, Nishi A, Yotsumoto K, et al. Midterm follow-up study of high-type imperforate anus after laparoscopically assisted anorectoplasty. *Journal of Pediatric Surgery* 2005;40:1923-6.

[38] Ichijo C, Kaneyama K, Hayashi Y, Koga H, Okazaki T, Lane GJ, et al. Midterm postoperative clinicoradiologic analysis of surgery for high/intermediate-type imperforate anus: prospective comparative study between laparoscopy-assisted and posterior sagittal anorectoplasty. *Journal of Pediatric Surgery.* 2008;43:158-62; discussion 162-3.

[39] Georgeson K. Laparoscopic-assisted approaches for the definitive surgery for Hirschsprungs disease. *Seminars in Pediatric Surgery* 2004;13:256-262.

[40] Georgeson KE, Cohen RD, Hebra A, Jona JZ, Powell DM, Rothenberg SS, et al. Primary laparoscopic-assisted endorectal colon pull-through for Hirschsprung's disease: a new gold standard. *Annals of Surgery* 1999;229:678.

[41] Craigie RJ, Conway SJ, Cooper L, Turnock RR, Lamont GL, Baillie CT, et al. Primary pull-through for Hirschsprung's disease: comparison of open and laparoscopic-assisted procedures. *Journal of Laparoendoscopic and Advanced Surgical Techniques. Part A* 2007;17:809-12.

[42] Fujiwara N, Kaneyama K, Okazaki T, Lane GJ, Kato Y, Kobayashi H, et al. A comparative study of laparoscopy-assisted pull-through and open pull-through for Hirschsprung's disease with special reference to postoperative fecal continence. *Journal of Pediatric Surgery* 2007;42:2071-4.

[43] Mattioli G, Pini Prato A, Giunta C, Avanzini S, Della Rocca M, Montobbio G, et al. Outcome of primary endorectal pull-through for the treatment of classic Hirschsprung disease. *Journal of Laparoendoscopic and Advanced Surgical Techniques. Part A* 2008;18:869-74.

[44] Bax N, Zee DC. Laparoscopic removal of aganglionic bowel using the Duhamel-Martin method in five consecutive infants. *Pediatric Surgery International* 1995;10:226–228.

[45] Travassos DV, Bax NM a, Van der Zee DC. Duhamel procedure: a comparative retrospective study between an open and a laparoscopic technique. *Surgical Endoscopy* 2007;21:2163-5.

[46] Muensterer OJ, Chong A, Hansen EN, Georgeson KE. Single-Incision Laparoscopic Endorectal Pull-Through (SILEP) for Hirschsprung Disease. *Journal of Gastrointestinal Surgery* 2010;14:1950-4.

[47] Garey CL, Laituri C a, Ostlie DJ, St Peter SD. A review of single site minimally invasive surgery in infants and children. *Pediatric Surgery International* 2010;26:451-6.

[48] Rothenberg SS, Shipman K, Yoder S. Technical Report : Experience with Modified Single-Port Laparoscopic Procedures in Children. *Journal of Laparoendoscopic and Advanced Surgical Techniques* 2009;19:695-8.

[49] Hansen EN, Muensterer OJ, Georgeson KE, Harmon CM. Single-incision pediatric endosurgery: lessons learned from our first 224 laparoendoscopic single-site procedures in children. *Pediatric Surgery International* 2011; 27:643-8.

[50] Muensterer OJ. Single-incision pediatric Endosurgical (SIPES) versus conventional laparoscopic pyloromyotomy: a single-surgeon experience. *Journal of Gastrointestinal Surgery* 2010;14:965-8.

[51] Muensterer OJ, Puga Nougues C, Adibe OO, Amin SR, Georgeson KE, Harmon CM. Appendectomy using single-incision pediatric endosurgery for acute and perforated appendicitis. *Surgical Endoscopy* 2010;24:3201-4.

[52] Tam YH, Lee KH, Sihoe JDY, Chan KW, Cheung ST, Pang KKY. Initial experience in children using conventional laparoscopic instruments in single-incision laparoscopic surgery. *Journal of Pediatric Surgery* 2010;45:2381-5.

[53] Dutta S. Early experience with single incision laparoscopic surgery: eliminating the scar from abdominal operations. *Journal of Pediatric Surgery* 2009;44:1741-5.

[54] Chandler NM, Danielson PD. Single-incision laparoscopic appendectomy vs multiport laparoscopic appendectomy in children: a retrospective comparison. *Journal of Pediatric Surgery* 2010;45:2186-90.

[55] Oltmann SC, Garcia NM, Ventura B, Mitchell I, Fischer AC. Single-incision laparoscopic surgery: feasibility for pediatric appendectomies. *Journal of Pediatric Surgery* 2010;45:1208-12.

[56] Emami CN, Garrett D, Anselmo D, Nguyen NX. Pediatric single incision laparoscopic cholecystectomy: lessons learned in the first 25 cases. *Pediatric Surgery International*. 2011; 27: 743-6.

[57] Bertozzi M, Prestipino M, Nardi N, Appignani A. Preliminary experience with a new approach for infantile hypertrophic pyloric stenosis: the single-port, laparoscopic-assisted pyloromyotomy. *Surgical Endoscopy*. 2011;25:2039-2043.

[58] Gaur DD. Retroperitoneoscopy : the balloon technique. *Annals of the Royal College of Surgeons of England* 1994;76: 259-263.

[59] El-Ghoneimi A, Farhat W, Bolduc S, Bagli D, McLorie G, Khoury A. Retroperitoneal laparoscopic vs open partial nephroureterectomy in children. *British Journal of Urology International* 2003;91:532-5.

[60] Valla J-S. Retroperitoneoscopic surgery in children. *Seminars in Pediatric Surgery* 2007;16:270-7.

[61] Lee RS, Retik AB, Borer JG, Diamond D, Peters C. Pediatric retroperitoneal laparoscopic partial nephrectomy: comparison with an age matched cohort of open surgery. *The Journal of Urology* 2005;174:708-11; discussion 712.

[62] Kawauchi A, Fujito A, Naito Y, Soh J, Ukimura O, Yoneda K, et al. Retroperitoneoscopic heminephroureterectomy for children with duplex anomaly: Initial experience. *International Journal of Urology* 2004;11:7-10.

[63] Kawauchi A, Naitoh Y, Soh J, Hirahara N, Okihara K, Miki T. Transvesical laparoscopic cross-trigonal ureteral reimplantation for correction of vesicoureteral reflux: initial experience and comparisons between adult and pediatric cases. *Journal of Endourology* 2009;23(11):1875–1878.

[64] Blackburn S, Smeulders N, Michalski A, Cherian A. Retroperitoneoscopic para-aortic lymph node sampling in bladder rhabdomyosarcoma. *Journal of Pediatric Urology* 2009; 6: 185-187.

[65] Traxel EJ, Minevich E a, Noh PH. A review: the application of minimally invasive surgery to pediatric urology: upper urinary tract procedures. *Urology* 2010;76:122-33.

[66] Mahomed A. Technique of laparoscopic transperitoneal lower pole heminephroureterectomy. *Journal of Laparoendoscopic and Advanced Surgical Techniques. Part A* 2009;19 Suppl 1: S201.

[67] Mahomed A, Hoare C, Welsh F, Driver CP. A two-center experience with the exclusive use of laparoscopic transperitoneal nephrectomy for benign renal disease in children. *Surgical Endoscopy* 2007;21:1532-6.

[68] Kim C, McKay K, Docimo SG. Laparoscopic nephrectomy in children: systematic review of transperitoneal and retroperitoneal approaches. *Urology* 2009;73:280-4.

[69] Castellan M, Gosalbez R, Carmack a J, Prieto JC, Perez-Brayfield M, Labbie a. Transperitoneal and retroperitoneal laparoscopic heminephrectomy-what approach for which patient? *The Journal of Urology*. 2006;176:2636-9; discussion 2639.

[70] Koyle MA, Woo HH, Kavoussi LR. Laparoscopic nephrectomy in the first year of life. *Journal of Pediatric Surgery* 1993;28:693-5.

[71] Jordan GH, Winslow BH. Laparoendoscopic upper pole partial nephrectomy with ureterectomy. *The Journal of Urology* 1993;150:940-3.

[72] Valla J. Treatment of Ureterocele on Duplex Ureter: Upper Pole Nephrectomy by Retroperitoneoscopy in Children Based on a Series of 24 Cases. *European Urology*. 2003;43:426-429.

[73] Janetschek G, Seibold J, Radmayr C, Bartsch G. Laparoscopic heminephroureterectomy in pediatric patients. *The Journal of Urology* 1997;158:1928-30.

[74] Lee RS, Retik AB, Borer JG, Diamond DA, Peters CA. Pediatric retroperitoneal laparoscopic partial nephrectomy: comparison with an age matched cohort of open surgery. *The Journal of Urology* 2005;174:708-11; discussion 712.

[75] Piaggio L, Francguimond J, Figueroa T, Barthold J, Gonzalez R. Comparison of Laparoscopic and Open Partial Nephrectomy for Duplication Anomalies in Children. *The Journal of Urology* 2006;175:2269-2273.

[76] Chertin B, Ben-Chaim J, Landau EH, Koulikov D, Nadu A, Reissman P, et al. Pediatric transperitoneal laparoscopic partial nephrectomy: comparison with an age-matched group undergoing open surgery. *Pediatric Surgery International* 2007 ;23:1233-6.

[77] Robinson B, Snow B, Cartwright P, Devries C, Hamilton B, Anderson J. Comparison of Laparoscopic Versus Open Partial Nephrectomy in a Pediatric Series. *The Journal of Urology*. 2003; 169:638-640.

[78] Sweeney DD, Ost MC, Schneck FX, Docimo SG. Laparoscopic Pyeloplasty for Ureteropelvic Junction Obstruction in Children. *Journal of Laparoendoscopic and Advanced Surgical Techniques. Part A* 2011: 21;261-265.

[79] Penn H, Gatti JM, Hoestje SM, DeMarco RT, Snyder CL, Murphy JP. Laparoscopic versus open pyeloplasty in children: preliminary report of a prospective randomized trial. *The Journal of Urology* 2010;184:690-5.

[80] Canon SJ, Jayanthi VR, Lowe GJ. Which is better--retroperitoneoscopic or laparoscopic dismembered pyeloplasty in children? *The Journal of Urology* 2007;178:1791-5; discussion 1795.

[81] Tan H. Laparoscopic Anderson-Hynes dismembered pyeloplasty in children. *The Journal of Urology* 1999;162:1045-1048

[82] Ravish IR, Nerli RB, Reddy MN, Amarkhed SS. Laparoscopic pyeloplasty compared with open pyeloplasty in children. *Journal of Endourology* 2007;21:897-902.

[83] Tanaka ST, Grantham J a, Thomas JC, Adams MC, Brock JW, Pope JC. A comparison of open vs laparoscopic pediatric pyeloplasty using the pediatric health information system database--do benefits of laparoscopic approach recede at younger ages? *The Journal of Urology* 2008;180:1479-85.

[84] Puri P, Granata C. Multicenter survey of endoscopic treatment of vesicoureteral reflux using polytetrafluoroethylene. *The Journal of Urology* 1998;160:1007-11; discussion 1038.

[85] Lipski B, Mitchell ME, Burns MW. Voiding dysfunction after bilateral extravesical ureteral reimplantation. *The Journal of Urology* 1998;159:1019-21.

[86] Tsai YC, Wu CC, Yang SSD. Minilaparoscopic nerve-sparing extravesical ureteral reimplantation for primary vesicoureteral reflux: a preliminary report. *Journal of laparoendoscopic and advanced surgical techniques. Part A* 2008;18:767-70.

[87] Okamura K, Yamada Y, Tsuji Y, Sakakibara T, Kondo a, Ono Y, et al. Endoscopic trigonoplasty in pediatric patients with primary vesicoureteral reflux: preliminary report. *The Journal of Urology* 1996;156: 198-200.

[88] Atala A, Kavoussi LR, Goldstein DS, Retik AB, Peters CA. Laparoscopic correction of vesicoureteral reflux. *The Journal of Urology* 1993;150:748-51.

[89] Yeung C, Sihoe J, Borzi P. Endoscopic cross-trigonal ureteral reimplantation under carbon dioxide bladder insufflation: a novel technique. *Journal of Endourology* 2005 ;19:295–299.

[90] Kawauchi A, Naitoh Y, Soh J, Hirahara N, Okihara K, Miki T. Transvesical laparoscopic cross-trigonal ureteral reimplantation for correction of vesicoureteral reflux: initial experience and comparisons between adult and pediatric cases. *Journal of Endourology* 2009;23:1875–1878.

[91] Kutikov A, Guzzo TJ, Canter DJ, Casale P. Ureteral Reimplantation at the Children's Hospital of Philadelphia. *Journal of Urology* 2006;176:2222-2226.

[92] Kaouk JH, Palmer JS. Single-port laparoscopic surgery: initial experience in children for varicocelectomy. *British Journal of Urology International* 2008;102:97-9.

[93] Jeon HG, Kim DS, Jeoung HB, Han SW, Hong CH, Im YJ, et al. Pediatric laparoendoscopic single-site partial nephrectomy: initial report. *Urology* 2010;76:138-41.

[94] Tugcu V, Ilbey Y, Polat H et al. Early experience with laparoendoscopic single-site pyeloplasty in children. *Journal of Pediatric Urology* 2011;7: 187-191.

[95] Jacobeus H. The practical importance of thoracoscopy in surgery of the chest. *Surg. Gynecol. Obset.* 1921;4289-296.

[96] Rodgers BM, Moazam F, Talbert JL. Thoracoscopy in children. *Annals of Surgery* 1979;189:176-80.

[97] Jaureguizar E, Vazquez J, Murcia J, Diezpardo J. Morbid musculoskeletal sequelae of thoracotomy for tracheoesophageal fistula. *Journal of Pediatric Surgery.* 1985 ;20:511-514.

[98] Rothenberg SS. Thoracoscopic pulmonary surgery. *Seminars in Pediatric Surgery* 2007;16:231-7.

[99] Bishay M, Giacomello L, Retrosi G, Thyoka M, Nah S a, McHoney M, et al. Decreased cerebral oxygen saturation during thoracoscopic repair of congenital diaphragmatic hernia and esophageal atresia in infants. *Journal of Pediatric Surgery* 2011;46:47-51.

[100] Lobe TE, Rothenberg SS, Waldschmitt J et al. Thoracoscopic repair of esophageal atresia in an infant: a surgical first. *Pediatr. Endosurg. Innov. Tech.* 1999 ;3:141-8.

[101] Rothenberg SS. Thoracoscopic Repair of a Tracheoesophageal Fistula in a Newborn Infant. *Pediatr. Endosurg. Innov. Tech.* 2000 Sep ;4:289-94.

[102] MacKinlay GA. Esophageal atresia surgery in the 21st century. *Seminars in Pediatric Surgery.* 2009 Feb ;18(1):20-2.

[103] Holcomb GW, Rothenberg SS, Bax KM a, Martinez-Ferro M, Albanese CT, Ostlie DJ, et al. Thoracoscopic Repair of Esophageal Atresia and Tracheoesophageal Fistula. *Annals of Surgery* 2005;242:422-430.

[104] Al T, Zamakhshary M, Aldekhayel S, Mandora H, Sayed S, Alharbi K, et al. Thoracoscopic repair of tracheoesophageal fistulas : a case – control matched study. *Journal of Pediatric Surgery* 2008;43:805-809.

[105] Van Der Zee DC, Bax KNM. Thoracoscopic treatment of esophageal atresia with distal fistula and of tracheomalacia. *Seminars in Pediatric Surgery* 2007; 16: 224-30.

[106] Lisle RM, Nataraja RM, Mahomed AA. Technical aspects of the thoracoscopic repair of a late presenting congenital H-type fistula. *Pediatric Surgery International* 2010;26:1233-6.

[107] Kawahara H, Okuyama H, Mitani Y, Nomura M, Nose K, Yoneda A, et al. Influence of thoracoscopic esophageal atresia repair on esophageal motor function and gastroesophageal reflux. *Journal of Pediatric Surgery* 2009;44:2282-6.

[108] Decou JM, Parsons DS, Gauderer MWL. Thoracoscopic Aortopexy for Severe Tracheomalacia. *Pediatric Endosurgery & Innovative Techniques* 2001;5:205-208.

[109] Zee DC van der, Bax NM. Thoracoscopic tracheoaortopexia for the treatment of life-threatening events in tracheomalacia. *Surgical Endoscopy* 2007;21:2024-5.

[110] Lima M, Dòmini M, Libri M, Morabito A, Tani G, Dòmini R. Laparoscopic repair of Morgagni-Larrey hernia in a child. *Journal of Pediatric Surgery* 2000;35:1266-8.

[111] Dutta S, Albanese CT. Use of a prosthetic patch for laparoscopic repair of Morgagni diaphragmatic hernia in children. *Journal of Laparoendoscopic and Advanced Surgical Techniques. Part A* 2007;17(3):391-4.

[112] Ponsky TA, Rothenberg SS. Minimally invasive surgery in infants less than 5 kg : experience of 649 cases. *Surgical Endoscopy* 2008;22:2214-2219.

[113] Ponsky TA, Lukish JR, Nobuhara K, Powell D, Newman KD. Laparoscopy is useful in the diagnosis and management of foramen of Morgagni hernia in children. *Surgical Laparoscopy, Endoscopy and Percutaneous Techniques* 2002;12:375-7.

[114] Harting MT, Lally KP. Surgical management of neonates with congenital diaphragmatic hernia. *Seminars in Pediatric Surgery* 2007;16:109-14.

[115] Becmeur F, Reinberg O, Dimitriu C, Moog R, Philippe P. Thoracoscopic repair of congenital diaphragmatic hernia in children. *Surgical Endoscopy* 2007;16:238-244.

[116] Yang EY, Allmendinger N, Johnson SM, Chen C, Wilson JM, Fishman SJ. Neonatal thoracoscopic repair of congenital diaphragmatic hernia: selection criteria for successful outcome. *Journal of Pediatric Sugery* 2005;40:1369 - 1375.

[117] Arca MJ, Barnhart DC, Lelli JL, Greenfeld J, Harmon CM, Hirschl RB, et al. Early experience with minimally invasive repair of congenital diaphragmatic hernias: results and lessons learned. *Journal of Pediatric Surgery* 2003;38:1563-8.

[118] Nguyen TL, Lee AD. Thoracoscopic repair for congenital diaphragmatic hernia: lessons from 45 cases. *Journal of Pediatric Surgery* 2006;41:1713-5.

[119] Guner YS, Chokshi N, Aranda A, Ochoa C, Qureshi FG, Nguyen NX, et al. Thoracoscopic repair of neonatal diaphragmatic hernia. *Journal of Laparoendoscopic and Advanced Surgical Techniques. Part A* 2008;18:875-80.

[120] Cho SD, Krishnaswami S, Mckee JC, Zallen G, Silen ML, Bliss DW. Analysis of 29 consecutive thoracoscopic repairs of congenital diaphragmatic hernia in neonates compared to historical controls. *Journal of Pediatric Surgery* 2009;44:80-86.

[121] Shah SR, Wishnew J, Barsness K, Gaines BA, Potoka DA, Gittes GK, et al. Minimally invasive congenital diaphragmatic hernia repair: a 7-year review of one institution's experience. *Surgical Endoscopy* 2009;23:1265-71.

[122] Liem NT, Dung LA, Nhat LQ, Ung NQ. Thoracoscopic Repair for Right Congenital Diaphragmatic Henia. *Journal of Laparoendoscopic and Advanced Surgical Techniques* 2008;18:661-663.

[123] Gourlay DM, Cassidy LD, Sato TT, Lal DR, Arca MJ. Beyond feasibility: a comparison of newborns undergoing thoracoscopic and open repair of congenital diaphragmatic hernias. *Journal of Pediatric Surgery* 2009;44:1702-7.

[124] Lansdale N, Alam S, Losty PD, Jesudason EC. Neonatal endosurgical congenital diaphragmatic hernia repair: a systematic review and meta-analysis. *Annals of Surgery.* 2010;252:20-6.

[125] Shah SR, Wishnew J, Barsness K, Gaines BA, Potoka DA, Gittes GK, et al. Minimally invasive congenital diaphragmatic hernia repair: a 7-year review of one institution's experience. *Surgical Endoscopy* 2009;23:1265–1271.

[126] Fishman JR, Blackburn SC, Jones NJ, Madden N, Caluwe DD, Haddad MJ, et al. Does thoracoscopic congenital diaphragmatic hernia repair cause a significant intraoperative acidosis when compared to an open abdominal approach? *Journal of Pediatric Surgery* 2011;46(3):458-61.

[127] Albanese CT, Sydorak RM, Tsao K, Lee H. Thoracoscopic lobectomy for prenatally diagnosed lung lesions. *Journal of Pediatric Surgery* 2003;38:553-5.

[128] Rothenberg SS. Experience with thoracoscopic lobectomy in infants and children. *Journal of Pediatric Surgery* 2003;38:102-4.

[129] Vu LT, Farmer DL, Nobuhara KK, Miniati D, Lee H. Thoracoscopic versus open resection for congenital cystic adenomatoid malformations of the lung. *Journal of Pediatric Surgery* 2008;43:35-9.

[130] Zallen G. Miniature access pectus excavatum repair: lessons we have learned. *Journal of Pediatric Surgery* 2004;39:685-689.

[131] Nuss D. Minimally invasive surgical repair of pectus excavatum. *Seminars in Pediatric Surgery* 2008;17:209-17.

[132] Bufo AJ, Stone MM. Addition of Thoracoscopy to Nuss Pectus Excavatum Repair. *Pediatric Endosurgery and Innovative Techniques* 2001;5:159-162.

[133] Saxena AK, Castellani C, Höllwarth ME. Surgical aspects of thoracoscopy and efficacy of right thoracoscopy in minimally invasive repair of pectus excavatum. *The Journal of Thoracic and Cardiovascular Surgery* 2007;133:1201-5.

[134] Ohno K, Nakamura T, Azuma T, Yamada H, Hayashi H, Masahata K. Modification of the Nuss procedure for pectus excavatum to prevent cardiac perforation. *Journal of Pediatric Surgery* 2009;44:2426-30.

[135] Schaarschmidt K, Kolberg-schwerdt A, Lempe M, Schlesinger F, Bunke K, Strauss J. Extrapleural, submuscular bars placed by bilateral thoracoscopy — a new improvement in modified Nuss funnel chest repair. *Journal of Pediatric Surgery* 2005;40:1407 - 1410.

[136] Ehrlich P. Lessons learned from a failed multi-institutional randomized controlled study. *Journal of Pediatric Surgery* 2002;37:431-436.

[137] Cribbs RK, Wulkan ML, Heiss KF, Gow KW. Minimally invasive surgery and childhood cancer. *Surgical Oncology* 2007;16:221-8.

[138] Holcomb GW, Tomita SS, Haase GM, Dillon PW, Newman KD, Applebaum H, et al. Minimally invasive surgery in children with cancer. *Cancer* 1995;76:121-8.

[139] Saenz NC, Conlon KC, Aronson DC, LaQuaglia MP. The application of minimal access procedures in infants, children, and young adults with pediatric malignancies. *Journal of Laparoendoscopic and Advanced Surgical Techniques. Part A* 1997;7:289-94.

[140] Iwanaka T, Arai M, Ito M, Kawashima H, Yamamoto K, Hanada R, et al. Surgical treatment for abdominal neuroblastoma in the laparoscopic era. *Surgical Endoscopy* 2001;15:751-4.

[141] Duarte RJ, Dénes FT, Cristofani LM, Odone-Filho V, Srougi M. Further experience with laparoscopic nephrectomy for Wilms' tumour after chemotherapy. *British Journal of Urology International* 2006;98:155-9.

[142] Duarte R, Denes F, Cristofani L, Giron a, Filho V, Arap S. Laparoscopic Nephrectomy for Wilms Tumor After Chemotherapy: Initial Experience. *The Journal of Urology.* 2004;172:1438-1440.

[143] Metzelder ML, Kuebler JF, Shimotakahara A, Glueer S, Grigull L, Ure BM. Role of diagnostic and ablative minimally invasive surgery for pediatric malignancies. *Cancer* 2007;109:2343-8.

[144] Yim APC. Video-assisted thoracoscopic management of anterior mediastinal masses. *Surgical Endoscopy* 1995;9:1184-1188.

[145] Spurbeck WW, Davidoff AM, Lobe TE, Rao BN, Schropp KP, Shochat SJ. Minimally Invasive Surgery in Pediatric Cancer Patients. *Annals of Surgical Oncology* 2004 ;11:340-343.

[146] Rescorla FJ, West KW, Gingalewski CA, Engum SA, Scherer III L, Grosfeld JL. Efficacy of primary and secondary video-assisted thoracic surgery in children. *Journal of Pediatric Surgery* 2000;35:134–138.

[147] Partrick D, Rothenberg SS. Thoracoscopic resection of mediastinal masses in infants and children: an evaluation of technique and results. *Journal of Pediatric Surgery* 2001 ;36:1165-7.

[148] Lima M, Ruggeri G, Dòmini M, Bertozzi M, Libri M, Federici S, et al. The role of endoscopic surgery in paediatric oncological diseases. *La Pediatria Medica e Cchirurgica : Medical and Surgical Pediatrics* 2002;24:41-4.

[149] Raza A, Turna B, Smith G, Moussa S, Tolley D. Pediatric urolithiasis: 15 years of local experience with minimally invasive endourological management of pediatric calculi. *The Journal of Urology* 2005;174:682-5.

[150] Sailhamer E, Jackson C-CA, Vogel AM, Sam K, Yeming W, Chwals WJ, et al. Minimally invasive surgery for pediatric solid neoplasms. *The American Surgeon* 2003 ;69:566-568.

[151] Nio M, Nakamura M, Yoshida S, Ishii T, Amae S, Hayashi Y. Thoracoscopic removal of neurogenic mediastinal tumors in children. *Journal of Laparoendoscopic and Advanced Surgical Techniques. Part A* 2005;15:80-3.

[152] Petty JK, Bensard DD, Partrick DA, Hendrickson RJ, Albano EA, Karrer FM. Resection of neurogenic tumors in children: is thoracoscopy superior to thoracotomy? *Journal of the American College of Surgeons* 2006 ;203:699-703.

[153] Esposito C, Lima M, Mattioli G, Mastroianni L, Riccipetitoni G, Monguzzi G, et al. Thoracoscopic surgery in the management of pediatric malignancies: a multicentric survey of the Italian Society of Videosurgery in Infancy. *Surgical Endoscopy* 2007 ;21:1772-5.

[154] Parekh K, Rusch V, Bains M, Downey R, Ginsberg R. VATS Port Site Recurrence : A Technique Dependent Problem. *Annals of Surgery* 2001;8:175-178.

[155] Kennith B, Sartorelli H, Partrick D, Meagher DP. Port-site recurrence after thoracoscopic resection of pulmonary metastasis owing to osteogenic sarcoma. *Journal of Pediatric Surgery* 1996;31:1443-1444.

[156] Castagnetti M, Delarue a, Gentet JC. Optimizing the surgical management of lung nodules in children with osteosarcoma: thoracoscopy for biopsies, thoracotomy for resections. *Surgical Endoscopy* 2004;18:1668-71.

[157] Waldhausen JHT, Tapper D, Sawin RS. Minimally invasive surgery and clinical decision-making for pediatric malignancy. *Surgical Endoscopy* 2000;14:250-253.

[158] Spurbeck WW, Davidoff AM, Lobe TE, Rao BN, Schropp KP, Shochat SJ. Minimally Invasive Surgery in Pediatric Cancer Patients. *Annals of Surgery* 2004;11:340-343.

[159] Clements RH, Goldstein RE, Holcomb GW. Laparoscopic left adrenalectomy for pheochromocytoma in a child. *Journal of Pediatric Surgery* 1999;34:1408-9.

[160] Schier, F, Mutter D, Benneck J, Brock D HW. Laparoscopic Bilateral Adrenalectomy in a Child. *European Journal of Pediatric Surgery* 1999 ;9:420-421.

[161] Radmayr C, Neumann H, Bartsch G, Elsner R, Janetschek G. Laparoscopic partial adrenalectomy for bilateral pheochromocytomas in a boy with von Hippel-Lindau disease. *European Urology* 2000;38:344-8.

[162] Mirallié E, Leclair MD, Lagausie P, Weil D, Plattner V, Duverne C, et al. Laparoscopic adrenalectomy in children. *Surgical Endoscopy* 2001;15:156-160.

[163] Castilho LN, Castillo O a, Dénes FT, Mitre AI, Arap S. Laparoscopic adrenal surgery in children. *The Journal of Urology* 2002;168:221-4.

[164] Stanford A, JS U, Nguyen N, E BJ, ES W. Surgical management of open versus laparoscopic adrenalectomy: Outcome analysis. *Journal of Pediatric Surgery* 2002 ;37:1027-1029.

[165] Miller K, Albanese C, Farmer H et al. Experience with laparoscopic adrenalectomy in pediatric patients. *Journal of Pediatric Surgery* 2002 ;37(7):979-982.

[166] Lagausie P de, Berrebi D, Michon J, Philippe-Chomette P, El Ghoneimi A, Garel C, et al. Laparoscopic adrenal surgery for neuroblastomas in children. *The Journal of Urology* 2003;170:932-5.

[167] Kadamba P, Habib Z, Rossi L. Experience with laparoscopic adrenalectomy in children. *Journal of Pediatric Surgery* 2004;39:764-767.

[168] Skarsgard ED, Albanese CT. The safety and efficacy of laparoscopic adrenalectomy in children. *Archives of Surgery* 2005; 140:905.

[169] Shanberg A, Sanderson K, Rajpoot D, Duel B. Laparoscopic retroperitoneal renal and adrenal surgery in children. *British Journal of Urology International* 2001;87:521–524.

[170] Varlet F, Stephan JL, Guye E, Allary R, Berger C, Lopez M. Laparoscopic radical nephrectomy for unilateral renal cancer in children. *Surgical Laparoscopy, Endoscopy and Percutaneous Techniques* 2009;19:148-52.

In: Laparoscopy: New Developments, Procedures and Risks   ISBN: 978-1-61470-747-9
Editor: Hana Terzic, pp. 43-70   © 2012 Nova Science Publishers, Inc.

Chapter II

Robotic Assisted Surgery in Endoscopy: The Problem of Learning Curve

*Andrea Tinelli[*1], Antonio Malvasi[2], Sarah Gustapane[3],*
Giorgio De Nunzio[4], Ivan DeMitri[8], Mario Bochicchio[5],
Lucio De Paolis[6] and Giovanni Aloisio[7]

[1] Department of Obstetrics and Gynecology, Vito Fazzi Hospital, Lecce, Italy.
[2] Department of Obstetrics and Gynaecology, Santa Maria Hospital, Bari, Italy.
[3] Department of Obstetrics and Gynaecology, SS. Annunziata Hospital, Chieti, Italy.
[4] Department of Materials Science, University of Salento, and INFN, Lecce, Italy.
[5] SET-Lab, Department of Innovation Engineering, University of Lecce, Italy.
[6] Department of Innovation Engineering, University of Salento, Lecce, Italy
[7] Information Processing Systems, Department of Innovation Engineering,
University of Salento, Lecce, Italy.
[8] Department of Physics, University of Salento, and INFN, Lecce (Italy).

Abstract

Robotic Surgery is a current procedure in endosurgery, but literature has not addressed the learning curve for the use of the robotic assisted surgery. The learning curve for robot surgical procedures varies widely.

Apart from innate skill, learning curves are composed of at least two fundamentals related to the volume of cases and the incidence rate. Commonly cited reasons include lack of adequate training in residency programs because of the time devoted to abdominal, vaginal, and obstetric procedures, lack of available and adequate training opportunities outside of dedicated fellowships, lack of proctors and mentor surgeons in communities to help to further advance the skills of younger surgeons, and lack of desire

[*] Andrea Tinelli MD Department of Obstetrics and Gynecology, Vito Fazzi Hospital, Lecce, Italy, Division of Experimental Endoscopic Surgery, Imaging, Minimally Invasive Therapy and Technology, 73100 Lecce, Italy, Tel-Fax +39/0832/661511, Cell. +39/339/207408, E-mail: andreatinelli@gmail.com

to leave established surgical practices to try to develop skills requiring long learning curves to master. Currently, the training involves practice with the surgical robot in either pig or human fresh tissue in a laboratory environment in order to become familiar with the functions of the robot, the attachment of the robotic arms to the robotic trocars, and the overall functions of the robotic console. In this chapter authors reviewed current literature on learning curve in robotic assisted surgery and screened problems linked to robotic surgical skills.

Keywords: Robotics, endoscopy, robotic assisted surgery, learning curve, training, complications, residency programs, surgical skills, cancers, oncology.

Introduction

To focus on the recent adoption, patents, experience, and future of Robotic assisted surgery (RAS) applications in surgery, a PubMed search and manual search for clinical and systematic reviews, randomized controlled trials, prospective observational studies, retrospective studies and case reports published between 1970 and April of 2010 has been performed.

RAS can be used in a wide field of endoscopic applications. Although individual studies may draw different conclusions, gynecological RAS is often associated with a longer operating room time, decreased blood loss, shorter hospital stay but leading to a similar clinical outcome.

However, RAS procedures have, their own limitations: the patented equipment is very large, bulky, and expensive, the staff must be trained specifically on draping and docking the instruments, the lack of surgical haptic feedback, a limited vaginal access, a limited specific instrumentation, and the need for larger port incisions requiring fascial closure.

Exchanging instruments become more troublesome and require a surgical assistant.

The RAS facilitates significantly endosurgery, even if well-designed, but prospective studies with well-defined clinical and long-term outcomes, including complications, cost, pain, return to normal activity and quality of life, are still needed to fully assess the value of this new technology.

Learning Curve and Teaching Problem in Robotics

The term 'learning curve' is used to describe the process of gaining knowledge and skills in the field of surgical technology.

As a minimum, reporting of learning should include the number and experience of the operators and a detailed description of data collection [1].

Still, current literature has not addressed the learning curve for the use of RAS by da Vinci System (Intuitive Surgical Inc., CA, USA) in gynecological surgery.

The learning curve for robot surgical procedures varies widely.

There are some questions about it:

- is there a specific 'number' of completed robotic-assisted procedures that would eliminate 'operative and console time'?
- is there a learning curve associated with this technology in gynecology?
- is there a statistically significant trend useful to establish a credentialing criterion for robotic training in gynecology?

Factors of influence are experience and expertise of the surgeon and type and volume of surgery.

There are several variables potentially useful to define the end-point of the learning curve [2].

It is important to identify objective variables for measuring the extent of proficiency.

Apart from innate skill, learning curves are composed of at least two fundamentals related to the volume and the absolute number of cases and incidence rate.

Several surgeons wandered why there would haven't been an earlier adoption of minimally invasive surgical approaches by rank-and-file gynecologists.

Commonly cited reasons include lack of adequate training in residency programs because of the time devoted to abdominal, vaginal, and obstetric procedures, lack of available and adequate training opportunities outside of dedicated fellowships, lack of proctors and mentor surgeons in communities to help to further advance the skills of younger surgeons, and lack of desire to leave established surgical practices to try to develop skills requiring long learning curves to master [3,4].

Currently, the training involves practice with the surgical robot in either pig or human fresh tissue in a laboratory environment in order to become familiar with the functions of the robot, the attachment of the robotic arms to the robotic trocars and the overall functions of the robotic console.

Several studies tried to define the best way for robotic skills learning assessment.

There is a significant difference between the learning curve of conventional laparoscopy and robot surgery.

Suturing and dexterity skills can be performed quicker in robot-assisted laparoscopy than in conventional laparoscopy [5].

The 3D view in robotic surgery improves surgical performance and learning as compared with the traditional 2D laparoscopy view [6].

The learning curve for robotic surgical techniques is relatively short and may be even shorter for new generations as residents have a greater ability to interact with the new robotic instruments [7].

A computerized assessment system (ProMIS) has been used to demonstrate the faster and more precise performance of the robotic system compared with conventional laparoscopy [8].

A major hurdle often early encountered in a surgeon's robotic experience is "docking time" intended as the time necessary for the attachment of the robotic device to the patient.

This is often perceived as excessively time-consuming.

Factors to be considered when choosing a robotic surgical approach, during a learning curve, may include type and extent of disease, preoperative imaging, stage, patient age, body mass index, parity, size of lesion(s), and equipment availability. So far there are no published guidelines on patient selection as it relates to robotic surgery.

The size and weight of the patient often plays a limited role in the decision to proceed with robotic surgery. The main factor is the ability of the patient to tolerate steep Trendelenburg, which is necessary to complete the surgery. Patients with multiple (non-pulmonary) co-morbidities can undergo a robotic surgical approach if anesthesia clears them [9].

Further training will allow the surgeon to learn how to perform simple manoeuvres such as grasping, cutting, and intracorporeal knot tying, the latter being very difficult with conventional laparoscopy.

In fact, the vast majority of laparoscopic surgeons perform extra corporeally knot tying.

Until recently relatively few data were available in the field of robotic learning curves for gynaecology. Two studies specifically looked at learning curves.

The former by Pitter et al compared blood loss and operative time in the first 20 cases of robotic hysterectomies and myomectomies versus the following 20 cases. All surgeries have been performed by a single surgeon. There was no significant difference in blood loss between the two groups, with 86 mL in the first group and 63 mL in the second group (p<0,05).

However, mean overall operative time was significantly shorter in the second group, with 212 minutes for the first group compared with 151 minutes for the second group (p<0,05). There were no conversions to laparotomy [10].

The latter by Lenihan et al evaluated 113 consecutive patients over a 22-month period. They found that the operative times for different benign surgical interventions stabilized after 50 cases. A similar learning curve was documented for the OR team to be able to set up the robot for surgery in 30 minutes. This break point was 20 cases [11].

Two other studies allude to learning curves.

The first, by Kho et al, addressed the issue of "docking times" by demonstrating decreasing times for subsequent groups of 10 patients in their series of 88 patients. Their mean docking time was 2.95 minutes [12].

Payne and Dauterive observed substantial improvement in mean operative time in their robotic cohort after 75 procedures. They reported a mean operative time for laparoscopic hysterectomy in the pre-robotic cohort of 100 procedures of 92.4 minutes versus 119 minutes in the immediate post-robotic cohort of 100 procedures. The authors noted shorter operative time (mean, 78.7 minutes) in the last 25 robotic procedures as compared with the prerobotic operative time.

As demonstrated by these studies, 20 to 75 procedures are required to transcend the early learning curves associated with RAS [13].

Authors affirmed that 18 radical prostatectomies were needed to achieve a level of efficiency superposable to that of experienced laparoscopic prostatectomy surgeons [14].

Vidovskzky cited the number of cases needed to decrease operative and console time in robotic-assisted cholecystectomies as in the range of 16–32 procedures [15].

For a skilled laparoscopic surgeon the learning curve for achieving proficiency with laparoscopic radical prostatectomy (LRP) is estimated at between 40 and 60 cases. For the laparoscopically naive surgeon the curve is estimated at 80 to 100 cases. The development of a robotic interface might significantly shorten the LRP learning curve for an experienced open yet naive laparoscopic surgeon.

A laparoscopically naive yet experienced open surgeon successfully transferred open surgical skills to a laparoscopic environment in 8–12 cases using a robotic interface.

This outcome is comparable to the reported experience of skilled laparoscopic surgeons after more than 100 LRP [16].

The RLRP learning curve for a fellowship-trained laparoscopic surgeon seems to be similar to that of laparoscopically naive yet experienced practitioners of open RRP.

The RLRP is safe and reproducible and even during the learning curve can produce results similar to those reported in large RRP series. The importance of assistance by an experienced open RRP surgeon during the learning curve should not be overemphasized [17].

However, most of comparative studies are from single institutions, and lack a high level of evidence.

Similar studies have been noted in cardiothoracic and general surgery.

Gynaecological surgeries appear not to be different.

Nowadays training programs exist for all disciplines of surgery, including general, cardiac, and thoracic surgeries as well as urologic and gynecologic surgeries [18].

Lenihan et al. realized that there were several learning curves to be estimated.

The first was the time required by the operating room (OR) team (nurses and technicians) to be able to prepare, activate, and use the elements of the robotic equipment necessary to perform the case (setup time). A second point of interest was the time required to complete the robotic portion of the operation. The third and most important parameter was the number of cases necessary to stabilize the surgeon's operative time. Other outcomes of interest included the effect of uterine weight on blood loss and the time required to perform the various procedures, the complications, the conversion rate from robotic to conventional procedures, the average patient length of staying in the hospital, and the average time required for patients to return to normal activities of daily living.

One hundred and thirteen patients were treated over a 22-month period with the "da Vinci Surgical System". Most procedures were hysterectomies, whereas other gynecologic procedures included supracervical hysterectomy, laparoscopic vaginal assisted hysterectomy, myomectomy, sacrocolpopexy, and oophorectomy. Total operative times for hysterectomies studied sequentially stabilized after 50 cases at approximately 95 minutes. The decrease in robotic time did not depend on uterine size. The mean length of hospital stay was 24 hours, and return to normal activities averaged 2.8 weeks.

The study concluded that RAS is an enabling technology that provides to gynecologic surgeons the ability to offer laparoscopic procedures to most of their patients. In the hands of surgeons with advanced laparoscopic skills, the learning curve to stabilize operative times for the various surgical procedures in women requiring benign gynecologic interventions reaches a plateau after about 50 cases [11].

Ali et al. described a gradual approach to their robotic curriculum that focused on completion of 3 discrete tasks of increasing difficulty in performing Roux-en-Y gastric bypass. Fellows were required to perform 10 cases of one operative segment before performing the next task [20].

Rashid et al required urology residents to assist in 12 cases before starting console training. Residents proceeded to the next step in performing a prostectomy only after showing proficiency on 3 separate occasions [21].

A recent research of Hayn MH et al. from a multicenter, contemporary, consecutive series on the learning curve of robot-assisted radical cystectomy (RARC), as a minimally invasive alternative to open radical cystectomy for patients with invasive bladder cancer, defined the learning curve for RARC and demonstrated an acceptable level of proficiency by the 30th case for proxy measures of RARC quality [22].

Mendevil et al utilized a process involving progressive involvement at University of North Carolina. At the start of both programs, a single surgeon developed procedures at the console with assistants at the bedside. Cases were scheduled according to the surgeon's level of comfort. With time, the involvement of assistants (residents and fellows) on the console increased. The observation of robotic cases by residents and fellows is important to familiarize them to the instrument.

At UNC, residents/fellows begin by learning the placement of trocars necessary for the particular case, followed by docking the robotic arms to the ports. It is also a goal for learners to gain the ability to trouble shoot the device/arms during the case as this can make a major difference in the ability of the console surgeon to the effectively complete the case.

Becoming familiar with the robot as the bedside surgeon also serves to teach the anatomy, surgical boundaries, and surgical procedures with vivid visualization. After case observation, residents and fellows train in the (dry) laboratory and practice specific tasks on the robot. The completion of such pre-surgical preparation is followed by performance of appropriate surgical procedures for patients under direct supervision [23].

While a training module has been established for attending, no standardized robotic training module exists for fellows and residents.

Hoekstra et al certified attending physicians, at their Institution, in robotics via the following training program: 1) completion of a department-sponsored porcine-based laboratory with a robotic proctor; 2) completion of a company-sponsored laboratory training program involving travel to distant site for a porcine-based laboratory with robotic proctors as well as a didactic teaching module; 3) 5 cases scheduled with an available proctor skilled in performing common gynecologic oncology procedures robotically [24].

Frumovitz et al, questioned, by a survey administered to full or candidate members of the Society of Gynecologic Oncologists, the proportion of gynecologic oncologists performing robotic surgery, to determine the level of fellows' training in robotic surgery.

The results showed that only 27% utilize the robot in their practice. Reasons for not using the robot included: hospital does not own a robotic system (32%); capable of performing all procedures with traditional laparoscopy (22%); robot limits laparoscopic exposure for trainees (9%).

Among robot users, 19% utilize it for more than 75% of their laparoscopic cases while 55% use it for less than 25% of their minimally-invasive surgeries. Thirty-seven percent felt the robot was appropriate for hysterectomy/staging in endometrial cancer, 33% felt it appropriate for radical hysterectomy/pelvic lymphadenectomy, and 15% as a diagnostic instrument for adnexal masses.

For procedures that respondents do not perform with traditional laparoscopy, 17% are able to perform laparoscopic radical hysterectomy and 10% perform hysterectomy/staging for endometrial cancer using the robot.

Two-thirds of respondents thought their use of the robot would increase in the next year while an additional 15% stated that although they do not currently utilize it, they were planning on beginning. For those respondents who train fellows, 75% allow the fellow to sit at the console although 73% do so in less than half their cases. For those who train residents, only 30% allow them to sit at the console although 79% do so in less than half their cases (25).

A study evaluated the operative time and estimated blood loss, as a function of experience in gynecological robotic surgery in a retrospective analysis of 40 consecutive cases (17 hysterectomies and 23 myomectomies) over a 1 year period using the da Vinci in two Institutions.

Authors demonstrate statistical improvement in operative time after the first 20 cases for a single surgeon [26].

Since currently, credentialing in robotic surgery for most surgeons requires off-site training followed by preceptor instruction, Gaddi et al tried to establish a foundation for and integration of formal da Vinci robotic surgical training into gynecology residency education. Authors used an observational analysis of residents in an obstetrics and gynecology residency program. Structured training sessions were split into two six-person groups, allotting about 6 hours per group. Each group was introduced to the da Vinci S Surgical System. The training modules included the following: overview of the robotic system, proper setting and docking of the system, skill set (docking practicum); timed evaluation of system docking overview of system controls, suturing overview, skill set (system manipulation and suturing); timed evaluation in various skills including rubber band manipulation on a peg board, suturing, and "peeling a grape".

For authors, robotic training using the da Vinci Surgical System can easily be integrated into a gynecology residency curriculum. The belief is that the earlier that gynecologists are exposed to formal training with the robotic platform, the more likely it is that the individual could be credentialed during residency. This pilot program is intended to promote progressive on-site robotic skill set mastering for gynecology residents [27].

A survey demonstrated that only the most senior laparoscopic surgeons found the robot to be frustrating [4].

In an analysis that specifically addressed suturing, expert surgeons required similar amounts of time when using the robot as compared with conventional laparoscopy; however, novice surgeons were able to suture faster with the robot [5].

Therefore, it seems that using the robot does result in an overall increase in precision and decrease in learning curves for performing laparoscopic skills in surgeons who are not expert laparoscopists.

Although these studies address specific surgical skills, they do not address whether the robot has an impact when used in actual surgical procedures.

Animal Model Learning

In contrast to open surgery, the basic laparoscopic and robotic skills can improve significantly in a relatively short-intensive course.

Robot-assisted surgery can be learned in different ways than conventional laparoscopy. At present, however, the only laboratory-based experience available for training with the da Vinci surgical system is to use the system on inanimate, cadaveric, or animate models [28].

Training on human cadavers still gives the best anatomic training, but fresh human cadavers are not always available [29].

The advantage of using fresh tissue models (like porcine intestine) is obvious in developing delicate tissue handling.

A complex sewing task, like a robotic-sutured intestinal anastomosis, can be reproduced successfully by residents [30].

Preclinical animal model training is effective in developing such skills and allows surgeons the opportunity to refine their surgical robotic technique prior to human application.

Robotic surgical simulators can be designed to represent surgical scenarios, allowing surgeons to become proficient at a particular operation before attempting it on a real patient.

Training consoles that can simulate haemorrhage, imitate skin turgor and organ reality are undergoing development and will better prepare the next generation of surgeons in this era of robotic surgery [31].

Most robotic live surgical procedures were first preformed in an animal model.

Robotic pyeloplasty was first performed by Sung and Gill in 1995 on a porcine model [32].

The learning curve associated with the introduction of a surgical robotic system into a surgeon's armamentarium is unknown. The systematic training on a surgical robotic system in an animal model would result in measurable improvement in robotic surgical skills, and that surgeons would benefit from such preclinical training.

Hanly et al. [33] reported that the direct costs associated with animal training protocol totaled $10,355. By delaying clinical use of the robotic system purchased by their department for the purpose of engaging in in-house animal model training, they were able to significantly reduce the $63,250 cost associated with da Vinci system training for 23 surgeons at designated Intuitive Surgical Training Centers ($5500 for two surgeons). Their model of ''on-site'' training resulted in a cost savings of approximately $52,895 and provided improved training opportunities for surgeons. While the cost savings are not as great for hospitals without dedicated animal operating room and veterinary support services, these and similar training protocols are recommended for institutions implementing clinical surgical robotics programs prior to clinical use.

However, some studies suggest that hospitals implementing clinical surgical robotics programs that institute preclinical surgical robotics training programs can expect to enjoy a 40% reduction in preclinical operative time and a 50% reduction in preclinical set-up time by allowing their surgeons and surgical teams to practice only three times.

At present, however, the only laboratory-based experience available for training with the da Vinci surgical system is to use the system on inanimate, cadaveric, or animate models [34].

Robotics Reported Injuries

Milad M et al determine the incidence, degree, and type of musculoskeletal injuries among surgeons performing conventional laparoscopy as compared to robotic assisted surgery, by a single institution cohort study involving surgeons who are proficient in both conventional laparoscopy and robotic assisted surgery.

Data was gathered from the administration of 3 surveys as well as from strength assessments performed on the individual surgeon. The first survey obtained basic demographic information, operative experience, and intra-operative decision making to limit strain from each surgeon.

This survey also includes a personal health information survey (PHI), or SF12, which helps to assess baseline physical fitness and activity. The second survey was completed both before and after each case, and was used to assess the degree of strain associated with each case. This survey includes a visual analog scale, which assesses the current level of pain/strain in the neck, wrist, back, and shoulder, as well as a Borg scale, which assesses the level of exertional strength.

Finally, both before and after the surgery, surgeons underwent physical examination, assessment of core body strength and posture, as well as manual muscle strength assessment via the use of a dynanometer, in order to evaluate strength and range of motion of key body regions of common injury.

A significant difference in musculoskeletal strain injuries exists amongst surgeons who perform Conventional Laparoscopic assisted Hysterectomy as compared to Robotic Assisted Hysterectomy [35]. Gaia et al [36] reported no statistical differences in vascular, urologic, or gastrointestinal intraoperative injuries for robotic-assisted surgeries compared with traditional laparoscopic or laparotomy techniques for the treatment of endometrial cancer. The vaginal cuff dehiscence rate was 1.5% for both robotic hysterectomy and laparoscopy in this analysis. In contrast, Kho et al [37] reported a 4.1% complete dehiscence rate for 510 patients undergoing a variety of gynecologic surgeries and hypothesized that the closure technique and thermal effect of electrocautery may have been contributory.

Koliakos et al reported, for the first time, a hardware malfunction of the tip of an instrument: a rare case of a da Vinci robotic arm failure during a laparoscopic robot-assisted radical prostatectomy.

The articulation joint of an Endowrist needle driver was broken and positioned at such an angle that made it impossible to remove through the trocar. In addition, it was later discovered that a small piece of the instrument was detached and remained inside the abdomen of the patient without even being identified on subsequent radiological evaluation.

In order to remove the broken instrument, authors had to uninstall it from the robot arm and a bigger incision had to be made in the abdominal wall of the patient. The operation was completed without any other incidents [38].

In the discussion, authors reported, in their experience of 5 years and 520 prostatectomies, three software malfunctions that just needed removal then reinstallation of the instruments, one loss of stereoscopic vision, and one complete malfunction of the system that made us convert the procedure to a laparoscopic prostatectomy. These numbers are in accordance with the numbers published in the literature report [39].

Zorn et al. reported four robot malfunctions that led to operation being postponed [40].

Costs-Effectiveness

The current cost of the da Vinci system is more than 2 million euro with the addition of the 10% annual maintenance fee for repair and service. The semi-reusable instruments cost $2000 and can be used for only 10 procedures. Finally, extra costs for training, delay in set-up and extraoperative time during the learning curve should be anticipated.

Basing on these costs, hospitals face a minimum of 3 to 4 years before seeing a positive cash flow. There are also periodic software upgrades that are required to maintain the fluid function of the system, the costs for any other accessories necessary for the particular case and there is the cost of training personnel to set up the system [41].

Several cost comparison studies exist that demonstrate the relative cost drivers of robotic surgery versus open surgery. The largest cost comparison study was recently published in European Urology by Bolenz, et al from the University of Texas Southwestern and Mannheim Medical Center at the University of Heidelberg. The study compared operating costs of robotic (RALP), laparoscopic (LRP), and open radical prostatectomy (RRP) for prostate cancer in a sample of 643 consecutive patients treated at Southwestern Medical Center in Dallas, Texas. Results showed that the cost of RALP was 50% higher than the cost of RRP even before the cost of purchasing and maintaining the robot was factored in to the calculations. The median cost for the RALP was US $6,752, followed by LRP at US $5,687 and RRP at US $4,437 (all adjusted to 2007 dollars). RALP had higher surgical supply costs and higher OR cost due to increased average length of procedure. The one cost benefit for RALP was the shorter average length of hospital stay (one day) relative to LRP and RRP (two days). However, the shorter RALP hospital stay relative to LRP and RRP did not make up for the RALP higher operating costs, even before considering the additional cost for the purchase and maintenance of the robot. The additional cost for the purchase and maintenance of the robot ($340,000 per year when amortized over a presumed 7yr life of the robot) would add an additional $2698 per patient undergoing a RALP (assuming 126 cases per year) [42].

Steinberg et al estimated that nearly 80 robotic prostatectomies per year were necessary for a hospital to pay for the robot, but in USA 85% of urologists do less than 30 prostatectomies per year. Given overall lower reimbursements for gynecologic procedures, even by combining gynecologic and urologic surgeries, most hospitals will not reach a cost-effective surgical volume [43].

A recent description of the cost patterns using a robotic system is given by Prewitt et al. They analyzed 224 procedures in different subspecialties in a single institution and found $1470 greater direct costs for the use of the robotic system [44].

Analyses of costs for different procedures are made: for robot-assisted laparoscopic rectopexy, there was an increase in operative costs of $557 or $745 (including material and time) [45].

For tubal anastomosis, the increase was $1,446 [46].

For myomectomy [47], pyeloplasty [48], cholecystectomy [49] and Nissen fundiplication [50] higher costs were also found for robot-assisted procedure.

Most, if not all, cost-effectiveness analyses do not or only partly take into account indirect costs.

Burgess et al. found significantly higher operative costs for the robot-assisted procedure, although these costs decreased after the learning curve was completed [51].

In relation to this, it is important to realise that the costs of hospital beds vary between hospitals, especially between community hospitals and academic medical centres.

So, a robotic program will be most competitive in a high-cost hospital combined with a high volume of cases [52].

Increased hospital market share evaporates as more hospitals acquire the da Vinci robot—in some cases without yet identifying a surgical team that has intention to use it.

Hospital administrators and surgeons must define the reasons for developing a robotic surgical program. Institutional commitments become much more solid when a surgeon organizes the program.

Costs remain in the forefront of issues to be addressed when implementing robotics in a gynecologic practice.

Each current robotic surgical system retails for approximately $1.6 million and is associated with an annual maintenance contract of at least $100,000.

The EndoWrist instruments, which retail for approximately $2000 each, have limited patient uses. A minimum of 3 or 4 Endo Wrist instruments are required for each case, that is, $200 per instrument = $600 to $800 per procedure, assuming 10 cases per instrument before replacement. In addition, there is the cost of drapes and other disposable equipment. Other costs to consider are the required training fees for surgeons and operating room personnel and the effect of learning curves on the costs involved with longer operative time and decreased productivity.

Advincula et al. evaluate cost in their comparison of robot-assisted laparoscopic myomectomy vs laparotomy. They found professional (mean, $5946.48 vs $4664.48) and hospital charges (mean, $3014.084.20 vs $1314.400.62) to be statistically higher in the robotic group.

Although professional reimbursement was not significantly different between the 2 groups, hospital reimbursement rates in the robotic group were significantly higher ($1314.181.39 vs $714.015.24) [47].

The total cost of laparoscopic vs abdominal surgical management was compared in a retrospective analysis by Scribner et al [53] and demonstrated no statistically significant difference. The cost savings of early hospital discharge in the laparoscopic group was offset by longer surgical time and higher anesthesia cost. Bell et al [54] published a larger case series comparing 40 robotic endometrial cancer surgeries with 40 laparotomies and 30 laparoscopic procedures. They concluded that while laparotomy was significantly more expensive than robotic surgery ($12 944 vs $8212; p , .001), the cost of laparoscopy was not statistically significantly different ($7570; p 5 .06). First, the lack of statistical significance may be explained by the large standard deviations in the laparoscopy ($1546) and robotic groups ($1150). Second, $642 per procedure is an economically significant difference even if not statistically so. If 100 procedures are performed at an institution in the absence of cost-saving benefits, robotic surgery could have an effect on overall hospital finances. Bell et al attempted to estimate the economic benefit gained by earlier return to work [54].

We did not try to replicate this analysis because we did not record the true date of return to work. Any future multicenter trial should include return to activity and economic effect as an outcome.

As evidenced by these studies, the issues surrounding costs as it relates to robotic technology can be complex and often include complex calculations geared toward depreciation factors. Although costs certainly are an obstacle to implementation of advanced technologies, strides have been made in the billing arena, in particular, on the facility's technical component side.

One such example is the implementation of a new *International Classification of Diseases, Ninth Revision, Clinical Modification subcategory code as of October 1, 2008: 17.42, Laparoscopic robot-assisted procedure.*

Hanly et al. characterized the learning curve associated with new use of advanced surgical robotics system among surgeons from multiple surgical disciplines in a more clinically relevant setting: same-member healthcare teams progressively improved their set-up times on average, by almost 30% each time they prepared the system.

Surgeons clearly benefited from participation in that study: their operative times decreased substantially (more than 20% each time they practiced) throughout the training period, and the absolute operative times achieved by many of the surgeons near the end of the training protocol were excellent.

Hanly et al. reported that the direct costs associated with animal training protocol totalled $10,355. By delaying clinical use of the robotic system purchased by their department for the purpose of engaging in in-house animal model training, they were able to significantly reduce the $63,250 cost associated with da Vinci system training for 23 surgeons at designated Intuitive Surgical Training Centers ($5500 for two surgeons) [55].

Their model of "on-site" training resulted in a cost savings of approximately $52,895 and provided improved training opportunities for surgeons.

Link et al. suggest that depreciation and maintenance costs can be minimised if the number of robotic cases is increased. They reported that for surgeons with intracorporeal suturing, dependence on the robot adds little speed or quality advantage to the LP procedure and results in substantially greater costs. Longer operative time combined with substantial expense for robot depreciation and consumables made robotic pyeloplasty (RLP) a much more expensive procedure than laparoscopic pyeloplasty (LP) (2.7 times).

One way sensitivity analysis holding RLP operative time constant projected that LP operative time must increase to 388 min (6.5 h) for RLP to be cost-equivalent with LP. da Vinci robot depreciation based on an estimated utilization of 150 cases per year (of all types) resulted in a $2000 premium for da Vinci use per case solely due to depreciation of capital equipment. This represented 46% of the total projected cost for RLP. However, even if da Vinci depreciation was eliminated from the model, RLP was still 1.7 times more costly than LP based on increased consumables and operative time costs [56].

Certainly, the impact of depreciation would be blunted if the total institutional volume of robot cases were to dramatically increase.

Over time the robot will become more financially favorable, but for general gynecology, the available alternative minimally invasive routes will likewise decline (as in the case of conventional laparoscopy) or remain low (as in the case of vaginal surgery).

Surgical innovation is necessary.

There are ethical and societal issues that remain incompletely understood about the use of robotic surgery. These include physician training, cost of health care, and rural medical practice. Is this new technology to usher in a brave new world or is the present technology tipping toward that grisly morning after? Evidence will, and should alone, answer this question.

In our current economic climate it is equally important for medical institutions and patients alike to consider the financial impact of treatment decisions.

Many observations emerge regarding the cost of robotic surgery and include: the fixed (equipment and maintenance) and variable (instruments) costs for robotic surgery higher than both conventional laparoscopic or open surgery, however when the total (fixed, variable, OR, and hospital stay) costs for robotic surgery and open surgery are comparable there is a considerable shortening of the length of hospital stay after the robotic surgery resulting in total cost savings.

Simulator Training

Training for specific procedures is possible in a cadaver or in a virtual-reality environment.

Conventional laparoscopic surgery requires different skills and training compared with open surgery. Basic laparoscopic skills can be obtained in a box trainer, in a cadaver or with virtual reality [57,58].

In conventional laparoscopy, the surgeon has a two-dimensional (2D) view, while in robotic surgery, the view is 3D, allowing tasks to be performed quicker and more efficiently [59].

Some protagonists of endoscopic surgery suggest that this increased complication is not a consequence of the surgical technique itself but rather a consequence of relative inexperience.

They point out that there is a significant learning curve associated with this type of surgery.

Robotic surgery is specifically suitable for virtual reality training, as the operation itself is computer guided.

Different companies are developing virtual reality simulators for robotic surgery and this is likely to be the training of choice for the surgeons of tomorrow [60].

Simulators help emulate with a high degree of accuracy the anatomy of "virtual" organs, "virtual" tissues, and "virtual" vessels not just in visualization but also in feel, now even possible using "virtual" instruments in a "virtual" operating theater with a "virtual" surgeon [61].

It has been suggested that this rather long learning curve may be overcome without increasing harm to patients by first exposing trainees to models of the procedures on virtual reality equipment [62].

A significant concern is how to incorporate robotic surgery into a training program without compromising teaching or patient safety and how to determine the ideal methodology for educating trainees to utilize this innovative technology [63].

The current generation of medical students has grown up in the age of computer technology and it has been shown that prior videogame experience can shorten the time to learn basic skills in virtual reality simulation for minimal invasive surgery [64], except for robotic suturing, where prior videogame experience had a negative impact on robotic performance [65].

New developments are the use of a mentoring console.

A recent consensus statement on robotic surgery was released by the Society of American Gastrointestinal and Endoscopic Surgeons and Minimally Invasive Robotic Association emphasizing guidelines for training and credentialing.

Guidelines for training included expert instruction, didactic experience, live case observation, and hands-on experience including simulation and clinical experience. The panel recommended that formal assessment of competency in specific procedures should be documented and an adequate number of cases be performed to allow proficiency under appropriate mentoring by an expert [66].

With the rapid incorporation of training fellows as console surgeons, the robotic platform may even allow faster acquisition of laparoscopic skills compared with traditional laparoscopy [4].

The development of computer-based simulators will allow surgeons in the future to more rapidly learn the skills required to efficiently and safely manipulate the robot before ever stepping into the OR with a live patient.

The dV-trainer robotic simulator (Mimic Technologies, Inc., Seattle, WA, USA) has modules for system training and for skill training [67].

Face, content and construct validity for the virtual reality dV-Trainer were established [68,69].

Another virtual reality trainer is the SEP, robotic surgery simulator (SimSurgery, Oslo, Norway, USA) [70].

Training on basic robot-assisted suturing skills using this simulator equaled training using a mechanical simulator [71].

At the University of Nebraska, a virtual reality trainer using da Vinci instruments and training task platform (dry lab) has been developed.

This 3D virtual reality program can be projected inside the actual console of the da Vinci robot.

Some tasks were adequately simulated but others need improvement in the complexity of the virtual reality simulation [72].

At the University of Hong Kong, a comprehensive computer-based simulator for the da Vinci robotic system is being developed. The simulator reproduces the behavior of the da Vinci system by implementing its kinematics and thus providing a promising tool for training and a way to plan operations [73].

Students of today easily and readily adopt virtual reality as part of their regular training program [74].

The prototype of the da Vinci mentoring system was tested by Hanly et al. It facilitates collaboration between the mentor and the resident during robotic surgery. It improves performance of complex three-handed tasks. This feature can also contribute to the patient's safety in hospitals with robotic surgical training programs.

On the other hand, it improves resident participation and resident education [75].

Other new developments in training robotics are the use of augmented visual feedback to enhance robotic surgical training [76].

Unlike open surgery, robotic surgery provides safe and easy opportunity to divide the operation into smaller segments, enabling participation as a console surgeon depending on the experience of the resident or fellow. It is advisable to develop a structured training program in advance. In this way, a complex operation can be incorporated in a residency or fellow training program and has less influence on the total operating time and patient safety [77].

Computer-based drills on simulators will allow surgeons to maintain skills between cases and to practice handling surgical emergencies just as pilots currently maintain their skills on aircraft simulators between actual flights [78,79].

To confirm this, Lee et al determined that a systematic approach to fellow training should included: [1] didactic and hands-on instruction with the robotic system in conjunction with the attending surgeons, [2] review of instructional videos, [3] patient-side first assistance, and [4] performance of segments of gynecologic procedures in tandem with the senior surgeon.

In their study, twenty-one robotic-assisted gynecologic procedures were performed from April 2006 to January 2007. Fellows participated as the console surgeon in 14/21 cases. Thirteen patients (62%) had prior abdominal surgery. Median values with ranges were age 51 years (range, 33 to 90); BMI 28 (range, 19.4 to 43.8); EBL 25 mL (range, 25 to 250); and hospital stay 1 day (range, 1 to 4). No significant difference existed between fellow and attending mean total operative and individual segment times. One conversion to laparotomy was necessary. No major surgical complications occurred. Lee et al strategy, with the use of a didactic program, instructional videos, repetitive drills on inanimate models followed by systematic surgical integration, with patient bedside assistance and tandem performance of progressively more difficult procedures, was successful in their fellowship training program [80].

Though many VR simulators with and without haptic feedback exist for training, especially in laparoscopic surgery from a general surgeon's requirement, unfortunately those with a specific gynecological software training module are limited [61].

Haptic feedback is incorporated in newer models like LapSimGyn (Immersion Medical and Surgical Science Ltd.), Lap Mentor (Simbionix), ProMIS (Haptica), Procedicus MIST (Mentice Medical), and VIRGY (Swiss Federal Institute of Technology).

LapSimGyn is equipped with the software for procedural tasks of laparoscopic salpingectomy for ectopic pregnancy removal [81,82], tubal occlusion, and laparoscopic suturing in a laparoscopic myomectomy. Tubal sterilization by cauterization procedural module has also been developed [83].

The LaHystotrain for training in both laparoscopy and hysteroscopy including hysteroscopic interventions was developed combining VR, multimedia technology, and the intelligent tutoring system [84,85].

Virtual hysteroscopy with forced feedback and lately with simulated bleeding models has also arrived [86-88]. The Hysteroscopy AccuTouch system (Immersion Medical) equipped with forced feedback simulates hysteroscopic procedures like cervical dilatation, endometrial ablation, and removal of intrauterine lesions. The fluid management monitor tracks fluid overload. Case histories with specific instructions and metric score analysis are also present.

Munz et al [89] compared LapSim with the classic box trainer and found no significant difference between the two. Also, training of novices using MIST VR yielded similar results as with conventional training [90]. Madan et al [91] found no statistically significant difference in the groups trained only with MIST VR or box trainer (LTS2000) when trainees were asked whether a specific trainer helped their skills. The group trained on both the trainers felt no statistically significant change except that 47% felt that VR was not realistic. VR trainers have some advantages, but most trainees felt the box trainers help more, are more interesting, and should be chosen over VR trainers if only one trainer is allowed. Surgeons who received VR simulation training showed significantly greater improvement in performance in the operating room versus those who did not [92,93]. Experienced laparoscopic surgeons performed the tasks significantly faster, with less error, more economy in movement and diathermy use, and with greater consistency in performance versus the inexperienced and novice laparoscopic surgeons after training on MIST VR [94-96].

Hart et al discussed the value of virtual reality–simulator training in improving the surgical skills of medical students and gynecologic trainees, by a prospective observational study. Authors assessed the changes observed in objectively measured surgical performance after VR training, and they undertaken on sheep standard gynecologic procedures before and after VR training. The procedures were video-recorded and edited to blind the scorer as to identity and seniority of the operator. The procedures were scored using a combination of operative time and penalties for surgical errors. The surgical scores were correlated with the VR scores. As measurements, operative skills were assessed using a combination score compiled from scores obtained while undertaking salpingectomy, salpingotomy, and tubal clipping. Virtual reality scores were also a combination score derived from summation of various computer calculated measures of time and accuracy in undertaking two standardized exercises. In the results, the baseline VR scores were significantly related to the overall pre-training scores, and a better initial VR score was also predictive of better surgical performance. In the conclusions, Hart et al suggest that serious consideration should be given to incorporating VR training into the training program of obstetricians and gynecologists at an early stage, since VR training is of value in improving surgical skills in the clinical environment [97].

The costs of the initial learning curve are high and can vary widely. A theoretical model of the expenses of the learning curve was made by including series of cases. The costs of the initial learning curve varied from $49,613 to $554,694 with an average of $217,034. To overcome these high costs, the concept of high-volume centers is of great importance. In such centers, the learning curve can be rapidly traversed and costs minimized [98].

Credentialing and Ethical Issues

The increasing complexity of modern surgical technology will require more stringent guidelines for operation and practice similar to the discipline exercised in aviation.

When surgeons adopt a new surgical technique, they should be supervised or assisted by a more experienced colleague, whenever feasible, until satisfactory competency has been demonstrated [99].

Credentialing for robotic-assisted surgery within and across specialties is based on training, experience, and documented current competency.

Using a surgical robot implies that the surgeon is no longer in direct physical of visual contact with the patient. The surgeon not only operates through computer commands but there is also a physical distance to the assistants attending the operation table.

Unfortunately, the current systems lack a satisfactory way to communicate between the operator and the assistants. As with many new technological advances, communication might appear the Achilles' heel of robotic surgery.

More appropriate equipment of communication and more strict discipline in follow up of the commands from the primary responsible person, the surgeon, will be essential for a safe and successful procedure.

With the possibility of telemedicine and robotics new legal and ethical issues arise. Telemedicine makes cross-border treatment possible. How to deal with liability and licensure across borders?

Cross-border care should not change usual medical ethics but makes treatment possible of patients in areas the specialist cannot reach in person.

In this way, underserved regions and countries could be helped.

Also, the security of the transmitted data between the surgeon and the (distant) robot is at stake.

Should data be treated the same way as written medical records? Who is responsible if complications arise due to transmission cuts, a breakdown of the system or instability of the software? Malfunction of the robotic system will occur more frequently with its increasing use; fortunately, it appeared that less than 5% of device failures resulted in patient complications.

With the adoption of new technologies into our surgical armamentarium, a structured curriculum and formal assessment of competency will need to be defined for trainees at various levels of surgical skills [100].

Valid concerns exist on the proper use and allocation of health care resources with new technologies. Although the issue of whether every resident ''needs'' to know how to perform robotic surgery is somewhat controversial, there is no doubt that most residents believe that robotic training is necessary and important to their future [101].

Beyond the point of training laboratories, residents must still be trained in the operating room on living patients. The necessity of robotic surgical training during residency is a matter of debate among surgical educators. With the recent boom in technology and an ever-increasing number of specialized procedures to teach, it is becoming ever more difficult to train a ''jack of all trades'' urologist. It is possible that elective additional training in more advanced techniques will be needed in the future, depending on interest and aptitude. The problem with placing robot-assisted surgery in a category by itself, however, is that the current system, like its predecessor laparoscopy, can be used for a multitude of procedures involving various organ systems [102].

Thus, robot-assisted surgery is not a technique, it is a means to an end.

With the introduction of robotic surgery, hospitals and departments have been challenged to establish credentialing requirements for this advanced surgical technique.

There are no universally established credentialing guidelines.

Visco et al recently proposed a set of guidelines that require as a prerequisite that the surgeon be fully credentialed in laparoscopic surgery.

About the basic system training, authors recommend that the surgeon show evidence of at least 8 hours of hands-on training in the use of the robotic surgical system.

A significant portion of this training must include console time as the primary surgeon performing surgical procedures on either anesthetized pigs or fresh cadavers.

For surgeons who are already familiar with the robotic surgical system, usually having completed a residency or fellowship that included training in robotic surgery or having performed robotic surgical procedures at another institution, demonstration of such experience is required.

Authors recommend that the requesting surgeon demonstrate proof of a minimum of 10 robotic surgical procedures of the same type to waive the basic system training [103].

The surgeon is required to perform a minimum of two robotic surgical procedures of each type for which privileges are being requested in the presence of an expert preceptor. Some institutions are using four as the minimum number of proctored robotic surgeries necessary for independent robotic privileges.

An expert preceptor is defined as a surgeon who has current Robotic Surgical Privileges and has been approved as an expert preceptor by the Chair of the Department of the individual applying for privileges.

Ideally, a preceptor will be from the same institution and will have full privileges at that institution. The ability to sit at the console occasionally during the first few surgical procedures is a valuable educational opportunity that is generally not possible when the preceptor is chosen from another institution or state.

The Intellectual Process of a
Robotic Program into Institutions

The most important characteristics in developing a robotic program are intellectual curiosity, and commitment which must be present throughout the institution, from top to bottom, including the department chairperson or group leader.

The potential is greatest when the surgical team and hospital administration can work together for patient care and institutional advancement.

In academic institutions or in University-affiliated Hospitals, there is much greater opportunity for collaborative work.

The intellectual process associated with a robotics program can promote grant writing and scientific publishing. New programs may be developed within these working interest groups, and realistic timelines should be strictly enforced. This is a potentially great source for resident training, offering many areas for research projects. It is important for new robotics programs to provide educational programs within the community.

Program initiation is based on two key players: surgeons and administrators. Surgeon interest and commitment to a robotic program is key in the successful implementation, whereas administrators have to protect the financial interests of an institution and thus must be convinced that robotics offers benefits and is marketable.

Moreover, there are multiple ways to obtain the skills necessary to become a successful robotic surgeon. One way is to participate in a dry (inanimate) lab session practicing suturing, and performing simple dexterity skills with the robotic surgical system. Furthermore, it is useful to participate in a formal porcine training lab in order to practice handling tissue, tissue dissection, cautery, and tissue resection to become proficient with the instrumentation.

However, this has proven financially impractical for multiple residents. It is important to formulate an early plan with mentors, the departmental chairperson, or a trusted colleague. This helps to solidify support and offers constructive comments in preparation for the development of a structured business plan. In developing a business plan and timeline, it is important to collect the necessary data, including the potential increase in referrals as well as savings from reduced hospital lengths of stay and faster recovery. During this phase, it is important not to forget the cost of the yearly service contract for the robotics system as well as instruments and disposables for each case. When negotiating with hospital administrators, it is most important to show them that robotics will add a dimension that will benefit the hospital through patient care.

In addition to potential benefits to patients, programmatic growth potential and institutional recognition should be emphasized.

Once the institution has decided to make the initial investment in a system, the next key step is to find a physician or small group of physicians within the institution who will take charge in building the program: a surgical champion.

This individual should not only have the training necessary to operate the robot, but also the support of the respective departments. Often the start of a robotic program meets resistance because initially the cases may take longer to complete, there may be high rates of conversion from robotic to open surgery, or there may be a lack of support from the operating room staff. Regardless, it is important for the robot program leader to assemble a team that will feel invested in the program and feel that the success of the program depends upon them.

The robot team should consist of individuals that are open to change, are willing to learn a whole new instrument, and do not mind enduring the growing pains of implementing a new system [23].

The transition period of an Institutional fellowship program into robotics is both challenging and beneficial; this period is characterized by the loss of participation of trainees in open and laparoscopic cases as first assistant, and the capitalization of surgical participation in robotic cases by attending being proctored for their own certification.

It is also characterized by a significant broadening of fellow surgical education.

The traditional perception of trainees is that participating in the case as first-assist is most beneficial. However, the first assistant in robotic surgery has minimal participation as compared to laparoscopic and traditional surgery.

Barriers to fellow training in robotics must be balanced by the benefits it provides.

To manage this period of transition, the surgeon (faculty and fellows) must accept several other aspects of participation as legitimate methods of learning, most notably: 1) learning a new technology; 2) learning to be an assistant for robotics and troubleshoot for the operative team; and 3) observation of others, which teaches the trainee what to do and, at times, what not to do. The commitment to robotics must cross all levels of training to successfully move through this transition period [24].

Future Developments and New Frontiers

The frontiers of surgery as we know them are expanding at an astounding pace. As medical students, it is essential that we brace ourselves for what this field may have in store for us when we take our places as surgeons.

Developments in technology coupled with the demand for improved patient safety and surgical finesse are fuelling a revolution in the field of surgery.

Despite the significant expense and learning curve associated with the new technology, the potential short- and long-term benefits for both patients and surgeons seem to outweigh the investment and technical issues.

It may be expected that wider availability of such systems will lead to more and more conventional laparoscopic procedures to be performed with robot assistance.

In this respect, it should also be appreciated that the next generations of doctors will have been raised with computer technology as part of daily life and will therefore more readily adopt computer-guided surgical techniques.

To overcome some of the current limitations of robotic surgery, creation of operating room suites with permanent, ceiling-mounted, robotic arms would be the next logical step.

This would resolve issues concerned with the bulkiness of the robotic set-up and make undocking and redocking the robot to operate on different parts of the body easier.

Apart from more compact systems, other technologic improvements may also include the development of tactile feedback and the incorporation of imaging techniques such as magnetic resonance imaging to more precisely locate lesions and achieve cleaner margins during cancer surgery.

The first adaptations to be expected are the development of tactile feedback and the use of cardanic transmission that will allow even more precise tissue handling.

Also, fusion with imaging techniques like computed tomography and magnetic resonance imaging (MRI) are likely to be introduced allowing more precise and safer surgery and thus more radical oncologic surgery with minimal trauma.

Newer applications of robotic surgery include routinely using the ability to telementor, both on site and off site.

Off-site mentoring where one expert can communicate with the surgeon and operating room team in real time from remote locations will also become more important as more surgeons are being credentialed in robotic surgery.

Da Vinci robot has high cost of purchasing and the maintaining the instruments of the robotic system is one of its many disadvantages. Moreover, the absence of haptic feedback remains an important issue, but this technology may well be introduced in the near future. The current da Vinci system is still sizeable and requires a team of trained staff to set it up over a lengthy time period. Nevertheless, the availability of the robotic systems to only a limited number of centers reduces surgical training opportunities.

The industry needs to develop a new product, more feasible, light and small, that provides enhanced functionality over conventional laparoscopic instruments to apply on new robots.

This enhanced functionality is accomplished by providing articulated motion at the end of the instrument to offer better manoeuvrability of the instrument tip.

The articulating motion is primarily controlled with finger and thumb controls which actuate small motors. The surgeon would remain at the patient's side, similar to current laparoscopic techniques.

Further future developments will focus on mobile in vivo robots to support minimal invasive surgery in remote locations (battlefield, space). For example, the in vivo robots can be placed in the abdominal cavity during surgery and perform wireless imaging or task assistance.

Another interesting feature of robotics is Telesurgery.

This allows the surgeon and the console to be at a different location to the patient and the robot.

This concept caught the attention of NASA and the American army. The military could use robotics to perform surgery on injured soldiers on the front line with the surgeon at a safer location. This concept can also be used to perform surgeries in locations without the surgeon having to travel to the patient.

Although robotic technology was initially developed to allow telesurgery to be performed in areas difficult or dangerous to access, this has not yet fully been implemented.

Sure enough surgeons from the European Institute of Telesurgery (IRCAD)/Louis Pasteur University in Strasbourg, France, have performed in 2001 the first transatlantic telerobotic laparoscopic cholecystectomy using the Zeus robot [104].

Another problem is the increased number and size of ports required from robotic surgery: the typical robotic surgical procedure will use three 8-mm ports and two 12-mm ports.

Single-port laparoscopy, also known as Laparo-Endoscopic Single Site (LESS) surgery, is an attempt to further enhance cosmetic benefits and reduce morbidity of minimally invasive surgery.

Initial laboratory experience with robotic LESS was reported by Haber et al [105].

Subsequently, Kaouk et al reported the first robotic single-port transumbilical surgery in urology by performing a successful radical prostatectomy and nephrectomy [106].

Escobar et al described their initial clinical experience and technique with robotic-assisted single-port surgery in gynecology.

They successfully performed a risk-reducing bilateral salpingo-oophorectomy and total hysterectomy in a 60-year-old woman, by a one 3-cm incision in the umbilicus: the procedure was performed through a multichannel single port and by Da Vinci system [107].

Single Port Laparoscopy (SPL) did not become a standard surgical technique in gynecologic surgery for several reasons including lack of "triangulation," need for special instrumentation, instrument crowding or clashing, challenging ergonomic positions, and need for advanced laparoscopic skill.

In the last decade, technology has advanced tremendously, and surgeons have overcome some of these limitations.

For example, flexible endoscopes help to ameliorate the loss of depth perception that occurs when the camera lines up with the shaft of a working channel. Triangulation, which is easily accomplished in traditional laparoscopy with 3 or 4 ports, can now be achieved during SPL using flexible or curved laparoscopic instruments. Nevertheless, SPL currently is not user friendly or practical in the gynecologic surgical community. The primary disadvantage of single-port surgery without the robot is the collision of instruments and limited degrees of freedom of the instruments. Furthermore, the technique is not ergonomically friendly.

The ability of the robotic arms to enable more degrees of freedom and triangulation at the surgical site, and the improved ergonomics facilitated the surgical success of robotic by LESS.

Some technical challenges merit further discussion. Triangulation is needed for proper dissection while providing effective traction and counter traction, a task that is difficult with SPL. Even though the da Vinci instruments are placed in parallel, the combination of a uterine manipulator with the superior range of motion of the robotic system arm wrist enables proper tissue dissection. Instrument crowding is perhaps the most frustrating aspect of SPL. This has improved somewhat with the development of streamlined profile camera systems and by using instruments of different lengths.

Furthermore, the major problem with the various single-port devices is gas leaking and structural integrity in response to the movement of robotic arms. There are also some patient-related limitations.

In conclusion, robotics may improve surgical capabilities during single-port laparoscopy, feasible in selected cases and a safe cosmetic alternative to conventional multiport robotic procedures.

Conclusion

The feasibility and safety of applying this technology is clearly demonstrated in such specialty, such as gynecology, reproductive surgery, urology and Urogynecology, surgical oncology, cardiosurgery, thoracic surgery, orthopaedics, neurosurgery and head-neck surgery [108].

Limitations such as the absence of tactile (haptic) feedback, bulky design of the instrumentation, and high cost will need to be addressed.

The current robotic technology should be considered an early prototype. Smaller, cheaper, and easier to use robots will be needed to make robotic surgery both faster and more cost efficient than the traditional techniques.

This technology, however, has exciting potential for future applications, especially in long-distance telesurgery, which could deliver the expertise of advanced laparoscopic surgeons to different areas of the world.

It is imperative that future research addresses the questions of cost-effectiveness of learning curve, its effect on resident training, and whether this technology is best made available to all surgeons or to a limited number of surgeons with high surgical volume who develop particular robotic expertise and are able to maintain proficiency with this evolving technology.

The future of robotic surgery in gynecology may be bright, but currently, caution is advisable and clinically meaningful long-term outcomes are needed. These outcomes include effect on quality of life and patient satisfaction associated with RAS.

Many questions still remain, in particular, related to the credentialing and privileging process and the appropriate training method for transference of skills to residents, fellows, and peers. Overall, RAS will likely be an important surgical resource for the minimally invasive surgery.

References

[1] Ramsay CR, Grant AM, Wallace SA, Garthwaite PH, Monk AF, Russell IT. Assessment of the learning curve in health technologies. A systematic review. *Int. J. Technol Assess Health Care* 2000;16:1095–108.

[2] Herrell SD, Smith JA Jr. Robotic-assisted laparoscopic prostatectomy: what is the learning curve? *Urology* 2005;66:105–7.

[3] Kolkman W, Wolterbeek R, Jansen FW. Implementation of advanced laparoscopy into daily gynecologic practice: difficulties and solutions. *J. Minim. Invasive Gynecol.* 2006;13:4–9.

[4] Sarle R, Tewari A, Shrivastava A, Peabody J, Menon M. Surgical robotics and laparoscopic drills. *J. Endourol.* 2004;18:63–67.

[5] Yohannes P, Rotariu P, Pinto P, Smith AD, Lee BR. Comparison of robotic versus laparoscopic skills: is there a difference in the learning curve? *Urology* 2002;60:39–45.

[6] Blavier A, Gaudissart Q, Cadie` re GB, Nyssen AS. Comparison of learning curves and skill transfer between classical and robotic laparoscopy according to the viewing conditions: implications for training. *Am. J. Surg.* 2007;194:115–21.

[7] DiLorenzo N, Coscarella G, Faraci L, Konopacki D, Pietrantuono M, Gaspari AL. Robotic systems and surgical education. *JSLS* 2005;9:3–12.

[8] Narula VK,Watson WC, Davis SS, Hinshaw K, Needleman BJ, Mikami DJ, et al. A computerized analysis of robotic versus laparoscopic task performance. *Surg. Endosc.* 2007;21:2258–61.

[9] Abaid LN, Boggess JF. Current applications of laparoscopy in gynecologic oncology: a literature review. *Women's Oncol. Rev.* 2005;5(4):193–201.

[10] Pitter MC, Anderson P, Blissett A, Pemberton N. Robotic assisted gynaecological surgery-establishing training criteria; minimizing operative time and blood loss. *Int. J. Med. Robot* 2008;4:114–20.

[11] Lenihan JP Jr, Kovanda C, Seshadri-Kreaden U. What is the learning curve for robotic assisted gynecologic surgery? *J. Minim. Invasive Gynecol* 2008;15:589–94.

[12] Kho RM, Hilger WS, Hentz JG, Magtibay PM, Magrina JF. Robotic hysterectomy: technique and initial outcomes. *Am. J. Obstet. Gynecol.* 2007;197:113. e1–113.e4.

[13] Payne TN, Dauterive FR. A comparison of total laparoscopic hysterectomy to robotically assisted hysterectomy: surgical outcomes in a community practice. *J. Minim. Invasive Gynecol.* 2008;15:286–291.

[14] El-Hakim AE, Tewari A Robotic prostatectomy – a review. *Medscape Gen. Med.* 2004; 6(4): 20.

[15] Vidovszky J Robotic cholecystectomy: learning curve, advantages, and limitations. *J. Surg. Res.* 2006; 136(2): 172–178.

[16] Ahlering TE, Skarecky D, Lee D, Clayman RV. Successful transfer of open surgical skills to a laparoscopic environment using a robotic interface: initial experience with laparoscopic radical prostatectomy. *J. Urol.* 2003;170(5):1738e41.

[17] Zorn KC, Orvieto MA, Gong EM, Mikhail AA, Gofrit ON, Zagaja GP, et al. Robotic radical prostatectomy learning curve of a fellowship-trained laparoscopic surgeon. *J. Endourol.* 2007; 21(4):441e7.

[18] Chitwood Jr WR, Nifong LW, Chapman WH, Felger JE, Bailey BM, Ballint T, et al. Robotic surgical training in an academic institution. *Ann. Surg.* 2001;234:475e84.

[19] 19.

[20] Ali MR, Rasmussen J, Bhasker Rao B. Teaching robotic surgery: a stepwise approach. *Surg. Endosc.*. 2007;21:912–915.

[21] Rashid HH, Leung YY, Rashid MJ, et al. Robotic surgical education: a systematic approach to training urology residents to perform robotic-assisted laparoscopic radical prostatectomy. *Urology.* 2006;68:75–79.

[22] Hayn MH, Hussain A, Mansour AM, Andrews PE, Carpentier P, Castle E, Dasgupta P, Rimington P, Thomas R, Khan S, Kibel A, Kim H, Manoharan M, Menon M, Mottrie A, Ornstein D, Peabody J, Pruthi R, Palou Redorta J, Richstone L, Schanne F, Stricker H, Wiklund P, Chandrasekhar R, Wilding GE, Guru KA. The learning curve of robot-assisted radical cystectomy: results from the international robotic cystectomy consortium. Eur Urol. 2010 Apr 23. Epub ahead of print.

[23] Mendivil A, Holloway RW, Boggess JF. Emergence of robotic assisted surgery in gynecologic oncology: American perspective. *Gynecol. Oncol.* 2009; 114:S24–S31.

[24] Hoekstra AV, Morgan JM, Lurain JR, Buttin BM, Singh DK, Schink JC, Lowe MP. Robotic surgery in gynecologic oncology: Impact on fellowship training. *Gynecol. Oncol.* 2009;114:168–172.

[25] Frumovitz M, Greer M, Soliman PT, Schmeler KM, Moroney J, Ramirez PT. Robotic surgery practice and training in gynecologic oncology. *J. Minim.ally Invasive Gynecol* 2008; 15:S1eS159.

[26] Pitter MC, Andreson P, Blissett A, Pemberton N. Robotic-assisted gynaecological surgery – establishing training criteria; minimizing operative time and blood loss. *Int. J. Med. Robotics Comput Assist. Surg.* 2008; 4: 114–120.

[27] Gaddi A, Panagiotakis A, Ginsburg F, Bruck L Integration of structured robotic surgical training into gynecology residency education. *J. Minimally Invasive Gynecol* 2009; 16: S52eS102.

[28] Chou DS, Abdelshehid CS, Uribe CA, Khonsari SS, Eichel L, Boker JR, et al. Initial impact of a dedicated postgraduate laparoscopic mini residency on clinical practice patterns. *J. Endourol.* 2005;19:360e5.

[29] Vlaovic PD, Sargent ER, Boker JR, Corica FA, Chou DS, Abdelshehid CS, et al. Immediate impact of an intensive one-week laparoscopy training program on laparoscopic skills among postgraduate urologists. *JSLS* 2008;12:1–8.

[30] Marecik SJ, Chaudhry V, Jan A, Pearl RK, Park JJ, Prasad LM. A comparison of robotic, laparoscopic, and hand-sewn intestinal sutured anastomoses performed by residents. *Am. J. Surg.* 2007;193: 349–55.

[31] Hanly EJ, Talamini MA. Robotic abdominal surgery. *Am. J. Surg.* 2004 Oct;188 (Suppl. 4A):19S–26S.

[32] Sung G, Gill I. Robotic laparoscopic surgery: a comparison of the da Vinci and Zeus systems. *Urology* 2001;58:893e8.

[33] Hanly EJ, Marohn MR, Bachman SL, Talamini MA, Hacker SO, Howard RS, et al. Multiservice laparoscopic surgical training using the daVinci surgical system. *Am. J. Surg.* 2004;187:309e15.

[34] Chou DS, Abdelshehid CS, Uribe CA, Khonsari SS, Eichel L, Boker JR, et al. Initial impact of a dedicated postgraduate laparoscopic mini-residency on clinical practice patterns. *J. Endourol.* 2005;19:360e5.

[35] Milad M, Nayak S, Fitzgerald C. A comparison of musculoskeletal injuries in conventional laparoscopy as compared to its incidence in robotic assisted laparoscopic surgery. *J. Minim. Invasive Gynecol.* 2009; 16: S1eS51.

[36] Gaia G, Holloway RW, Santoro L, Ahmad S, Di Silverio E, Spinillo A. Robotic-assisted hysterectomy for endometrial cancer compared with traditional laparoscopic and laparotomy approaches: a systematic review. *Obstet. Gynecol.* 2010;116:1422-31.

[37] Kho RM, Akl MN, Cornella JL, Magtibay PM, Wechter ME, Magrina JF. Incidence and characteristics of patients with vaginal cuff dehiscence after robotic procedures. *Obstet Gynecol* 2009;114:231–5.

[38] Koliakos N, Denaeyer G, Willemsen P, Schatteman P, Mottrie A. Failure of a robotic arm during da Vinci prostatectomy: a case report. *J. Robotic Surg.* 2008;2:95–96.

[39] Borden LS Jr, Kozlowski PM, Porter CR et al. Mechanical failure rate of da Vinci robotic system. *Can J. Urol.* 2007;14: 3499–3501.

[40] Zorn KC, Gofrit ON, Orvieto MA et al (2007) Da vinci robot error and failure rates: single institution experience on a single three-arm robot unit of more than 700 consecutive robot-assisted laparoscopic radical prostatectomies. *J. Endourol.* 2007;21: 1341–1344.

[41] Patel HR, Linares A, Joseph JV. Robotic and laparoscopic surgery: cost and training. *Surg Oncol.* 2009 Sep;18(3):242-6.

[42] Bolenz C, Gupta A, Hotze T, et al. Cost comparison of robotic, laparoscopic, and open radical prostatectomy for prostate cancer. *Eur. Urol.* 2010;57(3):453–458.

[43] Steinberg PL, Merguerian PA, Bihrle W 3rd, Heaney JA, Seigne JD. A da Vinci robot system can make sense for a mature laparoscopic prostatectomy program. *JSLS* 2008;12:9–12.

[44] Prewitt R, Bochkarev V, McBride CL, Kinny S, Oleynikov D. The patterns and costs of the Da Vinci robotic surgery system in a large academic institution. *J. Robotic Surg.* 2008;2:17–20.

[45] Heemskerk J, de Hoog DE, van Gemert WG, Baeten CG, Greve JW, Bouvy ND. Robot-assisted vs. conventional laparoscopic rectopexy for rectal prolapse: a comparative study on costs and time. *Dis. Colon Rectum* 2007;50:1825–30.

[46] Rodgers AK, Goldberg JM, Hammel JP, Falcone T. Tubal anastomosis by robotic compared with outpatient minilaparotomy. *Obstet. Gynecol.* 2007;109:1375–80.

[47] Advincula AP, Xu X, Goudeau S IV, Ransom SB. Robot-assisted laparoscopic myomectomy versus abdominal myomectomy: a comparison of short-term surgical outcomes and immediate costs. *J. Minim. Invasive Gynecol.* 2007;14:698–705.

[48] Link RE, Bhayani SB, Kavoussi LR. A prospective comparison of robotic and laparoscopic pyeloplasty. *Ann. Surg.* 2006;243:486–91.

[49] Breitenstein S, Nocito A, Puhan M, Held U, Weber M, Clavien PA. Robotic-assisted versus laparoscopic cholecystectomy: outcome and cost analyses of a case-matched control study. *Ann. Surg.* 2008;247:987–93.

[50] Nakadi IE, Me´ lot C, Closset J, DeMoor V, Be´ troune K, Feron P, et al. Evaluation of da Vinci Nissen fundoplication clinical results and cost minimization. *World J. Surg.* 2006;30:1050–4.

[51] Burgess SV, Atug F, Castle EP, Davis R, Thomas R. Cost analysis of radical retropubic, perineal, and robotic prostatectomy. *J. Endourol.* 2006;20:827–30.

[52] Scales CD Jr, Jones PJ, Eisenstein EL, Preminger GM, Albala DM. Local cost structures and the economics of robot assisted radical prostatectomy. *J. Urol.* 2005;174:2323–9.

[53] Scribner DR Jr, Mannel RS, Walker JL, Johnson GA. Cost analysis of laparoscopy versus laparotomy for early endometrial cancer. *Gynecol. Oncol..* 1999;75:460–463.

[54] Bell MC, Torgerson J, Seshadri-Kreaden U, Suttle AW, Hunt S. Comparison of outcomes and cost for endometrial cancer staging via traditional laparotomy, standard laparoscopy and robotic techniques. *Gynecol. Oncol..* 2008;111:407–411.

[55] Hanly EJ, Marohn MR, Bachman SL, Talamini MA, Hacker SO, Howard RS, et al. Multiservice laparoscopic surgical training using the daVinci surgical system. *Am. J. Surg.* 2004;187:309e15.

[56] Link RE, Bhayani SB, Kavoussi LR. A prospective comparison of robotic and laparoscopic pyeloplasty. *Ann. Surg.* 2006;243:486e91.

[57] Munz Y, Kumar BD, Moorthy K, Bann S, Darzi A. Laparoscopic virtual reality and box trainers: is one superior to the other? *Surg. Endosc.* 2004;18:485–94.

[58] Blavier A, Gaudissart Q, Cadiere GB, Nyssen AS. Impact of 2D and 3D vision on performance of novice subjects using da Vinci robotic system. *Acta Chir. Belg.* 2006;106:662–4.

[59] Albani JM, Lee DI. Virtual reality-assisted robotic surgery simulation. *J. Endourol.* 2007;21:285–7.

[60] Hyltander A, Liljegren E, Rhodin PH, Lonroth H. The transfer of basic skills learned in a laparoscopic simulator to the operating room. *Surg. Endosc..* 2002;16:1324 –1328.

[61] Mettler LL, Dewan P. Virtual reality simulators in gynecological endoscopy: a surging new wave. *JSLS* 2009;13:279-86.

[62] Seymour NE, Gallagher AG, Roman SA, et al. Virtual reality training improves operating room performance: results of a randomized, double- blinded study. *Ann. Surg.* 2002;236:458–463.

[63] Blavier A, Gaudissart Q, Cadiere GB, et al. Comparison of learning curves and skill transfer between classical and robotic laparoscopy according to the viewing conditions: implications for training. *Am. J. Surg.*. 2007;194:115–121.

[64] Shane MD, Pettitt BJ, Morgenthal CB, Smith CD. Should surgical novices trade their retractors for joysticks? Videogame experience decreases the time needed to acquire surgical skills. *Surg. Endosc.* 2007;22:1294–7.

[65] Harper JD, Kaiser S, Ebrahimi K, Lamberton GR, Hadley HR, Ruckle HC, et al. Prior video game exposure does not enhance robotic surgical performance. *J. Endourol.* 2007;21:1207–10.

[66] Herron DM, Marohn M. A consensus document on robotic surgery. *Surg. Endosc.*. 22:313–325, 2008; discussion 1–2.

[67] Mimic Technologies, Inc. [www.mimic.ws]. Accessed 16 June 2008.

[68] Lendvay TS, Casale P, Sweet R, Peters C. VR robotic surgery: randomized blinded study of the dV-Trainer robotic simulator. *Stud Health Technol Inform* 2008;132:242–4.

[69] Lendvay TS, Casale P, Sweet R, Peters C. Initial validation of a virtualreality robotic simulator. *J. Robotic Surg.* 2008;2:145–9.

[70] SimSurgery AG. [www.simsurgery.com]. Accessed 16 June 2008.

[71] HalvorsenFH, Elle OJ,DalininVV,MørkBE, SørhusV,Røtnes JS, et al.Virtual reality simulator training equals mechanical robotic training in improving robot-assisted basic suturing skills. *Surg. Endosc.* 2006;20:1565–9.

[72] Katsavelis D, Siu KC, Brown-Clerk B, Lee IH, Lee YK, Oleynikov D, et al. Validated robotic laparoscopic surgical training in a virtual-reality environment. *Surg. Endosc.* 2008.

[73] Sun LW, Van Meer F, Schmid J, Bailly Y, Thakre AA, Yeung CK. Advanced da Vinci Surgical System simulator for surgeon training and operation planning. *Int. J. Med Robot* 2007;3:245–51.

[74] Fiedler MJ, Chen SJ, Judkins TN, Oleynikov D, Stergiou N. Virtual reality for robotic laparoscopic surgical training. *Stud Health Technol. Inform* 2007;125:127–9.

[75] Hanly EJ, Miller BE, Kumar R, Hasser CJ, Coste-Maniere E, Talamini MA, et al. Mentoring console improves collaboration and teaching in surgical robotics. *J. Laparoendosc Adv. Surg. Tech. A.* 2006;16:445–51.

[76] Judkins TN, Oleynikov D, Stergiou N. Enhanced robotic surgical training using augmented visual feedback. *Surg. Innov.* 2008;15:59–68.

[77] Thiel DD, Francis P, Heckman MG, Winfield HN. Prospective evaluation of factors affecting operating time in a residency/fellowship training program incorporating robot-assisted laparoscopic prostatectomy. *J. Endourol.* 2008;22:1331–8.

[78] Cosman PH, Cregan PC, Martin CJ, Cartmill JA. Virtual reality simulators: current status in acquisition and assessment of surgical skills. *ANZ J. Surg.* 2002;72:30–34.

[79] Kavic M. Simulators: a new use for an old paradigm. *JSLS.* 2006;10: 281–283.

[80] Lee PS, Bland A, Valea FA, Havrilesky LJ, Berchuck A, Secord AA. Robotic-assisted laparoscopic gynecologic procedures in a fellowship training program. *JSLS.* 2009 Oct-Dec;13(4):467-72.

[81] Aggarwal R, Tully A, Grantcharov T, et al. Virtual reality simulation training can improve technical skills during laparoscopic salpingectomy for ectopic pregnancy. *BJOG.* 2006;113(12):1382–1387.

[82] Larsen CR, Grantcharov T, Aggarwal R, et al. Objective assessment of gynecologic laparoscopic skills using the Lap- SimGyn virtual reality simulator. *Surg. Endosc..* 2006;20(9):1460– 1466.

[83] Sung WH, Fung CP, Chen AC, Yuan CC, Ng HT, Doong JL. The assessment of stability and reliability of a virtual realitybased laparoscopic gynecology simulation system. *Eur. J. Gynaecol Oncol.* 2003;24(2):143–146.

[84] Voss G, Bockholt U, Los Arcos JL, Muller W, Oppelt P, Stahler J. LAHYSTOTRAIN intelligent training system for laparoscopy and hysteroscopy. *Stud. Health Technol. Inform.* 2000; 70:359 –364.

[85] Muller-Wittig WK, Bisler A, Bockholt U, et al. LAHYSTOTRAIN development and evaluation of a complex training system for hysteroscopy. *Stud. Health Technol. Inform.* 2001;81:336– 340.

[86] Levy JS. Virtual reality hysteroscopy. *J. Am. Assoc. Gynecol. Laparosc.* 3 (4,Supplement):25–26, 1996.

[87] Harders M, Bajka M, Spaelter U, Tuchsmid S, Bleuler H, Szekley G. Highly realistic, immersive training environment for hysteroscopy. *Stud. Health Technol. Inform.* 2006;119:176 –181.

[88] Zatonyi J, Paget R, Szekely G, Grassi M, Bajka M. Real-time synthesis of bleeding for virtual hysteroscopy. *Med. Image Anal.* 2005;9(3):255–266.

[89] Munz Y, Kumar BD, Moorthy K, Bann S, Darzi A. Laparoscopic virtual reality and box trainers: is one superior to the other? *Surg. Endosc..* 2004;18(3):485– 494.

[90] Torkington J, Smith SGT, Rees BI, Darzi A. Skill transfer from virtual reality to a real laparoscopic task. *Surg. Endosc..* 2001; 15(10):1076 –1079.

[91] Madan AK, Frantzides CT, Tebbit C, Quiros RM. Participants' opinions of laparoscopic training devices after a basic laparoscopic training course. *Am. J. Surg..* 2005;189(6):758 –761.

[92] Grantcharov TP, Kristiansen VB, Bendix J, Bardram L, Rosenberg J, Funch-Jensen P. Randomised clinical trial of virtual reality simulation for laparoscopic skills training. *Br. J. Surg.* 2004;91(2):146 –150.

[93] Seymour NE, Gallagher A, Anthony G, et al. Virtual reality training improves operating room performance: results of a randomized, double blinded study. *Ann. Surg.* 2002;236(4):458– 464.

[94] Gallagher AG, Satava RM. Virtual reality as a metric for the assessment of laparoscopic psychomotor skills. *Surg. Endosc..* 2002;16(12):1746 –1752.

[95] Gallagher AG, Karen R, McClure N, McGuigan J. Objective psychomotor skills assessment of experienced, junior, and novice laparoscopists with virtual reality. *World J. Surg.* 2001;25(11): 1478–1483.

[96] McNatt SS, Smith CD. A computer-based laparoscopic skills assessment device differentiates experienced from novice laparoscopic surgeons. *Surg. Endosc..* 2001;15(10):1085–1089.

[97] Hart R, Doherty DA, Karthigasu K, Garry R. The value of virtual reality–simulator training in the development of laparoscopic surgical skills. *J. Minim. Invasive Gynecol.* 2006;13, 126–133.

[98]   Steinberg PL, Merguerian PA, Bihrle IW, Seigne JD. The cost of learning robotic-assisted prostatectomy. *Urology* 2008;72:1068–72.

[99]   Patient safety in the surgical environment. ACOG Committee Opinion No. 328. American College of Obstetricians and Gynecologists. *Obstet. Gynecol.* 2006;107:429–33.

[100] Ferguson JL, Beste TM, Nelson KH, et al. Making the transition from standard gynecologic laparoscopy to robotic laparoscopy. *JSLS.* 2004;8:326 –328.

[101] Guru KA, Kuvshinoff BW, Pavlov-Shapiro S, et al. Impact of robotics and laparoscopy on surgical skills: A comparative study. *J. Am. Coll Surg.* 2007;204:96 –101.

[102] De Ugarte DA, Etzioni DA, Gracia C, et al. Robotic surgery and resident training. *Surg. Endosc..* 2003;17:960 –963.

[103] Visco AG, Advincula AP. Robotics in gynecologic surgery. *Obstet. Gynecol* 2008;112:1369 84.

[104] Lanfranco AR, Castellanos AE, Desai JP, Meyers WC. Robotic surgery: a current perspective. *Ann. Surg.* 2004 Jan;239(1):14–21.

[105] Haber GP, Crouzet S, Kamoi K, et al. Robotic NOTES (natural orifice translumenal endoscopic surgery) in reconstructive urology: initial laboratory experience. *Urology.* 2008;71:996–1000.

[106] Kaouk JH, Goel RK, Haber GP, Crouzet S, Stein RJ. Robotic single-port transumbilical surgery in humans: initial report. *BJU Int.* 2009;103:366–369.

[107] Escobar PF, Fader AN, Paraiso MF, Kaouk JH, Falcone T. Robotic-Assisted Laparoendoscopic Single-Site Surgery in Gynecology: Initial Report and Technique. *J. Minim.ally Invasive Gynecol.* 2009;16, 589–91.

[108] Schreuder HWR, Verheijen RHM. Robotic Surgery. *BJOG* 2009;116:198–213.

In: Laparoscopy: New Developments, Procedures and Risks   ISBN: 978-1-61470-747-9
Editor: Hana Terzic, pp. 71-90   © 2012 Nova Science Publishers, Inc.

Chapter III

The Utilization of Novel Technology in Risk Reducing Laparoscopic Gynecological Complications

Andrea Tinelli[*1], *Antonio Malvasi*[2], *Sarah Gustapane*[3],
Giorgio De Nunzio[4], *Ivan DeMitri*[8], *Mario Bochicchio*[5],
Lucio De Paolis[6], *Giovanni Aloisio*[7] *and Daniel A. Tsin*[8]*

[1] Department of Obstetrics and Gynecology, Vito Fazzi Hospital, Lecce, Italy.
[2] Department of Obstetrics and Gynaecology, Santa Maria Hospital, Bari, Italy.
[3] Department of Obstetrics and Gynaecology, SS. Annunziata Hospital, Chieti, Italy.
[4] Department of Materials Science, University of Salento, and INFN, Lecce, Italy.
[5] SET-Lab, Department of Innovation Engineering, University of Lecce, Italy.
[6] Department of Innovation Engineering, University of Salento, Lecce, Italy.
[7] Information Processing Systems, Department of Innovation Engineering,
University of Salento, Lecce, Italy.
[7] Division of Gynecological Endoscopy and Minimally Invasive Treatment,
Department of Obstetrics and Gynecology,
The Mount Sinai Hospital of Queens, Long Island City, New York, U.S.A.
[8] Department of Physics, University of Salento, and INFN, Lecce (Italy).

Abstract

Laparoscopy is the standard of treatment for many gynecological diseases, it is a very common procedure in gynaecology and it is widely accepted as the method of first choice for many gynaecological problems. A meta-analysis of 27 randomized controlled

* Andrea Tinelli MD Department of Obstetrics and Gynecology, Vito Fazzi Hospital, Lecce, Italy, Division of Experimental Endoscopic Surgery, Imaging, Minimally Invasive Therapy and Technology, 73100 Lecce, Italy, Tel-Fax +39/0832/661511, Cell. +39/339/207408, E-mail: andreatinelli@gmail.com

trials comparing laparoscopy and laparotomy for benign gynaecological procedures concluded that the risk of minor complications after gynaecological surgery is 40% lower with laparoscopy than with laparotomy, although the risk of major complications is similar. Laparoscopy has been considered a real alternative to laparotomy with numerous advantages: short hospital stay, less need of analgesia, low intraoperative blood loss and faster recovery time. Many researchers are in pursuit of new technologies and new tools of minimally invasive technologies for reducing laparoscopic complications. The industry responded to these demands with many innovations, such as new optical instruments and digital images, virtual and augmented reality, robotic assisted surgery, etc. In this chapter, authors discussed the possible utilization of novel technologies to reduce the risk of laparoscopic gynecological complications.

Keywords: Robotics, endoscopy, robotic assisted surgery, learning curve, training, complications, residency programs, surgical skills, cancers, and oncology.

Introduction

Endoscopy is a modern surgical method that allows a look inside the body for medical reasons using an endoscope, an instrument used to examine the interior of a hollow organ or cavity of the body. The first endoscope was developed in 1806 by Philipp Bozzini in Mainz with his introduction of a "Lichtleiter" (light conductor) "for the examinations of the canals and cavities of the human body". However, the Vienna Medical Society disapproved of such curiosity. An endoscope was first introduced into a human in 1822 by William Beaumont, an army surgeon at Mackinac Island, Michigan. The use of electric light was a major step in the improvement of endoscopy. The first such lights were external. Later, smaller bulbs became available making internal light possible, as in a hysteroscope by Charles David in 1908.

Hans Christian Jacobaeus has been given credit for early endoscopic explorations of the abdomen and thorax with laparoscopy (1912) and thoracoscopy (1910) [1].

Laparoscopy was used in the diagnosis of liver and gallbladder disease by Heinz Kalk in the 1930s.

Hope reported on the use of laparoscopy to diagnose ectopic pregnancy in 1937.

In 1944, Raoul Palmer placed his patients in the Trendelenburg position after gaseous distention of the abdomen and was able to perform gynecologic celioscopy [2].

Discussing on the origin of modern endoscopy, Georg Wolf (1873-1938) a Berlin manufacturer of rigid endoscopes, established in 1906, produced the Sussmann flexible gastroscope in 1911 [3].

Karl Storz began producing instruments for specialists in 1945. His intention was to develop instruments which would enable the practitioner to look inside the human body.

The technology available at the end of the Second World War was still very modest: the area under examination in the interior of the human body was illuminated with miniature electric lamps; alternatively, attempts were made to reflect light from an external source into the body through the endoscopic tube.

Karl Storz pursued a plan: he set out to introduce very bright, but cold light into the body cavities through the instrument, thus providing excellent visibility while at the same time allowing objective documentation by means of image transmission. With more than 400 patents and operative samples to his name, which were to play a major role in showing the way ahead, Karl Storz played a crucial role in the development of endoscopy.

It was however, the combination of his engineering skills and vision, coupled with the work of optical designer Harold Hopkins that ultimately would revolutionize the field of medical optics.

The science progress in surgery developed the modern laparoscopic surgery, also called minimally invasive surgery (MIS), band aid surgery, keyhole surgery. This is a modern surgical technique in which operations in the abdomen are performed through small incisions (usually 0.5–1.5 cm) as compared to the larger incisions needed in laparotomy.

Keyhole surgery uses images displayed on TV monitors for magnification of the surgical elements.

Laparoscopic surgery includes operations within the abdominal or pelvic cavities, whereas keyhole surgery performed on the thoracic or chest cavity is called thoracoscopic surgery.

Laparoscopic and thoracoscopic surgery belong to the broader field of endoscopy.

There are a number of advantages to the patient with laparoscopic surgery versus an open procedure. These include reduced pain due to smaller incisions and hemorrhaging, and shorter recovery time. The key element in laparoscopic surgery is the use of a laparoscope.

Currently, laparoscopy represents the best choice in modern general and specialized surgery: today, 80% of the common benign disease, on average, can be peacefully treated by endoscopy, so as 30% of malignant neoplasm. Nevertheless, this continual enthusiastic interest in developing the endoscopic borders lead to complications, argument of medical legal issues and subject of review of the possible employment of endoscopy. Gynaecologic endoscopy has three important surgical modalities: laparoscopy, hysteroscopy and culdoscopy.

Laparoscopy is a very common procedure in general surgery and it is widely accepted as the method of treatment for many gynecological problems including patients with history of previous surgery. Patients with previous abdominal surgeries have an increased incidence of complications during laparoscopic surgery.

Modern laparoscopy, if routinely used in common diseases is a safe procedure with few major complications [4-7].

Complications associated with laparoscopic entry have not changed significantly in the last 25 years and are often related to the access technique when the trocar passes through the abdominal wall during the first step of the procedure.

The Problem of the First Laparoscopic Entry

Vascular and bowel surgical complications are rare and major problems of the first laparoscopic access. During laparotomies bowel and bladder injures were reported, but major vessel complications were not described in the open abdominal surgery literature, while in laparoscopy all of the three complications were reported One of the pioneering examples of detailed surgical audit was the Confidential Enquiry into Gynaecological Laparoscopy conducted on behalf of the Royal College of Obstetricians and Gynaecologists (RCOG) by

Professor GVP Chamberlain, which revealed an overall complication rate of 34/1000 and a mortality rate of 0.08/1000 [8].

A much larger survey from West Germany reporting operative laparoscopies drew attention to the safety of laparoscopic surgery in the hands of experienced operators; major complications requiring laparotomy or re-laparoscopy were four times greater with operative procedures than with diagnostic procedures, but the rate was only 3.8/1000 with an overall mortality for all procedures of 0.05/1000 [8].

Currently, there is no clear evidence as to the best laparoscopic entry and there is no proof that any single technique or instrument used to enter the abdomen helps to prevent complications [9]. This problem is more relevant in patients who had previous surgery.

It is a common fact that the access in laparoscopic surgery is more difficult in women with previous abdomino-pelvic surgery, since adhesions and viscera could be close to the point of trocar insertion. The reported incidence of intra-abdominal adhesions after laparotomy ranges between 30% and 90% [9].

A dangerous time for direct trauma is when the Veress needle and the first trocar cannula are being introduced blindly (closed laparoscopy), especially in a patient who has had previous surgery [11].

Another high risk group is post-menopausal patients or very thin athletic women of whom the typical thickness of different layers of the abdominal wall is lost; the great vessels, which lie as close as 2.5cm below the skin at the umbilicus can be injured unless great care is taken [12].

Another group with an increased risk of complication is the morbidly obese where there is an increased risk of visceral injury because of thick abdominal wall, often unyielding increasing the chance of surgical emphysema making subsequent attempts at entry more difficult and often requiring longer instruments [13].

Major direct trauma injuries and diathermy accidents to the bowel are one of the most serious complications of operative laparoscopy that are associated with mortality and a high rate of surgical interventions associated with a temporary de-functioning colostomy, particularly if unrecognized at the time of surgery [14]. These surgical accidents can occur even in patients with no predisposing factors. All patients should be warned of the possibility of proceeding to laparotomy in the event of major hemorrhage or perforation or laceration of the bowel or urinary tract [15].

A thoroughly prepared bowel and the evacuated recto sigmoid facilitate laparoscopy and the potential injury repairs [16].

Injuries to the bowel, urinary tract and pelvic organs contributed 1.8/1000, 0.2/1000 and 3.4/1000 complications in the RCOG series, respectively [17].

In order to avoid these injuries with the primary trocar many laparoscopists have advocated the open approach with the Hasson cannula. In this technique the abdominal wall is elevated by two sutures or skin graspers, the layers of the abdominal wall are opened by a scalpel under direct vision. Once the peritoneum has been opened, the blunt end of the Hasson trocar is inserted and the cone is sutured in place to produce an airtight seal. Bowel laceration can occur with open laparoscopy, in 6 of 11000 cases as reported by Penfield [18].

A safety first entry surveillance step via a secondary port is adviced for early recognition and timely repair of complications [19].

Remote Operated Instruments

Some minimally invasive surgeons are looking beyond traditional laparoscopy to gradually reduce the size and numbers of abdominal ports till the eventual zero. To achieve such a task with no additional abdominal ports, a concept of Secured Independent Tools (SIT) for the deployment of miniature instruments may solve some issues, such as: direct current powered engines, electronic transmission devices, exposure, illumination, mobilization, retraction, traction and triangulation. SIT deploys mini instruments and engines in peritoneoscopy by replacing trocars and cannulas with threads for none motorized tools and narrow cables to power engines and lights. This technique provides sufficient strength for grasping and pulling, it also has the potential to power wired machines and signal transmissions using fiber optic micro cables for remote operated devices. The future is focusing on wireless and battery operated micro robotics instruments [19].

Today's available and affordable motorized technology is with wired DC power [20].

The advances in micro devices allow us to foresee multiple application for lights, cameras, engines, electro surgery, locomotives, graspers, small hands, etc. Laparoscopy and minilaparoscopy use a port per instrument. The diameter of a port is larger than the diameter of the instruments used for each particular entrance. The micro devices could be introduce via a single port umbilical or natural orifice using one entrance for multiple instruments avoiding the potential complication of multiple ports.

The strings or cables do not occupy the single or natural orifice port. The cables are exteriorized and held outside the skin. The authors try to limit the number of needle entrances per device, yet some earlier tools will require more than one string or cables for DC power. The surgeon or assistant working at the operating table or from a distant console could control the power-plugged devices.

The unobstructed entrance could be used for the placement of other rigid, flexible or large instruments needed in different procedures and for the extraction of specimens.

The use of remote operated magnets has been successfully done in humans [21].

The technique uses a hand-held external magnet to direct an internal magnet with a tandem device. The number of magnets that can be used per case is not known. There is no problem using one magnet, but placing more than one magnet per case raises the possibility of magnet attraction limiting the number. The distance among magnets is problematic. Distance less than 3 cm are at risk of coupling either the external or internal magnet. This technique precludes the use of additional ports.

Novel Technologies in Pelvic Laparoscopy and the Problem of Interactivity of Research

The current opinion in the different scientific groups is that a great difference occurs between Biomedical Engineering and Medical Surgery, especially in using new instruments. Most of these differences arise in Italy between Biomedical Engineers and Medical Doctors for various different experiences in different places (in Hospitals Medical Doctors and in Bio-Institutes Biomedical Engineers), different scientific languages, different knowledge, mural and extra mural university and post-university studies. Lack of co-operation between Biomedical Engineers and Specialist Medical Doctors, the Biomedical Industries interpose themselves between Biomedical Engineers and Medical Doctors with the purpose of invention and profits, without listening to the medical necessities. On the other hand , the main objective of a surgeon is to safely and efficiently operate with no complications. Traditionally the surgeon as a leader conceives a procedure and the industry will later provide the technology that enables and facilitates the operation. It is therefore our opinion that the doctors should be the leaders and the industry the facilitators and not the other way around.

Advantages of Gynecological Laparoscopy and Unsolved Problems

Gynaecological endoscopy permits to operate a patient by a minimal invasive access and to treat her by using small instruments. Reducing peritoneal damages made by laparoscopy decreases pelvic and abdominal pain, hospital stay, and reduces infections and peritoneal post-surgical adhesions [22,23].

Furthermore, it decreases the use of drugs during general anesthesia.

Endoscopic abdomino-pelvic surgery and in particular, the laparoscopic procedures have three important problems:

- *THE LAPAROSCOPIC ENTRY*: As we discussed before, the dangerous moment for direct trauma is when the Verres needle and the first trocar cannula are being introduced blindly (closed laparoscopy) specifically in patients with previous abdominal and pelvic surgeries.
- *THE BIDIMENSIONAL VISION AND THE IMPOSSIBILITY TO PALP DIRECTLY THE PATHOLOGY*: The current laparoscopic surgery is done in bidimensional vision and the tissue palpation is entrusted to an instrument and not one's finger; so direct evaluation of disease is not tridimensional or tactil and is different with respect to the open traditional abdominal surgery.
- *THE MEDICAL LEGAL ISSUES*: Laparoscopic complications cause medico-legal and forensics issues and require major malpractice insurance coverages by hospitals and endo-surgeons are obliged to organize their activity with private and expensive insurances.

The Industry Open Questions in Laparoscopic Gyneacology

Many researchers questions about the help of new technologies and new tools of minimally invasive technologies in reducing gynecologic endoscopic complications.

The key points to reduce laparoscopic complications are:

- to improve the first access in abdomen
- to reduce the learning curve of laparoscopic surgeons
- to use new instruments useful in laparoscopic surgical maneuvers
- to show the pathologic tissue modifications under the peritoneal and endometrial surfaces through endoscopic vision
- to detail the histological patterns in the uterine cavity during the hysteroscopy examination, differentiating the normal endometrial patterns by pathologic diseases such as polyps, endometrial hyperplasia or endometrial cancer
- to map in presurgical steps the abdominal and pelvic tissue to excise (ovary, fallopian tube, uterus, bowel, vessels)

Another question is if Virtual or Augmented Reality can really improve the medical training in endoscopy and reduce costs.

Virtual or Augmented Reality techniques showed in educational and experimental fields a promise to elevate the quality of training; in fact, the main cost of endoscopy, a part of the instrumental purchase, is the learning curve of the surgical endo-training, too expensive because of time spent and expert teaching.

Although great enthusiasm exists for developing skills in laparoscopic gynecology in the scientific surgical world, training opportunities are limited. Thus, another problem is the lack of approved, certified and not auto-referenced gynecology/laparoscopy fellowships, as should exist in the principal surgical school.

Since laparoscopy allows surgeons to operate through a tiny hole in the abdomen, young surgeons should be trained in this field at University and successively in the General Hospital.

The industry is gradually developing new surgical video-simulation systems.

A new and very promising technology is the use of computers and robots in medical education and training, so called "Virtual reality training systems" (VRTS); it generally consists of: a computer, a force-feedback-device, a display system, and the surgeon interacts with the training system via an input device that resembles the handles of instruments as they are used in real patient treatment.

A specialized medical simulation software is fed with digital models of a real patient's anatomy derived from computer tomography (CT) or magnetic resonance (MR) data. The computer also receives the position of the virtual instruments pretended by the current position of the handles while they are manipulated as they would be during a real procedure.

The software simulates physics such as gravity and behavior of fluids as well as optical appearance, like shadows and glossiness of a virtual scenario.

The challenging function of the software is to compute the interaction between the model of the virtual patient and the virtual instruments without noticeable delays and as close to reality as possible. Methods usually utilized in surgical simulation are spring-mass-damper models, finite-element methods or particle systems for computation of the physical behavior.

A realistic visual impression is mostly achieved by shader technology which means specialized software that runs for performance reasons on the processor of high-end graphic cards instead of the main unit processor. The force-feedback unit consists of one or more handles that resemble the tool-holders of a real procedure; each handle is connected to a mechanical system that is able to measure the current position of the handle, does some pre-processing and forwards it to the main computer. After computation in the simulation software, information with the new position and the needed forces is sent back to the force-feedback device where electric motors are moving the tool-handle actively to the desired position. If this is done fast enough, the user feels no delay and gets the illusion of touching, for example a deformable organ; a force-feedback device is usually limited by the number of motors needed to achieve all degrees of freedom as well as the maximal and minimal forces that are needed for the simulation of surgical interaction.

As a result of a VRTS, the user can train basic tasks as well as complex surgical procedures under very realistic conditions. Furthermore, sophisticated computer-based training systems like the Simbionix "LAP Mentor" are providing standardized training cases but still allow in detail individual surgical treatment during the simulation to compare individual skills.

Each training session can be recorded, various parameters such as for example speed, accuracy, blood loss or cauterization time are measured, evaluated and presented in an individual session score [24-29].

The Utilization of Virtual Reality in Risk Reducing Complications in Laparoscopy

Currently, research is in progress to improve mathematical models to simulate biological tissue and human organs as realistically as possible and to go forward to even more complex virtual procedures.

Examination of the of a training session scoring and a long-term follow-up allows better supervision and an optimized setup for the next training sessions, based on the individual skills and knowledge of the trainee.

New force-feedback devices will develop more degrees of freedom and stronger forces; active work is also done to determine which scoring parameters are most significant for a precise evaluation of skills and knowledge. Simulators already cover a large variety of simulated procedures, especially in gynecology, such as hysteroscopy, laparoscopy and others [30-32].

Laparoscopical Trainer is usually integrated with a Video technology, producing a highly portable and innovative laparoscopic video trainer; this technology is a simulated laparoscope with unsurpassed graphics displayed by leveraging PC technology and requires usually from 1.3 GHz processor to greater, 4 Gb RAM or greater, USB 2.0 slots or spare PCMCIA or PCI slot.

The Video technology has a boom mounted digital camera which allows the users to reposition the field of view within the operative cavity and zoom in on the operative site; in this way an affordable and portable platform is created, compatible with LapTop or Desktop PCs, that effectively demonstrates or trains laparoscopic skills and techniques outside of the operating room [33].

Simulation is routinely incorporated into programs designed to facilitate video endoscopic technical skill training. The impact of this training is difficult to discern because different types of simulation are often employed during the same course, and clinical performance after the course has not been assessed objectively [34].

Some of the earliest and most thorough analysis of simulation training showed significant correlation between the performance at three skill stations and the ability to perform a laparoscopic suturing exercise on pig intestine [35-38].

Another question of the researchers is the real utility of Virtual and of Augmented Reality (AR) in the first laparoscopic access. Mory et al define feedback as presented information that allows comparison between an actual first laparoscopic access outcome and the desired first access outcome [39].

Navab et al describe a novel technique for automatically providing elaborate feedback to Augmented Reality and Virtual Reality trainees; the focus is on teaching 3D manipulation of tools in an Augmented Reality enhanced simulators [40].

The feedback is a critical part of any learning procedure and this is also true for VR and AR for teaching system. Researchers propose a new method for providing feedback without time consuming authoring of possible mistakes and advice on improvements, since 3D movements cannot be trivially compared to each other, so the dynamic synchronization of expert and trainee performances is a crucial part of our system. Showing a synchronized replay of the expert and the trainee's movement, the system reveals differences without requiring the presence of the expert.

The authors studies are directed to the human delivery simulator of Obst et al. [41].

The potential for 3-dimensional vision should improve the dexterity and precision of both fine and broad movements; motion scaling can translate large, coarse hand motions into fine movement by the instruments, and electronic filtering could remove all tremors from the instrument.

Discomfort of Conventional Laparoscopy and the Use of Robotic Assisted Surgery in Gynecologic Laparoscopy to Reduce Complications

Studies have clearly shown that laparoscopic surgery allows faster recovery with shorter hospitalization, improved cosmetics, decreased blood loss, and reduced postoperative pain.

One major obstacle to the more widespread acceptance and application of minimally invasive surgical techniques to gynecologic surgery has been the steep learning curve for surgeons and longer operative times associated with many of these advanced procedures.

Moreover, the learning curve for standard advanced laparoscopy is steep and long, particularly with regard to suturing and intraabdominal knotting. Conventional laparoscopic instruments that have counterintuitive hand movements and amplification of hand tremor present significant technical challenges that the majority of practicing gynecologists cannot easily master [42].

Other limitations encountered with conventional laparoscopy include two-dimensional visualization, and limited degrees of instrument movement within the body as well as ergonomic difficulty. Fatigue and physical discomfort can become limitations during any surgical procedure [43].

The main disadvantages of the conventional laparoscopic procedures include:

- two-dimensional imaging
- lack of sensory feedback
- the limited mobility of the instruments
- tremor amplification
- the long learning curve
- fatigue and physical discomfort in long time operation
- working on a virtual operation site (as the hands and the tip of the instruments cannon be seen at the same time)

Therefore, much attention is now being paid to the expected advantages of robotic surgery. The future of telerobotic surgery and remote operated instruments could enable surgeons to operate at a distance from the operating table [19,20]. Furthermore, Agarwala et al. tried to compare the outcomes of laparoscopic and robotic operations at a single institute, evaluating intra-/post-operative parameters, comparing 20 laparoscopic and robotic operations by one surgeon for length of surgery, blood loss, hospital stay and short-term complications. In the conclusions, the authors reported that laparoscopic and robotic approaches to gynecological surgery have equal outcomes as long as the skill level is similar. Robotic surgery adds about 30 min. additional OR time for all types of cases, with no added disadvantages to the patient or complications [44].

The improved visualization and dexterity may offer some advantages over conventional laparoscopy for complex procedures such as those required for gynecologic malignancies or invasive endometriosis [45,46].

Based on these data, computer-enhanced technology is enabling more surgeons to do laparoscopic procedures especially in the field of gynecology. Robotic software allows camera and instrument movement to be direct and intuitive, electronically removing the fulcrum effect at the trocar sites; perhaps most importantly, robotic instrumentation can place a joint or a wrist near the tip of the instrument, producing deflection of the effectors tip of the instrument vertically (pitch) and/or laterally (yaw), resulting in 1 or 2 degrees of motion at the point of impact that are not available in traditional laparoscopic or open instruments.

Robotic instruments respond as though the surgeon's fingertips were at the end of the instrument, directly holding the needle, scissor tips, scalpel blade, energy source, or grasping tips at the point of impact with the tissue; the cumulative effect of these robotic characteristics is a dexterity and precision that cannot be duplicated by human hands or traditional instruments.

The Da Vinci surgical system is equipped with a 3-dimensional vision system in which double endoscopes generate two images resulting in the perception of a 3D image.

In addition, with the development of endowrist, it reproduces the range of motion and dexterity of the surgeon's hand, providing high precision, flexibility and ability to rotate instruments 360 degrees. Thus, the learning curve of achievement for the surgeons using the Da Vinci surgical system was shortened. In 2001, a more advanced Da Vinci surgical system with four robotic arms gained US FDA approval and is now being used in many surgical procedures throughout the world.

The ongoing competition between the ZEUS and the "Da Vinci" surgical system ended when Computer Motion Inc. was merged into Intuitive Surgical Inc. in 2003 [47].

The Da Vinci robotic system has three main components: the robotic cart, the operating console and the endoscopic stack.

The robotic surgeon operates from the remote master console using a combination of hand controls and foot pedals. The robotic cart is 2 meters high, approximately 1 meter long and 1 meter wide with a sliding system on the base which enables the cart to be placed freely according to patient's position. It is composed of four mechanical arms attached to a mobile base, which is connected to the operating console through a cable. The robotic arms are mounted on a patient's side cart. The central arm contains the optic system consisting of an endoscope with two optical channels and two three-chip cameras. Three of these lateral arms hold surgical instruments. Each robotic arm has three or four joints enabling the arms to rotate freely. The surgeon, seated at the console, performs the procedure by manipulating specially designed joysticks.

The movement is translated from the surgeon's fingers to the tip of the special instruments, called Endowrist. There are six degrees of freedom at the instrument tip and a seventh degree of freedom is provided by the action of the instruments itself. Each instrument can be resterilized, but can be used only ten times. The computer is able to eliminate physiologic tremor and to downscale the amplitude of motions enabling a wide range of surgical procedures.

The operating console integrates the 3D viewing, the masters with two controllers (joysticks) and four foot pedals. The Da Vinci robotic surgical system replaces two-dimensional with three-dimensional imaging with the optical channels and enhances the precision of anatomic dissection.

An important optical component of the Da Vinci Surgical System is the InSite vision system, which provides 3D stereoscopic imaging via a 12-mm endoscope. Because the endoscope of the Da Vinci Surgical System is composed of 2 parallel 5-mm telescopes (0- or 30-degree lenses) that are each capable of sending individual images to the camera head, a 3D view of the surgical field is seen at the console as the 2 images are merged by a computer.

The video system provides 10X to 15X magnification and the option of high definition.

The images are also projected such that the surgeon's hands simulate operating instruments over an open surgical field. In addition, the endoscope is programmed to regulate the temperature at the tip to minimize fogging during surgery. One foot pedal controls the camera movement (right/left, up/down, in/out) and horizontal orientation, while a nearby pedal controls the focus. Another pedal provides a clutching mechanism that allows for repositioning of hand controls and provides the instruments a range of motion beyond the physical confines of the console. Another set of pedals controls both monopolar and bipolar energy sources. The patient-side cart is wheeled in between the patient's legs, and the robotic arms are attached to stainless steel robotic trocars through a process termed "docking". The hand controls operate either the camera or up to two robotic instruments at one time. The surgeon sits in an ergonomically comfortable position at the console and his/her hands fit into the master instrument controllers. The movement is converted and translated from the surgeon's fingers to the tip of the instruments.

A myriad of laparoscopic instruments are available including needle drivers, Debakey forceps, and monopolar scissors that are placed through specific telerobotic ports. These instruments enable the surgeon to manipulate, coagulate, dissect, and suture. Generally all patients are positioned in dorsal lithotomy. A uterine manipulator and a Foley catheter are placed. Four trocars are inserted: one 12-mm supra- or intraumbilical, two 8-mm lateral and one 5-, 10-, or 12-mm left paraumbilical or suprapubic trocars. Every procedure starts as a standard laparoscopy. All tissue suturing tasks are performed with the assistance of the robotic arm. Morcellation of uterus and fibroids, cystoscopies and sigmoidoscopies were done after its disassembly from patients. The operating console has four foot pedals which can be manipulated to electrocauterize for hemostasis or to control the movement of the camera. Furthermore, the computer also provides motion scaling and tremor elimination, facilitating complicated surgical procedures. This system also allows a greater variety of scaled motion for precise and accurate control (5:1, 3:1, or 1:1) while eliminating tremors.

Along with the robotic arms standing over the patient, at least three persons (the surgeon, a scrub nurse, and a scrub assistant) are involved in each robotic procedure. The surgeon controls the robotic arms remotely from the console while watching a high-definition highly magnified three-dimensional (3D) image. The paraumbilical or suprapubic port is used by the assistant to provide additional laparoscopic instruments, as required. A microphone located on the surgeon's console improves communication among the team members [48].

Clearly, robots are not essential for basic laparoscopic procedures, however, there is a paucity of data regarding costs and benefits of robotics versus conventional techniques. Robotic precision is most useful for extremely fine dissection, for precise suturing techniques, and for dissection and suturing in awkward or narrow anatomic locations. The most salient value of robotics is the enabling function of this technology and its potential to allow surgeons to perform complex tasks that exceed their abilities with traditional laparoscopy [49-52].

The Possible Advantages of Laparoendoscopic Single-Site Surgery (Less)

Minimally invasive surgery has become a standard of care for the treatment of many benign and malignant gynecologic conditions. Laparoscopy and robotic assisted surgery have impacted the entire spectrum of gynecologic surgery. Laparoendoscopic single-site surgery (LESS), also known as single-port surgery is awakened . LESS improves the cosmetic benefits of minimally invasive surgery by providing only one incision, which also minimizes the potential morbidity associated with multiple incisions. LESS procedures are typically performed via one of two approaches. The first is single-site surgery, where two or more conventional ports are placed through a single-incision. The second approach utilizes a single, multichannel device, through which multiple instruments and optics are passed. The access point for these surgeries is typically the umbilicus, although less cosmetic extra-umbilical incisions may occasionally be necessary to complete the surgery. Improvements in access devices, optics and instrumentation have driven the dissemination of this new format of laparoscopic surgery. These early reports indicate that LESS is a promising surgical innovation that results not only in improved cosmesis, but also, in many cases, a shorter convalescence period and decreased postoperative analgesia requirements when compared with patients treated with conventional laparoscopic approaches. Several publications in the gynaecology literature have demonstrated preliminary feasibility, safety and reproducibility of LESS in the treatment of both benign and oncological female conditions [53-63]. The recent surge in the number and variety of LESS cases has been facilitated by the introduction of new instrumentation and access devices. Potential advantages of single-port over conventional multiport laparoscopy include superior cosmesis from a relatively hidden umbilical scar, a possible decrease in morbidity related to visceral and vascular injury during trocar placement, as well as risk reduction of postoperative wound infection, hernia formation and elimination of multiple trocar site closures. Studies have also suggested that women who undergo LESS report improved postoperative pain profiles when compared with those receiving conventional laparoscopic surgery [64].

This may be due to the utilization of the umbilicus as the single site of the incision, as it is one of the thinnest regions on the abdominal wall, containing few blood vessels, muscle or nerves.

Comparative data and prospective trials are required to determine the clinical impact of LESS in treatment of gynecologic conditions [65].

The Possible Use of Optical Coherence Tomography in Gynecological Laparoscopy

Another open question is if the OCT (Optical Coherence Tomography) endoscopic applications could offer new capabilities in laparoscopy. The OCT is an emerging medical imaging modality that offers new capabilities in endoscopy; the OCT is capable of high resolution imaging of epithelium, with resolution in the range 1-10 micron. OCT provides cross-sectional, depth-resolved information, giving the ability to interrogate tissues with micrometer-scale resolution without destruction or required excision of the tissue [66].

The use of optical coherence tomography in the gynecological field is still experimental and is mainly about the in vitro e in vivo diagnosis of cervical cancer dysplasia, cervical cancer, ovary cancer, endometrial cancer and endometriosis [67].

In a study on 16 patients cervical OCT images were matched to biopsy specimens: it was found that OCT could be used to differentiate the nuclei of normal cells from VS CIN (cervical intraepithelial neoplastic) lesion of grade 3. The study also found that average epithelial intensities were significantly stronger in the abnormal tissue of pre- menopausal women, although they were in the normal tissue of post-menopausal women [68].

Escobar et al examined the OCT application in cancer of the cervix and vulva in the study of 50 patients undergoing colposcopic examination; during the OCT cervical evaluation, OCT images were acquired of both normal and abnormal areas. Each woman underwent multiple selective biopsies and the OCT pictures were correlated with histological examination. Results showed that OCT could be used to reliably identify normal squamous epithelium and a characteristic appearance for CIN grade 2 and 3 lesion [69].

Future studies may also include ultrasound guided transvaginal imaging, dual modality imaging (combining OCT imaging with either spectroscopic or confocal imaging), and potentially volumetric imaging [70].

At this point, after this short examination on OCT using in gynecology, as a new tool, the authors question about the real use ability of OCT in these fields [71].

In the next future should histological examinations of uterine epithelium be necessary after OCT application? Has the OCT any possibilities in high resolution imaging of endometrium during hysteroscopy or not? Does OCT offer any possibilities in high resolution imaging of ovarian borderline tumor tissue during laparoscopy? Does OCT offer any possibilities in high resolution imaging of peritoneal stroma and endometriosis during laparoscopy? Does OCT offer any possibilities in high resolution imaging of sub peritoneal endometriosis around the vessels and the bowel during laparoscopy?

The Possible Use of High Resolution Imaging in Gynecological Laparoscopy

High-resolution imaging of gynaecological tissue should offer the potential for identifying pathological changes at early stages when interventions are more effective. OCT and laser-induced fluorescence (LIF) spectroscopy are non-destructive optical imaging modalities. OCT provides architectural cross-sectional images at near histological resolutions and LIF provides biochemical information. Hariri et al utilize combined OCT-LIF to image ovaries in post-menopausal ovarian carcinogenesis rat models, evaluating normal cyclic, acyclic and neoplastic ovaries [70].

As previously said, OCT is a high resolution, high speed optical imaging technology which is analogous to ultrasound B-mode imaging, and uses detected reflections of light rather than sound.

The OCT technology is capable of being integrated with laparoscopy for real-time subsurface imaging [71].

In a report, the feasibility of OCT for differentiating normal and pathologic laparoscopically-accessible gynecologic tissue was already demonstrated.

Differentiation is based on architectural changes of in vitro tissue morphology.

OCT has the potential to improve conventional laparoscopy by enabling subsurface imaging near the level of histopathology [72].

The Possible Laser Utilization in Gynecological Laparoscopy

The researchers questioned moreover on the possible utilization of laser in endosurgery [73-75].

Over the past decade, the excimer laser has proved to be an effective tool in refractive surgery. This laser produces high energy radiation at a wavelength related to the dimer molecule it is based on. For example, ArF excimer lasers generate 193-nm radiation, and are used to produce photo-ablation of the cornea with submicron accuracy and minimal effect on adjacent tissue. By the assumption that the excimer laser in gynecologic laparoscopic utilization could have good future perspectives, the researchers asked on the possible strategy to minimize post-laparoscopic stripping or coagulation ovarian tissue injury and the possible laser utilization for ovarian tissue laparoscopic excision.

The CO_2-laser has become very popular in the field of gynaecology for the treatment of endometriosis and adhesions [76].

The Nd:YAG laser was used in gynecology for endometrial ablation and other hystersocopic and laparoscopic procedures the results were good. Due to time consuming and cost the Nd;YAG laser is now rarely employed.

Photorefractive keratectomy is performed by gradually modifying the diameter of a circular aperture, thus, reducing the convexity and hence, the spherical power of the cornea. The use of a slit aperture can produce a toric surface ablation and astigmatism correction results. [77,78].

Should we have a strategy to minimize post laparoscopic stripping and coagulation? Could lasers be used for ovarian tissue laparoscopic excision? Currently laser use in gynecologic surgery is experimental, in particular the as the excimer laser is concerned.

The excimer laser use in laparoscopic ovarian surgery [79,80], could be used in the future, to minimize the coagulation and stripping ovarian tissue [81] unpreventable injury, in particular in the poor responder women.

Conclusions

MIS (Minimally Invasive Surgery) allows performing a lot of complex operations with a short hospital stay, and it is safe, feasible, and patient-friendly. Gynaecological endoscopy is essentially a safe procedure and serious complications are rare. The learning curve problem could be overcome by using the new surgical video-simulation systems. Moreover, a new and very promising technology is the use of computers and robots in minimally invasive surgical education and skill training, so called "VRTS", that allows training in basic skills as well as complex surgical procedures under very realistic conditions. Currently, research is done to improve mathematical models to simulate biological tissue and human organs as realistically as possible and go forward to even more complex virtual procedures.

To solve the limitations of endoscopic surgery, some years ago the industry invented robotic systems that enable surgeons to operate faster and in difficult to reach areas of traditional laparoscopy. The advanced surgical robotic systems offer the promise of a unique combination of advantages over open and conventional laparoscopic approaches. The robotic system enables us to manipulate endoscopic instruments, as well as instruments during open surgical intervention, regarding both the operative field and operation techniques. Robotic surgery is often heralded as promise for the future of surgery, but the exorbitant costs creates problems of affordability, availability and for physicians who lack experience in robotic surgery.

References

[1]   Jacobaeus HC. The Cauterization of Adhesions in Artificial Pneumothorax Treatment of Pulmonary Tuberculosis under Thoracoscopic Control. *Proc. R. Soc. Med.* 1923;16 (Electro Ther Sect):45-62.

[2]   Palmer R. First attempts at photocinematography during gynecological celioscopy. *C. R. Soc. Fr. Gyncol.* 1956 Jan;26(1):43-4.

[3]   Modlin IM, Farhadi J. Rudolf Schindler-- a man for all seasons. *J. Clin. Gastroenterol.*, 2000; 31(2):95-102.

[4]   Johnson N, Barlow D, Lethaby A, Tavender E, Curr L, Garry R. Methods of hysterectomy: systematic review and meta-analysis of randomised controlled trials. *BMJ.* 2005 Jun 25;330(7506):1478-1481.

[5]   Reich H, Roberts L. Laparoscopic hysterectomy in current gynaecological practice. *Rev. Gynaecol. Pract.* 2003;3:32-40.

[6]   Claerhout F, Deprest J. Laparoscopic hysterectomy for benign diseases. *Best Pract Res Clin. Obstet. Gynaecol.* 2005 Jun;19(3):357-75.

[7]   Elkington N, Cario G, Rosen D, Carlton M, Chou D. Total laparoscopic hysterectomy: a tried and tested technique. *J. Minim. Invasive Gynecol.* 2005 May-Jun;12(3):267-74.

[8]   Tinelli A, Malvasi A, Schneider AJ, Keckstein J, Hudelist G, Barbic M, Casciaro S, Giorda G, Tinelli R, Perrone A, Tinelli FG. First abdominal access in gynecological laparoscopy: which method to utilize? *Minerva Ginecol.* 2006 Oct;58(5):429-440.

[9]   Ahmad G, Duffy JMN, Phillips K, Watson A. Laparoscopic Entry Techniques. *Cochrane Database Syst. Rev.* 2008; 16: CD006583.

[10]   Tinelli A, Malvasi A, Guido M, Tsin DA, Hudelist G, Stark M, Mettler L. Laparoscopic entry in women with previous abdomino-pelvic surgery. *Surgical Innovations* 2011 [*in press*].

[11]   Tinelli A, Malvasi A, Istre O, Keckstein J, Stark M, Mettler L. Abdominal access in gynaecological laparoscopy: a comparison between direct optical and blind closed access by Veress needle. *Eur. J. Obstet. Gynecol. Reprod. Biol.* 2010;148:191-4.

[12]   Tinelli A, Malvasi A, Guido M, Istre O, Keckstein J, Mettler L. Initial laparoscopic access in postmenopausal women: a preliminary prospective study. *Menopause* 2009; 16:966-70.

[13]   Altun H, Banli O, Karakoyun R, Boyuk A, Okuduku M, Onur E, Memisoglu K. Direct trocar insertion technique for initial access in morbid obesity surgery: technique and results. *Surg. Laparosc. Endosc. Percutan Tech.* 2010; 20(4):228-230.

[14]   Tinelli A, Malvasi A, Hudelist G, Istre O, Keckstein J. Abdominal access in gynaecological laparoscopy: a comparison between direct optical and open access. *J. Laparoendosc Adv. Surg. Tech. A.* 2009; 19:529-33.

[15]   Varma R, Gupta JK. Laparoscopic entry techniques: clinical guideline, national survey, and medico legal ramifications. *Surg Endosc.* 2008;22:2686–2697.

[16]   Kumakiri J, Kikuchi I, Kitade M, Kuroda K, Matsuoka S, Tokita S, Takeda S. Incidence of Complications during Gynecologic Laparoscopic Surgery in Patients after Previous Laparotomy. *J. Minim. Invasive Gynecol* 2010; 17(4):480-486.

[17]   Garry R. A consensus document concerning laparoscopic entry: Middlesbrough, March 19–20 1999. *Gynaecol. Endosc.* 1999;8: 403–6.

[18]   Hasson HM, Rotman C, Rana N, Kumari NA. Open laparoscopy: 29-year experience. *Obstet. Gynecol.* 2000; 96: 763-6.

[19]   Tsin DA, Tinelli A, Malvasi A, Davila F, Jesus R, Castro-Perez R. Laparoscopy and Natural Orifice Surgery: First Entry Safety Surveillance Step. *JSLS.* 2011; [Epub ahead of print].

[20]   Tsin DA, Davila F, Dominguez G, Manolas P. Secured independent tools in peritoneoscopy. *JSLS.* 2010 ;14(2):256-258.

[21] Dominguez G, Durand L, DeRosa J, Danguise E, Arozema C, Ferrina P. Retraction and triangulation with neodymium magnetic forceps for a single-pot laparoscopy cholecystectomy. *Surg. Endosc.* 2009;23:1660-1666.

[22] Curet MJ. Special problems in laparoscopic surgery. *Surg. Clin. North Am.* 2000;80:1093-110.

[23] Madan AK, Taddeucci RJ, Harper JL, Tichansky DS. Initial trocar placement and abdominal insufflation in laparoscopic bariatric surgery. *J. Surg. Res* 2008;148(2):210–213.

[24] Pareek G, Hedican SP, Bishoff JT, Shichman SJ, Wolf JS Jr, Nakada SY. Survey from skills-based hands on learning courses demonstrates increased laparoscopic caseload and clinical laparoscopic suturing. *Urology*. 2005 Aug;66(2):271-3.

[25] Teber D, Dekel Y, Frede T, Klein J, Rassweiler J. The Heilbronn laparoscopic training program for laparoscopic suturing: concept and validation. *J. Endourol.* 2005 Mar;19(2):230-8.

[26] Lorin S, Poumarat G, Memeteau Y, Wattiez A, Tostain J. Design of aprototype operating seat with SESAM (Ergonomic System of Mobile Forearm Rests) mobile armrests designed to optimize the surgeon's ergonomy during pelvic laparoscopy. *Prog. Urol.* 2004 Dec;14(6):1181-7.

[27] Tevaearai HT, Mueller XM, von Segesser LK. 3-D vision improves performance in a pelvic trainer. *Endoscopy*. 2000 Jun;32(6):464-8.

[28] Sun CC, Chiu AW, Chen KK, Chang LS. Assessment of a three-dimensional operating system with skill tests in a pelvic trainer. *Urol. Int.* 2000;64(3):154-8.

[29] Piechaud PT, Pansadoro A. Transfer of skills from the experimental model to the patients. *Curr. Urol. Rep.* 2006 Mar;7(2):96-9.

[30] Zatonyi J, Paget R, Szekely G, Grassi M, Bajka M. Real-time synthesis of bleeding for virtual hysteroscopy. *Med. Image Anal.* 2005;9(3):255–266.

[31] Sung WH, Fung CP, Chen AC, Yuan CC, Ng HT, Doong JL. The assessment of stability and reliability of a virtual reality based laparoscopic gynecology simulation system. *Eur. J. Gynaecol. Oncol.* 2003;24(2):143–146.

[32] Larsen CR, Grantcharov T, Aggarwal R, et al. Objective assessment of gynecologic laparoscopic skills using the Lap SimGyn virtual reality simulator. *Surg. Endosc.* 2006;20(9):1460–1466.

[33] Munz Y, Kumar BD, Moorthy K, Bann S, Darzi A. Laparoscopic virtual reality and box trainers: is one superior to the other? *Surg. Endosc.* 2004;18(3):485– 494.

[34] Kothari SN, Kaplan BJ, DeMaria EJ, Broderick TJ, Merrell RC. Training in laparoscopic suturing skills using a new computer-based virtual reality simulator (MIST-VR) provides results comparable to those with an established pelvic trainer system. *J. Laparoendosc. Adv. Surg. Tech. A*. 2002 Jun;12(3):167-73.

[35] Medina M. The laparoscopic-ring simulation trainer. *JSLS*. 2002 Jan-Mar;6(1):69-75.

[36] Rane A. A training module for laparoscopic urology. *JSLS*. 2005 Oct-Dec;9(4):460-2.

[37] Nakada SY, Hedican SP, Bishoff JT, Shichman SJ, Wolf JS Jr. Expert videotape analysis and critiquing benefit laparoscopic skills training of urologists. *JSLS*. 2004 Apr-Jun;8(2):183-6.

[38] Pilar Laguna M, de Reijke tm, Wijkstra h, de la Rosette j. Training in laparoscopic urology. *Current Opinion in Urology*. 2006, Vol. 16, No. 2: 65.

[39] Mory EA. Feedback Research Revisited. *Handbook of Research on Educational Communications and Technology.* 2005;745-783.

[40] Blum T, Sielhorst T, Navab N. Advanced Augmented Reality Feedback for Teaching 3D Tool Manipulation. In: New Technology Frontiers in Minimally Invasive Therapies. Casciaro S, Gersak B. Lupiensis Editor, 2007, Italy; pp:223-236.

[41] Obst T, Burgkart R, Ruckhaberle E, Reine R. Geburtensimulator mit multimodaler - Interaction Delivery Simulator with Multimodal Interaction. *Automatisierrungstechnilk* 2000;54:280-287.

[42] Stylopoulos N, Rattner D. Robotics and ergonomics. *Surg. Clin. North Am.* 2003;83:1321–1337.

[43] Scott DJ, Young WN, Tesfay ST, Frawley WH, Rege RV, Jones DB. Laparoscopic skills training. *Am. J. Surg* 2001;182: 137-42.

[44] Agarwala N. To compare outcomes of laparoscopic and robotic cases at a single institute. *J. Minim. Invasive Gynecol.* 2009;16:S52-S102.

[45] Veljovich DS, Paley PJ, Drescher CW, Everett EN, Shah C, Peters WA 3rd. Robotic surgery in gynecologic oncology: program initiation and outcomes after the first year with comparison with laparotomy for endometrial cancer staging. *Am. J. Obstet. Gynecol.* 2008;198:679.1–9.

[46] Advincula AP, Reynolds RK. The use of robot-assisted laparoscopic hysterectomy in the patient with a scarred or obliterated anterior cul-de-sac. *JSLS* 2005;9:287–91.

[47] Advincula AP, Wang K. Evolving role and current state of robotics in minimally invasive gynecologic surgery. *J. Minim. Invasive Gynecol.* 2009;16(3):291-301.

[48] Tinelli A, Malvasi A, Gustapane S, Buscarini M, Gill IS, Stark M, Nezhat FR, Mettler L. Robotic Assisted Surgery in Gynecology: Current Insights and Future Perspectives. *Recent Pat Biotechnol.* 2011 Apr 28. [Epub ahead of print].

[49] Diaz-Arrastia C, Jurnalov C, Gomez G, Townsend C Jr. Laparoscopic hysterectomy using a computer-enhanced surgical robot. *Surg. Endosc.* 2002; 16:1271–3.

[50] Molpus KL, Wedergren JS, Carlson MA. Robotically assisted endoscopic ovarian transposition. *JSLS* 2003;7:59–62.

[51] Reynolds RK, Advincula AP. Robot-assisted laparoscopic hysterectomy: technique and initial experience. *Am. J. Surg.* 2006 Apr;191(4):555-60.

[52] Advincula AP, Reynolds RK. The use of robot-assisted laparoscopic hysterectomy in the patient with a scarred or obliterated anterior cul-de-sac. *JSLS.* 2005 Jul-Sep;9(3):287-91.

[53] Fader AN, Escobar PF. Laparoendoscopic single-site surgery (LESS) in gynecologic oncology: Technique and initial report. *Gynecol. Oncol.* 2009;114:157–61.

[54] Escobar PF, Fader AN, Paraiso MF, Kaouk JH, Falcone T. Robotic-assisted laparoendoscopic single-site surgery in gynecology: Initial report and technique. *J. Minim. Invasive Gynecol.* 2009;16:589–91.

[55] Escobar PF, Bedaiwy M, Fader AN, Falcone T. Laparoendoscopic single site (LESS) in patients with benign adnexal diease. *Fert. Steril.* 2010;93:2071.

[56] Fader AN, Rojas-Espaillat L, Ibeanu O, Grumbine F, Escobar PF. Laparoendoscopic single-site surgery (LESS) in gynecology: A multi-institutional evaluation. *Am. J. Obstet. Gynecol.* 2010 [In Press].

[57] Lee YY, Kim TJ, Kim CJ, Kang H, Choi CH, Lee JW, Kim BG, et al. Single-port access laparoscopic-assisted vaginal hysterectomy: A novel method with a wound retractor and a glove. *J. Minim. Invasive Gynecol.* 2009;16:450–3.

[58] Yim GW, Jung YW, Paek J. Transumbilical single-port access versus conventional total laparoscopic hysterectomy: Surgical outcomes. *Am. J. Obstet. Gynecol.* 2010; 203:26.e1–6.

[59] Fanfani F, Fagotti A, Scambia G. Laparoendoscopic single-site surgery for total hysterectomy. *Int. J. Gynecol. Obstet.* 2010;109:76–7.

[60] Jung YW, Kim YT, Lee DW, Hwang YI, Nam EJ, Kim JH, et al. The feasibility of scarless single-port transumbilical total laparoscopic hysterectomy: Initial clinical experience. *Surg. Endosc.*2010;24:1686–92.

[61] Ghezzi F, Cromi A, Fasola M, Bolis P. One-trocar salpingectomy for the treatment of tubal pregnancy: A 'marionette-like' technique. *BJOG.* 2005;112:1317–419.

[62] Savaris RF, Cavazzola LT. Ectopic pregnancy: Laparoendoscopic single-site surgery-laparoscopic surgery through a single cutaneous incision. *Fertil. Steril.* 2009;92:1170–e5-e7.

[63] Yoon BS, Park H, Seong S. Single-port laparoscopic salpingectomy for the surgical treatment of ectopic pregnancy. *J. Minim. Invasive Gynecol.* 2010;17:26–9.

[64] Kim YW, Park BJ, Ro DY, Kim TE. TEComparison of single-port transumbilical laparoscopically assisted vaginal hysterectomy (SPLAVH) and laparoscopically assisted vaginal hysterectomy (LAVH) *J. Minim. Invasive Gynecol.* 2009;16:S103–57.

[65] Fader AN, Levinson KL, Gunderson CC, Winder AD, Escobar PF. Laparoendoscopic single-site surgery in gynaecology: A new frontier in minimally invasive surgery. *J. Minim. Access Surg.* 2011 Jan;7(1):71-7.

[66] Hariri LP, Bonnema GT, Schmidt K, Winkler AM, Korde V, Hatch KD, Davis JR, Brewer MA, Barton JK. Laparoscopic optical coherence tomography imaging of human ovarian cancer. *Gynecol. Oncol.*2009;114(2):188–194.

[67] Ascencio M, Collinet P, Cosson M, Mordon S. The role and value of optical coherence tomography in gynecology *J. Gynecol. Obstet. Biol. Reprod.* (Paris). 2007 Dec;36(8):749-55.

[68] Zuluaga AF, Follen M, Boiko I, Malpica A, Richards-Kortum R. Optical Coherence Tomography. A pilot study of a new imaging technique for noninvasive examination of cervical tissue. *Am. J. Obstet. Gynecol.* 2005;193:83-88.

[69] Escobar PF, Rojas-Espaillat L, Tisci S, Enerson C, Brainard J, Smith J, Tresser NJ, Feldchtein FI, Rojas LB, Belinson JL. Optical coherence tomography as a diagnostic aid to visual inspection and colposcopy for preinvasive and invasive cancer of the uterine cervix. *Int. J. Gynecol. Cancer.* 2006 Sep-Oct;16(5):1815-22.

[70] Hariri LP, Liebmann ER, Marion SL, Hoyer PB, Davis JR, Brewer MA, Barton JK. Simultaneous optical coherence tomography and laser induced fluorescence imaging in rat model of ovarian carcinogenesis. *Cancer Biol. Ther.* 2010 Sep;10(5):438-47.

[71] Vincent KL, Bell BA, Rosenthal SL, Stanberry LR, Bourne N, Cosgrove Sweeney YT, Patton DL, Motamedi M. Application of optical coherence tomography for monitoring changes in cervicovaginal epithelial morphology in macaques: potential for assessment of microbicide safety. *Sex Transm. Dis.* 2007 Dec 4.

[72] Boppart SA, Goodman A, Libus J, Pitris C, Jesser CA, Brezinski ME, Fujimoto JG. High resolution imaging of endometriosis and ovarian carcinoma with optical

coherence tomography: feasibility for laparoscopic-based imaging. *Br. J. Obstet. Gynaecol.* 1999 Oct;106(10):1071-7.

[73] Mac Laughlin RA, Sampson DD. Introduction to Optical Coherence Tomography for endoscopic imaging. In: New Technology Frontiers in Minimally Invasive Therapies. Casciaro S, Gersak B. Lupiensis Editor, 2007, Italy; pp: 122-127.

[74] Foulot H, Lefebvre G, Jagueux M, Darbois Y.Experimental study of CO2-laser-induced histological effects on human fallopian tube: determination of CO2 laser parameters to be used in microsurgery. *Lasers Surg. Med.* 1987;7(2):202-6

[75] Fayez JA, Jobson VW, Lentz SS, Payne DG, Westra DF, Martin DK.Tubal microsurgery with the carbon dioxide laser. *Am. J. Obstet. Gynecol.* 1983 Jun 15;146(4):371-3.

[76] Schmidt S, Decleer W, Kermani O, Koort HJ, Kindermann C, Dardenne MU, Krebs D. Excimer laser cold section technique for surgical gynecology. *Geburtshilfe Frauenheilkd.* 1989 Mar;49(3):305-6.

[77] Keckstein J, Sasse V, Roth A, Karageorgieva E, Tuttlies F. Laser techniques in gynaecology. *Endosc. Surg. Allied Technol.* 1994 Jun-Aug;2(3-4):176-80.

[78] Gabrieli CB, Pacella E, Abdolrahimzadeh S, Regine F, Mollo R.Excimer laser photorefractive keratectomy for high myopia and myopic astigmatism. *Ophthalmic Surg. Lasers.* 1999 Jun;30(6):442-8.

[79] Pacella E, Abdolrahimzadeh S, Gabrieli CB.Excimer laser photorefractive keratectomy for hyperopia. *Ophthalmic Surg. Lasers.* 2001 Jan-Feb;32(1):30-4.

[80] Abdolrahimzadeh S, Pacella E, Morgia P, Prencipe F., Pacella f., Balacco-Gabrieli C:Visual compliance after PRK. Abstract 4894-B841. ARVO March 15;2000.

[81] Tinelli A, Hudelist G, Malvasi A, Tinelli R. Laparoscopic management of ovarian pregnancy. *JSLS* 2008; 12(2): 169-172.

In: Laparoscopy: New Developments, Procedures and Risks   ISBN: 978-1-61470-747-9
Editor: Hana Terzic, pp. 91-113   © 2012 Nova Science Publishers, Inc.

Chapter IV

Laparoscopic Reconstructive Adnexal Surgery: A Practical Approach

Atef Darwish

Endoscopy Unit of the Woman's Health University Center,
Assiut University, Assiut, Egypt.
Obstetrics and Gynecology, Assiut University, Assiut, Egypt.
Minimally Invasive Surgery Society of Egypt,
Egptian Society of Laparoscopic Surgery, and
Egyptian Society of Hysteroscopy and Colposcopy.

Introduction

Reconstructive gynecologic surgery is performed to treat the primary disease as well as refashion abnormal genital organs to restore anatomy and more importantly improve function. It leads to reduce potential problems and side effects from primary surgery and improve patients' quality of life. Early discharge within 24 hours after the procedure with an excellent outcome is a common sequel to reconstructive gynecologic surgery even if done via laparotomy [1].

Nevertheless, reconstructive surgery requires high level of expertise, delicate instruments, fine maneuvers, longer time, and fine energy modalities. Reconstructive gynecologic surgery is a broad term covering a lot of gynecologic subsepecielities e.g. urogynaecology [2], infertility [3], onocology [4], breast reconstruction [5] and pelvic floor dysfunction [6]. Laparoscopic approaches have been dramatically changed and in many cases replaced most of the traditional approaches. Thus, adding endoscopic approach to the principles of reconstruction is expected to achieve best results for the women's health.

Laparoscopic Approach to Reconstructive Gynecologic Surgery

Since the early breakthroughs by its pioneers [7-10], laparoscopic gynecologic surgery is gaining popularity due to developments in illumination and instrumentation that led to the emergence of laparoscopy in the late 1980's as a credible diagnostic as well as therapeutic intervention. Performing reconstructive gynecological surgery is appreciated as it is cosmetically acceptable to patients due to small skin incisions with short hospital stay, low liability of ileus, fast recovery, minimal post-operative pain and discomfort, and early resumption of normal activities and employment [11]. Furthermore, there is reduced contamination of the surgical field with glove powder or lint, bleeding is reduced due to tamponade of small vessels by the pneumoperitoneum, and drying of tissues is minimal because surgery occurs in a closed environment [12]. All these factors contribute to reduced postoperative adhesion formation and its associated morbidity (eg, pain, impaired fertility, bowel obstruction) [13]. Of particular importance, laparoscopy offers easy intraoperative access to the pouch of Douglas and the posterior aspects of the genital organs with good magnification, and the ability to perform an underwater examination at the end of the procedure during which all blood clots are evacuated and meticulous hemostasis is obtained [14]. Nevertheless, the adage that no surgery is without risk also applies to laparoscopic surgery [15-18]. Out Of 25,764 laparoscopic procedures, 145 complications (rate 5.7 per 1000) were reported in one study [18]. The authors concluded that operative laparoscopic procedures are still hazardous and women with a previous laparotomy are particularly at risk. Nevertheless, most of these complications occur with blind insertion of instruments [19]. Continuous training and upgrading of the level of the laparoscopist as well as preoperative preventive measures of complications should be encouraged [20].

Fertility-Preserving Reconstructive Gynecologic Surgery

If future fertility is of concern, endoscopic reconstructive gynecologic surgery should follow microsurgical principles [21,22] which include avoidance of serosal insults e.g. tissue trauma, ischemia, hemorrhage, infection, foreign-body reaction, and leaving raw surfaces [25]. Other microsurgical principles include minimizing tissue trauma by using atraumatic techniques, meticulous hemostasis, complete excision of abnormal tissues and precise alignment and approximation of tissue planes [24]. With this so meticulous reconstruction of the gynecological structures, maximal possibilities of pregnancy without the utilization of other complex procedures of assisted reproduction can be achieved. It has been estimated by some enthusiastic proponents that microsurgery could results in double the pregnancy rate compared conventional macrosurgery [25]. However, a recent Cochrane review did not demonstrate any advantage of microsurgery over the conventional approach [23]. Laparoscopic microsurgeons should have enough experience in classical microsurgery as well as highly-developed two-handed laparoscopic skills for intracorporeal knotting [26,27].

Basic Diagnostic Aids for Reconstructive Laparoscopic Surgery

Of course diagnostic laparoscopy is the gold standard diagnostic aid for all adnexal lesions making it superior to old invasive diagnostic tools (Figure 1).

Nevertheless, alternative less invasive diagnostic procedures may be done in selected cases. For instance, saline infusion sonography (SIS) is commonly practiced in many centers. In 1999 we described a simplified approach [28]. The procedure starts with routine transvaginal sonogrphy (TVS) to explore the endometrial cavity as regards endometrial thickness or any evident lesion, myometrial architecture and the adnexae. Special emphasis on the presence of fluid in the Douglas pouch, particularly at the time of ovulation, should be made to avoid confusion at SIS. Then, the transvaginal probe is extracted and a special bivalve Collin's speculum is inserted into the vagina. Its blades are attached laterally at one side to allow its extraction without disturbing other instruments inserted inside the vagina. After proper disinfection using povidone iodine, gentle grasping of the cervix with a volsellum is performed. Then a Nelaton plastic catheter of different sizes is inserted inside the cervix after gentle sounding. This step is followed by reinsertion of the transvaginal probe alongside the catheter. Gradual injection of sterile saline into the endometrial cavity should be done until a clear view is achieved. At this step, comments on shape, any irregularities of the wall, polyps or filling defects should be reported. Then, an extra amount of sterile saline is injected to assess both fallopian tubes successively with comment on their visualization, shape and patency. Lastly, the Douglas pouch is looked at for the presence of fluid or adhesions. After completion of the procedure, the patients should be asked about their experience with the technique regarding pain during or after it as well as its convenience.

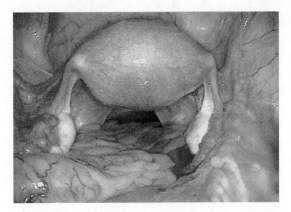

Figure 1. Normal laparoscopic findings.

Robotics in Reproductive Medicine

Along the road of refinement of endoscopic reconstructive gynecologic surgery, robotic technology, more specifically telerobotic surgical systems, has been used to bridge this gap between laparotomy and laparoscopy by enabling minimally invasive surgery with three-dimensional vision, ergonomically optimal positioning, tremor filtration, and laparoscopic instruments with intra-abdominal articulation [29,30]. This remarkable technology facilitates suturing and dissection [31]. Although the learning curve is steep, the robot may actually level the playing field among various skilled gynecologic surgeons performing laparoscopy for the management of complex pathology. Nevertheless, a skilled laparoscopic surgeon may not find any advantage in the meantime with the current robotic prototypes. Some major disadvantages of robot-assisted endoscopy include lack of tactile feedback or haptics and the high costs of the equipments. The size of some of the robotic systems may also be a limitation [32].

Overview on laparoscopic ovarian drilling in polycystic ovarian syndrome (PCO):

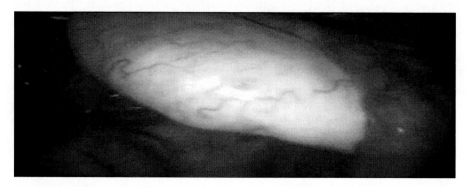

Figure 2. Typical polycystic ovary.

In modern practice, surgical methods of ovulation induction for women with clomifene citrate-resistant polycystic ovarian syndrome (PCOS) only include laparoscopic ovarian drilling (LOD). This technique is designed to create several ovarian stromal drills, which may help correct endocrine abnormalities and trigger ovulation. LOD, which has been evaluated in well-designed trials, may be an alternative to gonadotropins [33]. A systematic review of four RCTs found no significant differences between LOD after 6–12 months follow-up and 3–6 cycles of ovulation induction with gonadotrophins in cumulative pregnancy rate (OR 1.42; 95% CI 0.84 to 2.42) or miscarriage rate (OR 0.61; 95% CI 0.17 to 2.16) in women with clomifene citrate-resistant PCOS[34]. Multiple pregnancy rates were considerably reduced in those women who conceived following laparoscopic drilling (OR 0.16; 95% CI 0.03 to 0.98). Although gonadotropin treatment and LOD have demonstrated similar reproductive outcomes, LOD has some advantages over gonadotropin treatment such as lower cost per pregnancy, improvement in menstrual regularity, and better long-term reproductive performance [35]. However, ovarian reserve assessed by hormonal levels and sonography seems to be lower in the LOD than in the PCOS group without LOD in a recent study [36]. This risk of damaged ovarian reserve could be minimized if LOD is restricted to patients with high preoperative LH level as demonstrated in a retrospective cohort study [37]. One RCT showed a significant difference between the use of a fine or thick needle in the occurrence of adhesion formation (52% with fine needle versus 88% with a thick needle, RR 0.59, 95% CI 0.39 to 0.91) in LOD in patients with PCOS [38]. A retrospective study showed that three punctures per ovary appeared to be the plateau dose for laparoscopic ovarian diathermy [39]. Nevertheless, more punctures were recommended like 5 punctures [40] or even up to 15 punctures in another study [41]. In a recent RCT, unilateral ovarian drilling in PCOS was shown to be effective, less time-consuming and probably associated with fewer complications than bilateral drilling [42]. LOD can impose technical problems and anesthetic risks in obese women with PCOS [42]. Whether done via standard laparoscopy or microlaparoscopy, the efficacy of LOD in PCOS, estimated by ovulation and pregnancy rates within 12 months of follow-up is similar as well as the trends in hormonal changes. Ovarian electrocautery was significantly longer in microlaparoscopy, but the difference in time was of no practical impact [43]. Nevertheless, a small sample sized study demonstrated decreased adhesion formation following microlaproscopic LOD compared with conventional laparoscopic LOD. This finding may possibly be due to lack of or minimal adverse effects on peritoneal microcirculation and cell-protective systems, which are proposed mechanisms for adhesion formation and closely related to peritoneal injury [44]. In recent years, there is a growing interest in transvaginal hydrolaparoscopic LOD by some teams in France [45], Italy [46], and Belgium [47]. Utilizing fine bipolar electrode, LOD can be easily performed in a shorter time compared to the standard laparoscopy. They achieved high pregnancy rate within 6 months of the procedure (71% at 6 months [48], 76% at about 8 months [47]). Nevertheless, many gynecologists don't practice transvaginal hydrolaparoscopy as they consider it less informative than standard laparoscopy [49] or even minilaparoscopy. Therefore, further comparative studies of hydrolaparoscopy versus standard laparoscopy especially efficacy and cost effectiveness are badly needed. Recently, we tested the single puncture LOD using a disposable set (figure 2) and found it time consuming and sophisticated procedure for this minor laparoscopic technique and therefore omitted it from our endoscopic options for LOD.

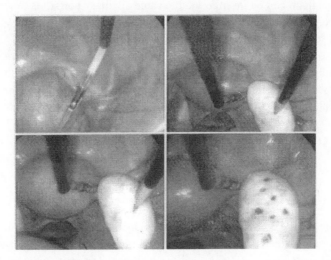

Figure 2. LOD via a single puncture approach.

Technical Tricks of Laparoscopic Ovarian Drilling (LOD)

The ovarian ligament should be grasped by atruamatic grasping forceps from the contralateral side. The ovary should be gently grasped and elevated towards the lateral pelvic wall. Multiple ovarian drilling should be done on the antimestic surface only to minimize the risk of subsequent adhesion formation. Drilling should be done with a thin needle while firing should be started after perforation of the capsule bluntly to be sure that stromal destruction starts with minimal capsular damage. Firing should never exceed 5 seconds at 30-40 Watt setting of the monopolar diathermy. Practically, the number of drills should tailored according to the ovarian size. The same steps are repeated on the other side after exchanging instruments. Proper hemostasis should be achieved. Repeated suction irrigation followed by leaving some fluid in the peritoneal cavity like lactated ringer's solution or even saline. Alternative drilling procedures including minilaparoscopy or single port laparoscopy, or bipolar drilling do need more studies to support these interesting ideas.

Complications of Ovarian Drilling

Short term complications include injuries and unintentional bleeding. Bleeding may come from the round ligament due to overtraction or excessive weight of the ovary. Control should be rapidly achieved with grasping of the bleeder with a bipolar forceps with taking care to avoid tubal damage. Sometimes, bleeding comes from the ovarian drills. This bleeding can be controlled by monopolar coagulation. Start with spray mode directed towards the bleeding points. If bleeding continues, try to get the bleeder from another adjacent drill. Rarely, bleeding occurs from the auxillary portals. Bleeding can be controlled by grasping the bleeder from the opposite auxillary portal and its coagulation. If no response was achieved, an intraabdominal balloon can be inserted via the same auxillary portal, its upward traction, and then inflation.

Long term complications are related to the procedure of drilling in the form of overdestruction of the ovarian stroma with subsequent reduction of the ovarian reserve and postoperative adhesion formation. In a previous study, it was reported that postoperative adhesions can occur even if microsurgical principles were followed. Moreover, adhesions were reported in a good number of the pregnant cases as examined at the time of cesarean section [50].

Overview on Laproscopic Reconstructive Surgery in Gynecologic Emergencies

The clinical situation in some gynecologic emergencies may oblige some gynecologists to rush in performing unneeded laparotomies. Emergency laparoscopic surgery allows both the evaluation of acute abdominal pain and the treatment of many common acute abdominal disorders. Laparoscopic surgery is firmly established as the best intervention in acute appendicitis, acute cholecystitis and most gynecologic emergencies but requires further RCTs to definitively establish its role in other conditions [51]. Many acute gynecologic disorders can be diagnosed and treated via laparoscopy [52]. Following conventional investigations, diagnostic laparoscopy is highly effective [53] and recommended [54].

Ectopic Pregnancy

One of the best examples is ectopic pregnancy (EP). There is a significant amount of high quality evidence regarding the role of laparoscopic surgery in ectopic pregnancy (EP). In confirmed EP, laparoscopy should be performed unless haemodynamic instability is present. The first case report of laparoscopic excision of a tubal ectopic pregnancy was published in 1973 [55]. Since then, much data has been published concerning the effectiveness of treatment as well as the fertility outcome of EP treated by laparoscopic salpingostomy and salpingectomy. Laparoscopy is fast, cheaper [56], and fertility outcome is comparable to laparotomy [57]. Furthermore, hospitalization and sick leave times are shorter, and adhesion development reduced when compared to laparotomy [58]. Laparoscopic salpingostomy in the treatment of EP has been associated with an 85% tubal patency rate; a subsequent intrauterine pregnancy rate of 55–61.2% and a recurrent EP rate of between 14 to 15.5% [59-62]. The rate of persistent EP after laparoscopic salpingostomy has been reported to range from 3.3% to 20% with a mean of 8.3%15. If tubal rupture has occurred, a laparoscopic salpingectomy should be performed. Data on laparoscopic salpingectomy is less extensive but investigators [63] have reported subsequent IUP rates of 50–54% and recurrent ectopic pregnancy (REP) rates of 7.7%–15.2%. However, in cases of unruptured tubal pregnancy, a tube preserving operation should be considered [64]. Compared to laparotomy, several authors have shown that for hemodynamically stable patients, the laparoscopic approach had similar operating times, less blood loss and significantly shorter hospital stays [57,65-67]. A RCT of cost-effectiveness [67] done on 109 patients subjected to either laparotomic or laparoscopic treatment of EP, reported that laparoscopic treatment was as effective as laparotomy but at lower costs. Laparoscopic surgery has improved our management of surgical emergencies and in certain conditions is now an essential part of recent practice. What is clear is that as surgical expertise and technology both continue to improve, so the remit for laparoscopic surgery will expand, to the benefit of patients [68].

In modern practice, there is a place for medical treatment of EP [69] thanks to the use of sensitive assays for hCG and the high definition of vaginal ultrasound. By using these sensitive diagnostic tools, we are now able to select those patients who are most likely to respond to medical management. A variable dosing methotrexate regimen is more effective if compared with single dose regimen. The fixed multiple regimen is associated with a high rate of side effects [70]. Besides being less invasive and associated with significantly lower risks, medical therapy with methotrexate (MTX) was found to be more cost effective than laparoscopic surgery, but the frequent need for second-line treatment should be assessed [71]. Thus, the main goal is to identify those patients with EP who are most likely to respond to MXT and least likely to develop significant side effects. Recent studies have helped us define the predictors of success with MXT treatment in women with ectopic pregnancy. The reported success rates of treating EP with methotrexate vary from 71% to 100%. The highest success rates have been reported from institutions that have detailed diagnostic and therapeutic protocols, readily available assays for serum hCG levels, high-resolution vaginal probe ultrasound, and support staff that can closely monitor clinical response. The importance of developing specific protocols to create a clinical environment that supports the effective use of medical therapy for ectopic pregnancy is confirmed by the associated cost savings, decreased morbidity, and patient preference. Modern diagnostic advances and minimally invasive treatments coupled with improved success rates for assisted reproductive technologies should reduce the morbidity and mortality associated with ectopic pregnancy and offers the affected couple a much more optimistic outlook for subsequent reproductive potential [71]. In the Netherlands, a controlled clinical trial was conducted to evaluate patient preferences for systemic MXT therapy relative to laparoscopic salpingostomy in the treatment of tubal pregnancy. They concluded that systemic methotrexate therapy would be preferred by most patients as part of a completely nonsurgical management strategy [72]. However, the same team found MXT to have a more negative impact on patients' health-related quality of life than did laparoscopic salpingostomy [73].

Technical Tricks of Laparoscopic Management of Ectopic Pregnancy (EP)

One of the keys of success is to achieve proper visualization of the pelvis after meticulous peritoneal wash. Better to insert a 10 mm left sided auxillary portal to be able to use a 10 mm suction cannula. It will help get rid of organized blood clots and debris. Mobilize the affected tube from the adjacent organs and take care of bleeding or perforation of a vital organ like a loop of intestine or the colon since tissues are congested and a bit friable. Start by evaluation of the sound tube and be sure that it is healthy and functioning. Evaluate the affected tube and make it away from any adjacent structure. If EP is seen, first localize its site and the state of the fallopian tube over it. If EP is fimbrial or distal ampulary, try tubal milking. To achieve excellent results, grasp the tube firmly proximal to the ectopic pregnancy with a blunt grasping forceps and try to milk the tubal contents with another blunt grasping forceps towards the fimbria. Each forward movement of the grasping forceps should be associated with distal movement of the proximally situated grasping forceps to be sure that the intratubal contents proceed towards the fimbria. Don't crush the tube aggressive to avoid mucosal damage. A tricky step at the end of milking is to inject saline (with little dye) via the cervix to ensure complete milking.

When salpingotomy is decided (figure 4), again grasp the tube just proximal to the EP firmly to het the EP bulging. Use a fine needle incise the tube on the antimesenteric side. Don't incise more than needed to minimize ooze from the edges and subsequent coagulation and to avoid the need for using sutures. Once the EP comes via the incision, use a toothed grasping forceps to catch the EP in mass and extract it immediately via a 10 mm auxillary portal. Ensure meticulous hemostasis and use minimal electrosurgery. Don't leave the abdomen withour prior repeated suction of blood clots with changing the position of the table to allow clots from the flanks to be suced. If hemostasis is metculous, no need for an intraperitoneal drain.

Whenever the tube is ruptured, a decision of salpingectomy should be made provided the other tube is Ok. Start by coagulation and cutting of the proximal part of the tube. This step should be followed by coagulation of the mesosalpnix from both side with a bipolar forceps just underneath the affected tube.

Use a hook scissors to cut the mesosalpnix. Control any bleeder with a hemostatic forceps till complete excision Immediately extract the pathologic tube and ensure secured hemostasis, An intraperitoneal drain should be left for few hours to allow drainage of any retained blood clots.

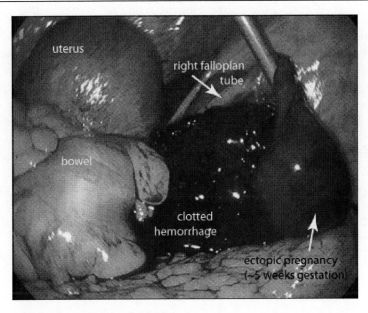

Figure 4. Right undisturbed ampullary ectopic pregnancy.

Adnexal Torsion

Ovarian cyst accidents include cyst rupture, haemorrhage and torsion. These accidents are considered organ-threatening conditions that cause patients to present with acute lower abdominal pain. Initially, pregnancy must be excluded, and transvaginal scan performed to exclude ovarian cyst formation. Torsion commonly occurs to the whole adnexa and is not necessarily associated with an ovarian cyst. Suspected adnexal torsion should always be managed with early laparoscopy and de-torsion of the twisted tube or ovary. Ovarian cyst rupture and haemorrhage usually occur in association with functional cysts and are generally self-limiting [74]. However, torsion of other types of benign cysts has been reported like dermoid cysts or paraovarian cysts [75]. Early diagnosis can help prevent irreversible structural damage and may allow conservative, ovary-sparing treatment. Laparoscopy may be necessary in cases where the diagnosis is in doubt or for haemodynamic compromise. If pain fails to settle, laparoscopy must be performed to exclude adnexal torsion [76]. Clinical features of ovarian cyst accidents are nonspecific. Ultrasound is the first-line investigation and is diagnostic in the case of haemorrhage. Typical ultrasound findings have been described for ovarian torsion, including an enlarged oedematous ovary with peripheral displacement of follicles. In adnexal torsion, the ovary, ipsilateral fallopian tube, or both twist with the vascular pedicle, resulting in vascular compromise. Unrelieved torsion is likely to cause hemorrhagic infarction as the degree of arterial occlusion increases. Therefore, early diagnosis is important to preserve the affected ovary. Adnexal torsion commonly accompanies an ipsilateral ovarian neoplasm or cyst but can also occur in normal ovaries, usually in children. Although ultrasonography is typically the initial emergent examination, computed tomography (CT) and magnetic resonance (MR) imaging may also be useful diagnostic tools. Common CT and MR imaging features of adnexal torsion include fallopian tube thickening, smooth wall thickening of the twisted adnexal cystic mass, ascites, and uterine deviation to the twisted side [77]. Doppler blood flow findings are variable and not diagnostic. If clinical suspicion for torsion is high, early diagnosis and treatment via laparoscopy is encouraged as a means of preserving ovarian and fallopian tube integrity and maintaining fertility, especially in reproductive-age women. Recurrent cyst rupture or haemorrhage should be prevented by suppression of ovulation, usually with the combined oral contraceptive. Fixation of the ovary by a variety of techniques should be considered to prevent recurrent torsion. Most of twisted ovarian cysts found during laparoscopy can be treated laparoscopically [78]. Laparoscopic surgery to repair ovarian torsion is superior to laparotomy [79] and is suitable even in pregnancy. Laparoscopic procedure for ovarian conservation is recommended to treat patients suffering from ovarian torsion owing to its shorter hospital stay, fewer postoperative complications and ovarian preservation [80]. Commonly both fallopian tube and ovarian cyst are involved in the process of torsion. Few studies on isolated fallopian tube torsion have been reported [81].

Acute Pelvic Infection

Pelvic inflammatory disease (PID) is one of the most common infections seen in nonpregnant reproductive-age women. It is a major public health problem associated with substantial medical complications (e.g., infertility, ectopic pregnancy, and chronic pelvic pain) and healthcare costs. Prevention of these long-term sequelae requires treatment strategies that are based on the microbiologic etiology of acute PID [82].

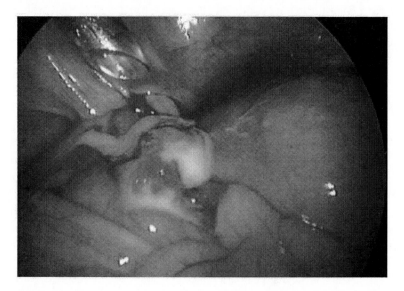

Figure 5. Acute PID.

Acute salpingo-oophoritis commonly causes acute pelvic and lower abdominal pain, and can mimic other surgical diagnoses. Diagnostic laparoscopy can be useful to exclude other common pathologies. If the diagnosis is correct, microbiological samples can be taken to target anti-microbial therapy, and in pyosalpinx, pus can be drained laparoscopically [83]. If gynecologic disorders are the suspected cause of pain, diagnostic laparoscopy should be performed, as frequently simultaneous therapy will be possible. Acute-phase operative laparoscopy provides a final diagnosis and prompt management of most cases with acute PID [84].

Many of these patients will undergo exploration for suspected appendicitis, but in 20-35% of cases a normal appendix is found. Because of the limited access provided by the gridiron incision, a definitive diagnosis may not be found. Other patients may be treated conservatively and discharged. In patients with acute abdominal pain, early laparoscopy is an accurate means of both making a definitive diagnosis and proper management [85] as seen in figure 5.

Laparoscopic Management of Distal Tubal Disease

Distal tubal occlusion may be due to hydrosalpnix, pyosalpnix or peritubal adhesions. Obstruction of the distal fallopian tube is one of the most common causes of female infertility [86]. Nowadays, it is perceived that the presence of hydrosalpinx is associated with a compromised outcome for IVF/ ICSI. Hydrosalpinx is associated with lower implantation and fecundibility rates even if the contralateral tube is sound which may be attributed to alteration in endometrial receptivity [87] or direct embryo toxic effect. Furthermore, it is liable to be unintentionally punctured at the time of egg retrieval or it may disturb access to the ovary if it is too big. In a meta-analysis, it has been demonstrated that there was a reduction by half in the probability of achieving a pregnancy in the presence of hydrosalpinx, and an almost doubled rate of spontaneous abortion [88]. In an animal study, hydrosalpinx fluid was shown to contain toxins that are potentially teratogenic [89]. Proposed mechanisms of impaired implantation rate due to hydrosalpinges are well addressed in the literature [90]. Selected patients with unilateral hydrosalpinges and a patent contralateral Fallopian tube may exhibit increased cycle fecundity after salpingectomy or proximal tubal occlusion of the affected tube, and may conceive without the need for IVF [91]. In a retrospective case-control study, bilateral salpingectomy due to hydrosalpinges restored a normal delivery as well as implantation rate after IVF treatment compared to controls [92]. Randomized controlled trials recommended performing laparoscopic salpingectomy prior to IVF, especially in patients with ultrasound-visible hydrosalpinges [93]. In a recent Cochrane review [94], it was concluded that further randomized trials are required to assess other surgical treatments for hydrosalpinx, such as salpingostomy, tubal occlusion or needle drainage of a hydrosalpinx at oocyte retrieval. Functionless hydrosalpinx can be defined as a large blocked tube with lost major and minor folds, as seen at salpingoscopy after laparoscopic salpingoneostomy.

On sonography, the dilated fallopian tube presents as a thin- or thick-walled tubular fluid-filled structure that may be elongated or folded (figure 6). Longitudinal folds that are present in a normal fallopian tube may become thickened in the presence of a hydrosalpinx. The dilated fallopian tube may or may not show longitudinal folds. These longitudinal folds are pathognomonic of a hydrosalpinx . If the elongated nature of these folds is not noted, they may be mistaken for mural nodules of an ovarian cystic mass. Identification of a separate ovary helps distinguish a hydrosalpinx from a cystic ovarian mass, an important distinction because malignancy is rare with an extraovarian cystic adnexal mass. A significantly scarred hydrosalpinx may present as a multilocular cystic mass with multiple septa creating multiple compartments. These septa are generally incomplete, and the compartments can be connected. However, with more pronounced scarring, differentiation from an ovarian mass may not be possible [95]. Potential pitfalls in the diagnosis of hydrosalpinx include paratubal, paraovarian, or perineural cysts. In some cases, CT or MRI may be helpful to differentiate these conditions from a hydrosalpinx [96].

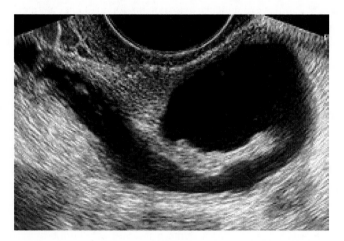

Figure 6. Sonographic appearance of a typical hydrosalpnix.

Technical Tricks of Laparoscopic Management of Hydrosalpnix

A. Salpingoneostomy: One of the keys of success is to evaluate the tube externally and internally. If peritubal adhesions exist, microsurgical adhesiolysis should be performed at first. Be sure that the tube is freely mobile. Imagine the site of the new ostium before dealing with the hydroslpnix. It should be directed towards the pouch of Douglas to help ovum pick-up. Start by salpingoneostomy using a fine monopolar or bipolar needle. The finest the needle, the better ostium. Incise the distended distal part of the tube " + shaped" (cruciate incision). Then, evaluate the tubal mucosa using a salpingoscopy. Practically, use the diagnostic hysteroscopy which consists of a 4 mm telescope and a 5 mm outer sheath. Connect it to a normal IV infusion set and use saline as an irrigating fluid. Grasp the new ostium with an atruamatic grasping forceps and insert the hysteroscope with comment on the major and minor folds till reaching the narrowest part of the tube. F major and minor folds are lost this means that the prognosis is poor even after proper refashioning. The next step is to grasp the tubal lumen with atruamatic forcpes and to evert it outside. Lastly, fix the edges of the new ostium either with monopolar spray coagulation just distal to the incised parts to evert them or with the aid of fine sutures.

B. Salpingectomy: This procedure is indicated if a pathologic unilateral huge hydrosalpnix is present to enhance spontaneous pregnancy or bilateral big hydrosalpnix before IVF/ICSI. It is performed in the same manner as mentioned in the section of EP.

C. Tubal occlusion: Once the peritoneal cavity is entered, a panoramic evaluation of the pelvis is performed. If the pelvis looked frozen or if access to the fallopian tubes is impossible, the patient is considered a failed laparoscopic approach. Those cases are subsequently treated by open laparotomic or hysteroscopic approach. If the procedure seems feasible, a third auxiliary puncture is carried out. Utilizing a bipolar forceps, the isthmic part of the fallopian tube is coagulated and incised to ensure complete tubal occlusion, as a case of tubal sterilization. The procedure is completed after securing hemostasis. The patient is discharged after 3-4 h under antibiotic prophylaxis.

Laparoscopic salpingectomy or bipolar proximal tubal occlusion yielded statistically similar responses to controlled ovarian hyperstimulation and IVF-ET cycle outcome. Proximal occlusion might be preferable in patients who present with dense pelvic adhesions and easy access only to the proximal fallopian tube [97]. Occlusion is considered a minimally invasive procedure, requires less experience, feasible in most cases, and has fewer burdens on the psychological status of those infertile women. Hysteroscopic approach is recently described by our team at Assiut University Institution [98]. The cervix is primed in all cases using misoprostol (200 mg) 8 h prior to the procedure. The procedure is carried out immediately postmenstrual without specific preparation. Local paracervical, spinal or general anesthesia could be used. Selection of the anaesthetic technique is chosen according to patient preference after proper explanation by the anaesthesiologist. The cervix is gently dilated with Hegar 10 and a rotatory continuous flow monopolar resectoscope is inserted. Once the peritubal bulge (the proximal part of the intramural segment of the tube [11]) was clearly seen, a roller ball electrode (size: 3 mm) is introduced inside it and activated at 50 Watts for about 8 seconds. A thorough comment on the fundus and the rest of the endometrial cavity should be reported. The patients are usually discharged immediately if the procedure is carried out under local paracervical anesthesia, while the remaining cases are discharged a few hours later.

Paratubal and Paraovarian Cysts

Introduction

Paratubal or paraovarian cysts represent approximately 10% of all adnexal masses [99,100]. They are usually derived from the mesothelial covering of the peritoneum or remnants of paramesonephric and mesonephric origin, so histologically they are covered by a single layer of ciliated columnar or flattened cells [101]. The concept of paramesonephric (Müllerian) origin is supported by a report of 6 women with paraovarian cysts who were exposed prenatally to diethylstilbestrol (DES[102]. Morgagni's hydatid cysts are usually under 1 cm and found along the course of the fallopian tube, but paratubal cysts are seen in the broad ligament and may be larger in size [103]. However, other paraovarian cystic lesions have been reported, for example cystadenoma and adenofibroma [104], lymphangioma diagnosed in 15 women [105], ependymoma [106], multicystic endosalpingiosis associated with tamoxifen therapy, if papillary projections are present [107]. Two cases of primary paraovarian serous cystadenocarcinoma have been reported [108]. Some case reports were published on paratubal cystic leiomyoma [109]. Malignant change has been reported in about 2% to 3% [110] and it has been reported in 2 postmenopausal women [111]. One case of transitional cell carcinoma that arose within a paratubal cyst has been clearly described [112]. The prevalence of paratubal or paraovarian cysts in a healthy population is not known due to the lack of data on healthy women [110].

Diagnosis of Paratubal and Parasovraina Cysts

Preoperative transvaginal ultrasonography (TVS) is usually performed as a routine examination in most patients. The ability to sonographically diagnose the paratubal or paraovarian cysts as a hypoechoic mass separate from the ovary should be put in mind and recorded (Figure 7).

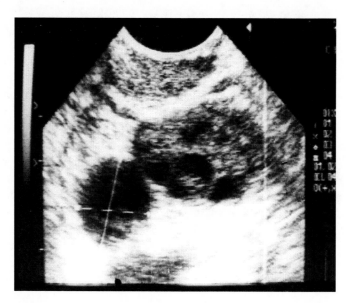

Figure 7. Typical appearance of a paraovarian cyst.

Meticulous evaluation of hysterosalpingography (HSG), whenever available, should be made in infertile patients to identify tubal shape and patency. At laparoscopy, a thorough visualization of the mesosalpinx is achieved. If a cyst is seen between the ovary and the tube, it is called a "paraovarian cyst." The term "paratubal cyst" is used if the cyst seen near the distal end of the tube. In all cases, observations should be made about its size and site in relation to the ovary, evidence of associated Morgagni's hydatid cysts, and vasculature over the cyst. The principal diagnostic laparoscopic criterion is the location of the cyst and the crossing of the blood vessels over the cyst that made differentiation from ovarian cysts easy (Figure 8). By this pathognomonic sign, differentiation from ovarian cyst (figure 9) would be easy. In all patients, tubal chromopertubation should be used to assess tubal patency, and the relation of the cyst to the tubal lumen should be recorded.

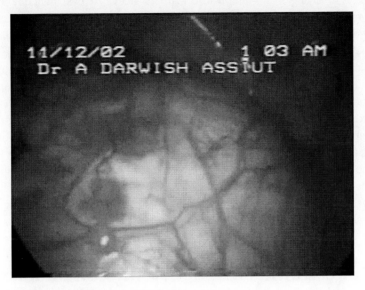

Figure 8. Crossing of blood vessels over paratubal cyst.

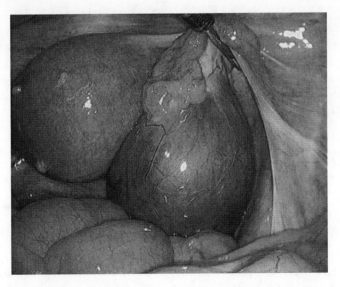

Figure 9. Laparoscopic appearance of ovarian cysts.

Operative Procedures

Operative treatment of these cysts varies according to cyst size. In cases of small cysts measuring less than 3 cm3, simple cyst puncture is performed with a microneedle followed by the cyst's coagulation with a bipolar forceps. In cases of larger cysts, complete extraction is performed. Complete extraction starts by making an antimesenteric linear incision over the cyst as far as possible from the tube by using microscissors or a microneedle with caution not to injure the cyst. Using a 5.5-mm trocar with its sleeve, a cyst puncture is performed followed by repeated suction irrigation. Meticulous endocystic visualization is achieved in all cases with a diagnostic hysteroscope loaded inside its diagnostic sheath to ensure its benign nature. The cyst is then distended with warm saline. The 5.5-mm hole in the cyst wall is closed with a blunt grasping forceps with traction of the cyst upwards. Unlike ovarian cysts, paratubal and paraovarian cysts are easily dissected with another blunt grasping forceps within a shorter time. The cyst wall usually appears thick and whitish that can be easily extracted. Extraction of the entire cyst wall is usually followed by gentle coagulation of the bed with bipolar diathermy after proper identification of the ureter. Closure of the mesosalpingeal defect with coagulation of the edges with bipolar forceps may be required. Sutures or monopolar diathermy should be limited to minimize the risk of peritubal adhesions or tubal damage. In all cases, histopathologic examination of the cyst is conducted. Copious peritoneal washing is done followed by leaving about 1 liter of lactated Ringer's solution intraperitoneally.

Take-Home Messages and Conclusions

Laparoscopic approach to reconstructive adnexal surgery is superior to conventional approach in most of the aspects including ovarian cysts, paratubal or paraovarian cysts. LOD is a controversial procedure that carries serious long term sequele. Intraoperative additional endocystic evaluation of ovarian or paraovarian cysts is a valuable quick prcedure and should be encourged. Laparoscopic reconstruction of DTO should be attempted provided at least major folds are preserved at salpingoscopy. In cases of acute abdomen, laparoscopy is a valuable diagnostic as well as therapeutic tool and should be tried at first provided the patient is hemodynamically stable.

References

[1]   Fayez JA, Dempsey RA. Short hospital stay for gynaecologic reconstructive surgery via laparotomy. *Obstet. Gynaecol.* 1993;81:598-600.
[2]   Miklos, JR. Laparoscopic Repair of Vesicouterine Fistula. *J. Am. Assoc. Gyn. Laparosc.* 1999;6(3):339-341.
[3]   Peacock LM, Rock JA. Distal tubal reconstructive surgery. In. Sanfilippo JS, Levine RL. Operative Gynaecologic Endoscopy. 2nd edition. New York, Springer Verlag Inc., 1996, Chapter 2.
[4]   Friedman RM, Gyemishi I, Robinson JB, Rohrich RJ. Saline made viscous with polyethylene glycol: a new alternative breast implant filler material. *Plastic and Reconstructive Surgery* 1996; 98: 1208.
[5]   Marcickiewicz J, Brannstrom M. Fertility preserving surgical treatment of borderline ovarian tumour: long-term consequence for fertility and recurrence. *Acta Obstet. Gynaecol. Scand.* 2006;85(12):1496-500.

[6]   Paraiso MF, Chen CC. Laparoscopic surgery for pelvic organ prolapse. *Minerva. Ginecol.* 2006;58(5):381-91.

[7]   Semm K: Tissue puncher and loop ligation: new side for surgical-therapeutic pelviscopy (laparoscopy). *Endoscopy* 1978;10:119-124.

[8]   Bruhat MA, Manhes H, Mage G, Pouly JL: Treatment of ectopic pregnancy by means of laparoscopy. *Fertil. Steril.* 1980; 33:411-414.

[9]   Daniell JF, Brown DH: Carbon dioxide laser laparoscopy: critical experience in animals and humans. *Obstet. Gynaecol.* 1982; 59:761-764.

[10]   Reich H, McGlynn F: Treatment of ovarian endometriosis using laparoscopic surgical techniques. *J. Reprod. Med.* 1986, 31:577-584.

[11]   Reich H, McGlynn F: Treatment of ovarian endometriosis using laparoscopic surgical techniques. J Reprod Med 1986, 31:577-584.Gynaecologic Laparoscopy. Principles and Techniques. 2nd edition, NewYork ,McGraw Hill., 2000,Ch 9.

[12]   Papp A, Vereczkei , Lantos J, Horváth OP. The effect of different levels of peritoneal CO_2 pressure on bleeding time of spleen capsule injury. *Surgical Endoscopy* 2003; 17(7);1125-1128.

[13]   Diamond, M.P. and Schwartz, L.B. (1998) Prevention adhesion development. In Sutton, C. and Diamond, M.P. (eds), Endoscopic Surgery for Gynaecologists , 2nd edn. Philadelphia, W.B.Saunders, pp. 398–403.

[14]   Garry R. Laparoscopic surgery. *Best Pract. Res. Clin. Obstet. Gynaecol..* 2006; 20(1):89-104.

[15]   Harkki-Siren P, Sjoberg J, Kurki T. Major complications of laparoscopy: a follow-up Finnish study. *Obstet. Gynecol.* 1999;94:94-98.

[16]   Chapron C, Querleu D, Bruhat MA, et al. Surgical complications of diagnostic and operative gynaecological laparoscopy: a series of 29,966 cases. *Hum. Reprod.* 1998;13:867-872.

[17]   Jansen FW, Kapiteyn K, Trimbos-Kemper T, Hermans J, Trimbos JB. Complications of laparoscopy: a prosepctive multicentre observational study. *Br. J. Obstet. Gynaecol..* 1997;104:595-600.

[18]   Jansen FW, Kolkman W, Bakkum EA, de Kroon CD, Trimbos-Kemper TC, Trimbos JB. Complications of laparoscopy: an inquiry about closed- versus open-entry technique. *Am. J. Obstet. Gynecol.* 2004;190(3):634-8.

[19]   Vilos GA, Ternamian A, Dempster J, Laberge PY, The Society of Obstetricians and Gynaecologists of Canada. Laparoscopic entry: a review of techniques, technologies, and complications. *J. Obstet. Gynaecol. Can.* 2007;29(5):433-65.

[20]   Cohen SM, Singer AJ. Preventing complications before the operation. In. Complications of Gynaecologic Endoscopic Surgery. Isaacson K Philadelphia, Saunders Elsevier. 2006,Ch 3.

[21]   Wiedermann R, Hepp H. Selection of patients for IVF therapy or alternative therapy methods. *Hum. Rep.* 1989.;4:23-27.

[22]   Watson A, Vandekerckhove P, Lilford R. Techiques for pelvic surgery in subfertility. *Cochrane Database Syst. Rev.* 2:CD00022, 2000.

[23]   Ahmad G, Watson A, Vandekerckhove P, Lilford R. Techniques for pelvic surgery in subfertility.*Cochrane Database Syst. Rev..* 2006 Apr 19;(2):CD000221.

[24] Sauer MV. Tubal infertility. The role of reconstructive surgery. In. Lobo RA, Mishell DR, Paulson RJ, Shoupe D. Infertility, Contraception and Reproductive Endocrinology. Boston, Blackwell Scientific Publications, 4th edition, 1997,Ch 36.

[25] Bateman BG, Nunley JW, Kitchen JD. Surgical management of distal tubal occlusion-are we making progress?. *Fertil. Steril* 1987;48;523.

[26] Gomel V, Taylor PJ (Ed). Fertility-promoting procedures and assisted reproductive technology. In. Diagnostic and Operative Gynaecologic Laparoscopy. St Louis, Mosby-Year Book, Inc., 1995,Ch 15.

[27] Koh CH. Anastomosis of the fallopian tube. In. Tulandi T. Atlas of Laparoscopic and Hysteroscopic Techniques for gynaecologists. 2nd edition, London, W.B. Saunders, 1999. Ch 7.

[28] Darwish AM, Youssef AA. Screening sonohysterography in infertility. *Gynecol. Obstet. Invest.* 1999;/48(1):/43_7.

[29] Nezhat FR, Shama Datta M, Liu C, Chunag L, Zakashansky K. Robotic radical hysterectomy versus total laparoscopic radical hysterectomy with pelvic lymphadenectomy for treatment of early cervical cancer. *JSLS* 2008;12:227-237.

[30] Ballantyne GH. Robotic surgery, telerobotic surgery, telepresence, and telementoring. *Surg. Endosc.* 2002;16:1389–402.

[31] Diaz-Arrastia C, Jurnalov C, Gomez G, Townsend Jr. Laproscopic hysterectomy using a computer enhanced surgical robot. *Surg. Endosc.* 2002;16:1271-1273.

[32] Advincula A.P, Falcone T, Laparoscopic robotic gynecologic surgery. *Obstet Gynecol* Clin N Am 2004;31:599– 609.

[33] Urman B, Yakin K.Ovulatory disorders and infertility. *J. Reprod. Med.* 2006;51(4):267-82.

[34] Farquhar C, Vandekerckhove P, Arnot M, Lilford R. Laparoscopic "drilling" by diathermy or laser for ovulation induction in anovulatory polycystic ovary syndrome. *Cochrane Database Syst. Rev.* 2000 ;(2):CD001122.

[35] Unlu C, Atabekoglu CS. Surgical treatment in polycystic ovary syndrome. *Curr. Opin. Obstet. Gynecol.* 2006;18(3):286-92.

[36] Weerakiet S, Lertvikool S, Tingthanatikul Y, Wansumrith S, Leelaphiwat S, Jultanmas R. Ovarian reserve in women with polycystic ovary syndrome who underwent laparoscopic ovarian drilling. *Gynecol. Endocrinol.* 2007;2;1-6.

[37] Hayashi H, Ezaki K, Endo H, Urashima M. Preoperative luteinizing hormone levels predict the ovulatory response to laparoscopic ovarian drilling in patients with clomiphene citrate-resistant polycystic ovary syndrome. *Gynecol. Endocrinol.* 2005;21(6):307-11.

[38] El Saeed M, Ezzat R, Hasan M, Elhelw B, Aboulmaaty Z, Aboulghar M. High incidence of pelvic adhesions detected by second look laparoscopy after laparoscopic ovarian drilling. *Middle East Fertility Society Journal* 2000;5:519–25.

[39] Amer SAK, Li TC, Cooke ID. Laparoscopic ovarian diathermy in women with polycystic ovarian syndrome: a retrospective study on the influence of the amount of energy used on the outcome. *Hum. Reprod.* 2002; 17:1046–51.

[40] Malkawi HY, Qublan HS. Laparoscopic ovarian drilling in the treatment of polycystic ovary syndrome: how many punctures per ovary are needed to improve the reproductive outcome?. *J. Obstet. Gynaecol. Res.* 2005;31(2):115-9.

[41] Tabrizi NM, Mohammad K, Dabirashrafi H, Nia FI, Salehi P, Dabirashrafi B, Shams S. Comparison of 5-, 10-, and 15-point laparoscopic ovarian electrocauterization in patients with polycystic ovarian disease: a prospective, randomized study. *JSLS.* 2005;9(4):439-41.

[42] Youssef H, Atallah MM. Unilateral ovarian drilling in polycystic ovarian syndrome: a prospective randomized study. *Reprod. Biomed. Online.* 2007;15(4):457-62.

[43] Muenstermann U. Long-term GnRH analogue treatment is equivalent to laparoscopic laser diathermy in polycystic ovarian syndrome patients with severe ovarian dysfunction. *Hum. Reprod.* 2000; 15:2526–30.

[44] Marianowski P, Kaminski P, Wielgos M, Szymusik I. The changes of hormonal serum levels and ovulation/pregnancy rates after ovarian electrocautery in microlaparoscopy and laparoscopy in patients with PCOS. *Neuro. Endocrinol. Lett.* 2006;27(1-2):214-8.

[45] Taskin O, Sadik S, Onoglu A, Gokdeniz R, Yilmaz I, Burak F, Wheeler J. Adhesion formation after microlaparoscopic and laparoscopic ovarian coagulation for polycystic ovary dis. *The Journal of the American Association of Gynecologic Laparoscopists* 1999; 6, 2,159-163.

[46] Fernandez H, Alby JD, Gervaise A, de Tayrac R, Frydman ROperative transvaginal hydrolaparoscopy for treatment of polycystic ovary syndrome: a new minimally invasive surgery. *Fertil. Steril.* 2001;75(3):607-11.

[47] Ferraretti AP, Gianaroli L, Magli MC, Iammarrone E, Feliciani E, Fortini D. Transvaginal ovarian drilling: a new surgical treatment for improving the clinical outcome of assisted reproductive technologies in patients with polycystic ovary syndrome. *Fertil. Steril.* 2001;76(4):812-6.

[48] Gordts S, Gordts S, Puttemans P, Valkenburg M, Campo R, Brosens I. Transvaginal hydrolaparoscopy in the treatment of polycystic ovary syndrome. *Fertil. Steril.* 2009 Jun;91(6):2520-6.

[49] Daraï E, Rouzier R, Ballester M. Transvaginal hydrolaparoscopy: practices in French teaching hospitals. *J. Minim. Invasive Gynecol.* 2008;15(3):273-6.

[50] Darwish AM, AbdelAleem MA, Ismail AM. Risk of adhesions formation following microsurgical monopolar laparoscopic ovarian drilling: a comparative study. *Gynecological Surgery* 2009,6 (2) 135-141.

[51] Taylor EW, Kennedy CA, Dunham RH, Bloch JH: Diagnostic laparoscopy in women with acute abdominal pain. *Surg. Laparosc. Endosc.* 1995; 5(2):125-128.

[52] Sallam HN, Garcia-Velasco JA, Dias S, Arici A. Long-term pituitary down-regulation before in vitro fertilization (IVF) for women with endometriosis. *Cochrane Database Syst. Rev..* 2006 25;(1):CD004635.

[53] Ma C, Qiao J, Liu P, Chen G. Ovarian suppression treatment prior to in-vitro fertilization and embryo transfer in Chinese women with stage III or IV endometriosis. *Int. J. Gynaecol. Obstet.* 2008;100(2):167-70.

[54] Gray DT, Thorburn J, Lundorff P, Strandell A, Lindblom B: A cost-effectiveness study of a randomised trial of laparoscopy versus laparotomy for ectopic pregnancy. *Lancet* 1995; 345(8958):1139-1143.

[55] Shapiro HI, Adler DH. Excision of an ectopic pregnancy through the laparoscope. *Am. J. Obstet. Gynaecol.* 1973; 117: 290-291.

[56] Lundorff P, Thorburn J, Lindblom B: Fertility outcome after conservative surgical treatment of ectopic pregnancy evaluated in a randomized trial. *Fertil. Steril.* 1992; 57(5):998-1002.

[57] Lundorff P, Thorburn J, Hahlin M, Kallfelt B, Lindblom B: Laparoscopic surgery in ectopic pregnancy. A randomized trial versus laparotomy. *Acta Obstet. Gynaecol. Scand* 1991; 70(4-5):343-348.

[58] Pouly JL, Mahnes H, Mage G, Canis M, Bruhat MA. Conservative laparoscopic treatment of 321 ectopic pregnancies. *Fertil. Steril.* 1986; 46: 1093-7.

[59] Vermesh M, Presser SC. Reproductive outcome after linear salpingostomy for ectopic gestation: a prospective 3-year follow-up. *Fertil. Steril.* 1992; 57: 682-4.

[60] Sultana CJ, Easley K, Collins RL. Outcome of laparoscopic versus traditional surgery for ectopic pregnancies. *Fertil. Steril.* 1992; 57:285-9.

[61] Yao M, Tulandi T. Current status of surgical and nonsurgical management of ectopic pregnancy. *Fertil. Steril.* 1997; 67:421-33.

[62] Silva PD, Schaper AM, Rooney B. Reproductive outcome after 143 laparoscopic procedures for ectopic pregnancy. *Obstet. Gynaecol.* 1993; 81:710-5.

[63] Dubuisson JB, Morice P, Chapron C, De-Gayffier A Mouelhi T. Salpingectomy - the laparoscopic surgical choice for ectopic pregnancy. *Hum. Reprod.* 1996; 11(6):1199-203.

[64] Vermesh M, Silva PD, Rosen GF, Stein AL, Fossum GT, Sauer MV: Management of unruptured ectopic gestation by linear salpingostomy: a prospective, randomized clinical trial of laparoscopy versus laparotomy. *Obstet. Gynaecol.* 1989; 73(3 Pt 1):400-404.

[65] Brumsted J, Kessler C, Gibson C, Nakajima S, Riddick DH, Gibson M. A comparison of laparoscopy and laparotomy for the treatment of ectopic pregnancy. *Obstet. Gynaecol.* 1988; 71:889-92.

[66] Baumann R, Magos A, Turnbull A. Prospective comparison of videopelviscopy with laparotomy for ectopic pregnancy. *Br. J. Obstet. Gynaecol.* 1991; 98:765-771.

[67] Murphy AA, Nager CW, Wujek JJ, Kettel LM, Torp VA, Chin HG. Operative laparoscopy versus laparotomy for the management of ectopic pregnancy: a prospective trial. *Fertil. Steril.* 1992; 57:1180-5.

[68] Warren O, Kinross J, Paraskeva P, Darzi A. Emergency laparoscopy – current best practice. *World Journal of Emergency Surgery* 2006, 1:24.

[69] Cheong Y, Li TC. Controversies in the management of ectopic pregnancy. *Reprod Biomed Online.* 2007;15(4):396-402.

[70] Vaissade L, Gerbaud L, Pouly JL, Job-Spira N, Bouyer J, Coste J, Glanddier PY. Cost-effectiveness analysis of laparoscopic surgery versus methotrexate: comparison of data recorded in an ectopic pregnancy registry. *J. Gynecol. Obstet. Biol. Reprod.* (Paris). 2003;32(5):447-58.

[71] Luciano AA, Roy G, Solima E. Ectopic pregnancy from surgical emergency to medical management. *Ann. N. Y. Acad. Sci.* 2001;943:235-54.

[72] Nieuwkerk PT, Hajenius PJ, Van der Veen F, Ankum WM, Wijker W, Bossuyt PM. Systemic methotrexate therapy versus laparoscopic salpingostomy in tubal pregnancy. Part II. Patient preferences for systemic methotrexate. *Fertil. Steril.* 1998;70(3):518-22.

[73] Nieuwkerk PT, Hajenius PJ, Ankum WM, Van der Veen F, Wijker W, Bossuyt PM Systemic methotrexate therapy versus laparoscopic salpingostomy in patients with tubal

pregnancy. Part I. Impact on patients' health-related quality of life. *Fertil. Steril.* 1998;70(3):511-517.

[74] Bottomley C, Bourne T.Diagnosis and management of ovarian cyst accidents. *Best Pract. Res. Clin. Obstet. Gynaecol.*. 2009 Oct;23(5):711-24

[75] K0ostov M, Mijović Z, Mihailović D. Giant paraovarian cyst in a child complicated with torsion. *Vojnosanit Pregl.* 2008 Nov;65(11):843-6.

[76] Sauerland S, Agresta F, Bergamaschi R, Borzellino G, Budzynski A, Champault G, Fingerhut A, Isla A, Johansson M, Lundorff P, Navez B, Saad S, Neugebauer EA: Laparoscopy for abdominal emergencies: evidence-based guidelines of the European Association for Endoscopic Surgery. *Surg. Endosc.* 2006; 20(1):14-29.

[77] Rha SE, Byun JY, Jung SE, Jung JI, Choi BG,Kim BS, Hyun Kim H, Lee JM. CT and MR Imaging Features of Adnexal Torsion. *Radiographics.* 2002;22:283-294.

[78] Mais V, Ajossa S, Piras B, Marongiu D, Guerriero S, Melis GB: Treatment of nonendometriotic benign adnexal cysts: a randomized comparison of laparoscopy and laparotomy. *Obstet. Gynaecol.* 1995; 86(5):770-774.

[79] Yuen PM, Yu KM, Yip SK, Lau WC, Rogers MS, Chang A: A randomized prospective study of laparoscopy and laparotomy in the management of benign ovarian masses. *Am. J. Obstet. Gynaecol.* 1997; 177(1):109-114.

[80] Lo LM, Chang SD, Horng SG, Yang TY, Lee CL, Liang CC. Laparoscopy versus laparotomy for surgical intervention of ovarian torsion. *J. Obstet. Gynaecol. Res.* 2008 Dec;34(6):1020-5.

[81] Phillips K, Fino ME, Kump L, Berkeley A. Chronic isolated fallopian tube torsion. *Fertil. Steril.*. 2009 Jul;92(1):394.e1-3.

[82] Sweet RL. Treatment strategies for pelvic inflammatory disease. *Expert Opin. Pharmacother.* 2009;10(5):823-37.

[83] Teisala K, Heinonen PK, Punnonen R: Laparoscopic diagnosis and treatment of acute pyosalpinx. *J. Reprod. Med.* 1990; 35(1):19-21.

[84] Molander P, Cacciatore B, Sjöberg J, Paavonen J. Laparoscopic management of suspected acute pelvic inflammatory disease. *J. Minimally Invasive Surgery* 2000; 7, 1,107-110.

[85] Golash V, Willson PD. Early laparoscopy as a routine procedure in the management of acute abdominal pain: a review of 1,320 patients. *Surg. Endosc.* 2005;19(7):882-5.

[86] Peacock LM, Rock JA. Distal tubal reconstructive surgery. In: Sanfilippo JS, Levine RL, editors. Operative gynecologic endoscopy. New York: Springer-Verlag Inc; 1996. p. 182_91.

[87] Seli E, Kayisli UA, Cakmak H, Bukulmez O, Bildirici I, Guzeloglu-Kayisli O. Removal of hydrosalpinges increases endometrial leukaemia inhibitory factor (LIF) expression at the time of the implantation window. *Hum. Reprod.* 2005;/ 20(11):/3012_7.

[88] Zeyneloglu HB, Arici A, Olive DL. Adverse effects of hydrosalpinx on pregnancy rates after in vitro fertilizationembryo transfer. *Fertil. Steril.*. 1998;/70:/492_9.

[89] Chan LY, Chiu PY, Cheung LP, Haines CJ, Tung HF, Lau TK. A study of teratogenicity of hydrosalpinx fluid using a whole rat embryo culture model. *Hum. Reprod.* 2003;/18(5):/955_8.

[90] Nackley AC, Muasher SH. The significance of hydrosalpinx in in vitro fertilisation. *Fertil. Steril.*. 1998;/69:/373_84.

[91] Sagoskin AW, Lessey BA, Mottla GL, Richter KS, Chetkowski RJ, Chang AS, et al. Salpingectomy or proximal tubal occlusion of unilateral hydrosalpinx increases the potential for spontaneous pregnancy. *Hum Reprod.* 2003;/ 18(12):/2634_7.

[92] Ejdrup H, Bredkjær, Ziebe S, Hamid B, Zhou Y, Loft A, et al. Delivery rates after in-vitro fertilization following bilateral salpingectomy due to hydrosalpinges: a case control study. *Human Reprod.* 1999;/14(1):/101_5.

[93] Strandell A, Lindhard A, Waldenstro¨m U, Thorburn J, Janson PO, Hamberger L. Hydrosalpinx and IVF outcome: a prospective, randomized multicentre trial in Scandinavia on salpingectomy prior to IVF. *Hum. Reprod.* 2001;/16(11):/ 2403_10.

[94] Johnson NP Mak W Sowter MC. Surgical treatment for tubal disease in women due to undergo in vitro fertilization (Cochrane Review). The Cochrane Library, Issue 2. Chichester, UK: John Wiley and Sons, Ltd; 2005.

[95] Atri M, Nazarnia S, Bret PM, Aldis AE, Kintzen G, Reinhold C. Endovaginal sonographic appearance of benign ovarian masses. *RadioGraphics*1994; 14:747 -76.

[96] Benjaminov O, Atri M. Sonography of the Abnormal Fallopian Tube *AJR* 2004; 183:737-742.

[97] Surrey ES, Schoolcraft WB. Laparoscopic management of hydrosalpinges before in vitro fertilization-embryo transfer: salpingectomy versus proximal tubal occlusion. *Fertil. Steril..* 2001;/75(3):/612_7.

[98] Darwish AM, ElSamam M. Is there a role for hysteroscopic tubal occlusion of functionless hydrosalpinges prior to IVF/ICSI in modern practice. *Acta Obstetricia et Gynecologica.* 2007; 86: 1484_1489.

[99] Azzena A, Quintieri F, Salmaso R. A voluminous paraovarian cyst. Case report. *Clin Exp. Obstet. Gynecol.* 1994;21(4):249-252.

[100] Barloon TJ, Brown BP, Abu-Yousef MM, Warnock NG. Paraovarian and paratubal cysts: preoperative diagnosis using transabdominal and transvaginal sonography. *J. Clin. Ultrasound.* 1996;24(3):117-122.

[101] Athey PA, Cooper NB. Sonographic features of paraovarian cysts. *AJR.* 1985;144:83-86.

[102] Haney AF, Newbold PR, Fetter BF, McLachlan JA. Paraovarian cysts associated with prenatal diethylstilbestrol exposure. Comparison of the human with a mouse model. *Am. J. Pathol.* 1986;124(3):405-411.

[103] Occhipinti KA. Computed tomography and magnetic resonance imaging of the ovary. In: Anderson JC, ed. *Gynecologic Endoscopy.* London: Churchill Livingstone; 1999:347-349.

[104] Korbin CD, Brown DL, Welch WR. Paraovarian cystadenomas and cystadenofibromas: sonographic characteristics in 14 cases. *Radiology.* 1998;208(2):459-462.

[105] Pellicano M, Iorio F, Fortunato N. Increase of paraovarian cysts. Differential diagnosis, macroscopic and microscopic aspects and role of laparoscopy. *Minerva Ginecol.* 1994;46(11): 597-600.

[106] Guerrieri C, Jarlsfelt I. Ependymoma of the ovary. A case report with immunohistochemical, ultrastructural, and DNA cytometric findings, as well as histogenetic considerations. *Am. J. Surg. Pathol.* 1993;17(6):623-632.

[107] McCluggage WG, Weir PE. Paraovarian cystic endosalpingiosis in association with tamoxifen therapy. *J. Clin. Pathol.* 2000;53(2):161-162.

[108] Carabias E, Lopez-Pino MA, Dhimes FP, Vargas J. Paratubal cystic leiomyoma: radiologic and pathologic analyses. *Eur. J. Radiol.* 1995;20(1):28-31.

[109] Stein AL, Koonings PP, Schlaerth JB, Grimes DA, d'Ablaing G 3rd. Relative frequency of malignant paraovarian tumors: should paraovarian tumors be aspirated? *Obstet. Gynecol.* 1990;75:1029-1031.

[110] Tailor A, Hacket E, Bourne T. Ultrasonography of the ovary. In: Anderson JC, ed. *Gynecologic Endoscopy*. London: Churchill Livingstone; 1999:334-349.

[111] Kim JS, Woo SK, Suh SJ, Morettin LB. Sonographic diagnosis of paraovarian cysts: value of detecting a separate ipsilateral ovary. *AMJ.* 1995;164(6):1441-1444.

[112] Altras MM, Jaffe R, Corduba M, Holtzinger M, Bahary C. Primary paraovarian cystadenocarcinoma: clinical and management aspects and literature review. *Gynecol. Oncol.* 1990;38(2): 268-272.

In: Laparoscopy: New Developments, Procedures and Risks   ISBN: 978-1-61470-747-9
Editor: Hana Terzic, pp. 115-139   © 2012 Nova Science Publishers, Inc.

Chapter V

Surgical Treatment of Deep Endometriosis by Laparoscopy

William Kondo[*1,2]*, Monica Tessmann Zomer*[1]*,*
Lorne Charles[1]* and Michel Canis*[2]

[1] Department of Gynecology, Sugisawa Hospital Medical Center,
Curitiba, Paraná, Brazil.
[2] Department of Gynecologic Surgery, CHU Estaing, Clermont-Ferrand, France.

Introduction

Endometriosis is a gynecologic disorder defined by the presence of endometrial glands and stroma outside the uterus [1]. The most common site of endometriotic implants is the peritoneal cavity, but occasionally lesions have been found in the pleural cavity, liver, kidney, gluteal muscles, bladder, and even in men. The anatomical location and the inflammatory response to these injuries appear to be responsible for the signs and symptoms associated with endometriosis [2].

Macroscopically, pelvic endometriosis can be subdivided into three distinct entities [3,4]: superficial peritoneal (and ovarian) endometriosis, cystic ovarian endometriosis and deeply infiltrating endometriosis.

Epidemiology

The prevalence in women of reproductive age is estimated at 10% [5]. In women with chronic pelvic pain that prevalence can approach 82% [6,7] and in those undergoing investigation for infertility it can reach 20 to 50% [5,8,9].

---
* William Kondo, Av. Getulio Vargas, 3163 ap. 21., Zip Code 80240-041, Curitiba – Paraná – Brazil, Phone number: (55) (41) 9222-1065, E-mail: williamkondo@yahoo.com

Symptomatology

Pelvic pain, represented by dysmenorrhea, dyspareunia, dysuria and dyschezia, is one of the most important symptoms of women with endometriosis. Typically in women of reproductive age who are affected by this disease, the onset of the pain is before the commencement of menses and continues throughout the entire menstrual period each month. The pain can also be referred in musculoskeletal regions such as the flanks, the lower lumbar region or the calves [2].

Another common symptom is infertility. In the event of moderate or severe disease, reduced fertility can occur as a result of mechanical obstruction of the fallopian tubes, or of the presence of adhesions or distortion of the normal pelvic anatomy which can impede the union between sperm and egg. Women with minimal or mild disease, however, also have decreased fertility compared to those without clinical evidence of endometriosis. The exact causes are still unknown, but several mechanisms have been postulated [10].

Many women with endometriosis seek treatment because of pelvic pain, infertility, or both [11]. Lesions penetrating deeply beneath the peritoneal surface (> 5mm) are found more frequently in patients who have chronic pelvic pain symptoms (with or without infertility) than in patients who have infertility alone (odds ratio = 3.9) [12]. However, endometriosis is a condition in which even minimal disease may be associated with severe pain whereas extensive disease may be clinically silent [13].

Deep Infiltrating Disease

The infiltrative forms of endometriosis penetrate more than 5mm below the peritoneal surface [14]. Deep lesions of endometriosis are responsible for painful symptoms with correlation between the intensity of the pain and the depth of the lesion [15]. The role of the lesions in the establishment of painful symptoms is confirmed by the phenomenon of hyperalgesia triggered by palpation and by the presence of nerve fibers in proximity to these lesions, with increased expression of nerve growth factor and transforming growth factor beta at the level of these nerve fibres [16,17]. The histological study conducted by Anaf et al. [18] demonstrated that there is a relationship between the severity of the chronic pelvic pain symptoms and the infiltration of nerves in the rectovaginal space by posterior deep infiltrating endometriotic lesions. Two prospective randomized double-blind studies have shown that surgical treatment of lesions of endometriosis is an effective treatment for chronic pelvic pain [19,20].

Anatomic Distribution and Symptoms of Deep Endometriotic Lesions

The distribution pattern of the deep infiltrating disease in the pelvis is: 55% at the base of the pouch of Douglas, 35% in the utero-sacral ligaments and 11% in the anterior peritoneal reflection [14]. Along with endometriomas, deeply infiltrative disease is considered the most severe form of endometriosis.

In a series of 241 women with histologically proven deep infiltrating endometriosis, Chapron et al. [21] found a total of 344 deep infiltrating lesions. They were located at the utero-sacral ligaments in 69.2%, at the vagina (infiltrating the anterior rectovaginal pouch, the posterior vaginal fornix and the retroperitoneal area in between) in 14.5%, at the bladder (infiltrating the muscularis propria) in 6.4%, and at the intestine (infiltrating the muscularis propria) in 9.9%.

The painful symptoms that are related to deep infiltrating endometriosis have particular characteristics[12]. There is a clear-cut relationship between posterior deep infiltrating endometriosis and deep dyspareunia [22-25]. Fauconnier et al. [26] demonstrated that in women with deep infiltrating endometriosis, the painful semiology is specific to the anatomical location or to the organ affected by the endometriotic implant: dyspareunia is associated with involvement of the utero-sacral ligaments, painful defecation during menses with involvement of the posterior wall of the vagina, non-cyclic pelvic pain and functional bowel signs with bowel involvement, and functional urinary tract signs with involvement of the bladder. Therefore, semiological evaluation of the chronic pelvic pain symptoms can also help in the definition of the surgical strategy [12].

Clinical Significance of Deep Infiltrating Lesions

Large posterior endometriotic lesions in the midline can extend laterally and involve one or both utero-sacral ligaments. This lateral extension has two important implications:

- Surgical implication: ureterolysis is indispensable at time of treatment of utero-sacral endometriotic lesions;
- Clinical implication: the preoperative evaluation in cases of surgical treatment or the follow-up in cases of surgical abstention should always include an ultrasound of the urinary tract.

These posterior lesions can also infiltrate the rectum and the vagina. Lateral lesions infiltrating one or two utero-sacral ligaments also have the potential risk of vaginal and rectal involvement, particularly when lesions are bulky.

The surgery for deep infiltrating endometriosis is a source of numerous debates. It has been agreed that surgical treatment of massive infiltrating lesions (greater than 1 cm in diameter) or lesions infiltrating organs such as the colon or the ureter, is often difficult and laborious. Surgical treatment of deep infiltrating endometriosis may require extensive surgery [27-30], which may include utero-sacral ligament resection [31], partial colpectomy [32,33], resection of rectal endometriosis [29,30,34,35], partial cystectomy [36], and ureteral surgery (ureterolysis, ureteral resection, and ureteral reimplantation) [37]. These kinds of procedures are best performed in specialized centers where a multi-disciplinary approach is possible. This may include the gynecologist, the colorectal surgeon and the urologist. It is important that this team is under the command of the gynecologist who has knowledge about the disease and may indicate surgical steps taking into account the technical consequences of the decisions [38].

The surgical treatment of deep lesions carries a high risk of serious complications, which has been estimated at between 4 and 6% [30,39,40]. Consequently, the patient should be aware that there is always a chance of development of such complications [41]. Most patients accept this risk because of the long duration and severity of pelvic pain.

Treatment should be as complete as possible. The choice of the limits of resection is difficult and requires extreme knowledge of the surgical semiology. Painful recurrences observed after this type of surgery are most often due to an incomplete treatment during the first intervention rather than a true recurrence. The operative difficulties are greater when the disease is severe, when the lesions are large and when the lesion has been previously surgically treated even if only partially. It is very difficult to differentiate postoperative fibrosis from fibrosis induced by the disease. The second intervention is more difficult and can lead to unnecessary and needlessly dangerous resection of fibrous scar. Therefore, surgery should be as complete as possible in the first intervention and a great caution should be exercised in determining the indications for re-intervention.

Preoperative Evaluation

Medical History

The key to diagnosis is careful elicitation of medical history. The French National College of Obstetricians and Gynaecologists recommended the use of a specific questionnaire and a scale measuring the severity of pain [42]. This is very important, since certain lesions are difficult to be visualized in preoperative imaging or during laparoscopy. Whatever the research method, we see better what we seek, and we especially seek lesions whose presence is suggested by the clinical examination. It is essential to investigate digestive or urinary symptoms during the peri-menstrual period. Certain patterns of painful symptoms are characteristic of lesions in specific locations, as described above [12]. However, these symptoms may be absent and infiltrative lesions should be sought in all women who present with complaints of severe dysmenorrhea that alters their quality of life in a meaningful way (away from work, school, etc.) or who necessitate the use of potent analgesics.

Physical Examination

Clinical examination is an essential step in the preoperative evaluation of these lesions. For the surgeon, whatever the result of imaging studies, nothing replaces the information obtained by digital vaginal and rectal examination. One must be patient and gentle when performing this exam. In women with severe pain, the vagina is often tense and constricted. It is sometimes advised to start the vaginal examination introducing just one finger. An endometriotic nodule can be palpated as a hardened zone beneath the mucosal surface of the vagina. When the examining finger touches the posterior vaginal fornix extreme pain may be felt by the patient. The volume, upper, lower and lateral extent of the lesion should be appreciated. Rectal examination can clarify the relationship between the lesion and the wall of the rectum, by assessing the mobility of the tunics of the rectal wall. The clinical record should describe the physical exam findings and its limitations with respect to particular areas that could not be assessed. For instance, the examiner may be unable to identify the upper limit of the lesion if it extends proximally along the rectum, beyond the reach of the examining finger.

Some authors suggest that re-examination of the patient during the menstrual period increase the diagnostic sensitivity of exam [42].

Laboratory Tests

The presence of high Ca-125 levels in a young patient with clinical suspicion of endometriosis increases the index of suspicion for the disease but a normal value does not exclude the possibility. Usually, no laboratory investigation is required for the diagnosis of endometriosis. The increase in the Ca-125 is related to the volume of the endometriomas or the extent of deep infiltrating disease [42]. Some authors [43] suggest that a panel of six plasma markers (interleukin 6, interleukin 8, tumor necrosis factor-alpha protein, high-sensitivity Ca-125 and Ca-19-9) obtained during the secretory phase or during menstruation allow the diagnosis of both minimal and mild endometriosis and moderate to severe disease, with high sensitivity and specificity that is clinically acceptable.

Kafala et al. [44] demonstrated that we can perhaps make a clinical diagnosis of endometriosis by evaluating the differences in the levels of Ca-125 during the menstruation compared to the rest of the menstrual cycle. In their study which included 28 women, there was a 22% increase in serum Ca-125 during the menstrual period (12.2 U / ml) compared with the rest of the menstrual cycle (10U/ml) in the control group. This increase was also observed in women with endometriosis, but levels varied by 198.3%. The Ca-125 levels in these patients during menstruation and the rest of the menstrual cycle were 35.8 and 12U/ml, respectively.

Imaging Studies

Magnetic resonance imaging (MRI), transrectal ultrasound (TRUS) and transvaginal ultrasound (TVUS) have been used to perform the evaluation of infiltrative endometriotic lesions. It seems that in the hands of experts, the TVUS examination is an important preoperative examination for the diagnosis of deep retrocervical and rectosigmoid endometriosis [45].

In the experience of Bazot et al. [46], MRI has similar results compared with TVUS and TRUS for the diagnosis of intestinal endometriosis, but has greater sensitivity and likelihood ratios for the diagnosis of utero-sacral ligament and vaginal endometriosis. Some authors [47] have shown that injection of ultrasound gel inside the vagina and rectum for the performance of MRI can enhance the identification of rectovaginal endometriosis with a sensitivity of 90.9% and specificity of 77.8%. For the presence of deep disease, the sensitivity approached 94.1% and specificity 100%. These findings were confirmed by Chassang et al. [48] who also showed that the opacification of the vagina and rectum with ultrasound gel significantly improved the sensitivity of MRI for the detection of deep endometriosis, allowing a better delineation of the pelvic organs. This was especially apparent for lesions in the vagina and rectovaginal septum.

A definitive conclusion about the comparative value of these three methods is not yet possible. It is important to remember that these methods are operator dependent. A close communication between surgeons and radiologists must be established so that they can gradually understand the needs of surgeons and better interpret the images of infiltrating endometriosis.

Surgical Technique

Under general anesthesia, the patient is placed in a supine position with lower limbs in abduction and with flexion of the thighs onto the pelvis of about 20°. This position allows concomitant abdominal and vaginal access without the need to re-position the patient. The use of a table that allows flexion of the thighs facilitates the placement of sutures in the vagina at the end of the operation.

These interventions are often long and it is appropriate to avoid problems due to prolonged compression or stretching of the nerve trunks. To avoid injuries of the brachial plexus, the two arms are positioned alongside the body. The placement of the lower limbs should avoid compression of the sciatic nerve, external popliteal nerve and calves.

The buttocks of the patient should project slightly beyond the edge of the operating table. The use of a system to prevent heat loss during surgery is recommended for these prolonged interventions.

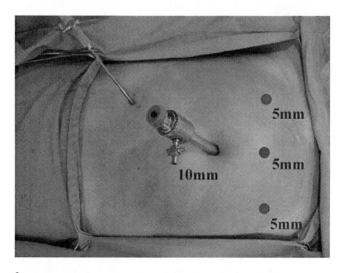

Figure 1. Position of trocars.

The classic laparoscopic setup is established, with an umbilical trocar for the 10mm zero degree laparoscope and three 5mm trocars in the suprapubic region. One trocar is positioned at the midline, 8 to 10 cm below the umbilical trocar, and two trocars are placed in the iliac fossae, about 2 cm medial to the anterior superior iliac spine and always lateral to the inferior epigastric vessels (Figure 1). If a bowel resection is planned, lateral trocars are positioned higher in the lateral-umbilical region, and a fifth trocar is inserted into the right upper quadrant if necessary.

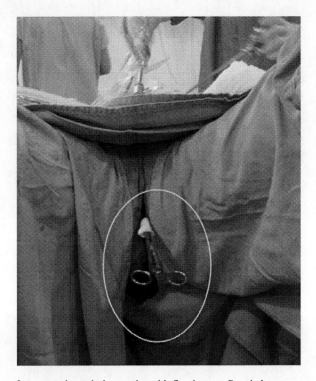

Figure 2. Positioning of a curette through the cervix, with fixation to a Pozzi clamp.

An effective uterine manipulation is necessary. This is achieved by the placement of a high caliber curette through the cervix, which is fixed to a Pozzi clamp. This allows anterior uterine flexion and limits the risk of perforation of the uterine fundus (Figure 2). When necessary, this method also allows the easy performance of a digital vaginal and/or rectal examination during surgery. In case of involvement of both utero-sacral ligaments, it is useful to place an Allis forceps fitted with gauze or a valve in the posterior vaginal fornix to facilitate the identification of the limits of the lesion.

Principles of Surgery

The principles of surgery for severe endometriosis are simple:

- Start with the dissection of healthy tissue in order to identify vulnerable structures (ureters and branches of the nerve plexus) and systematically progress towards the focus of pathological tissue.
- Excision of the entire lesions.
- Avoid unnecessary dissection and displacement of the surrounding organs.

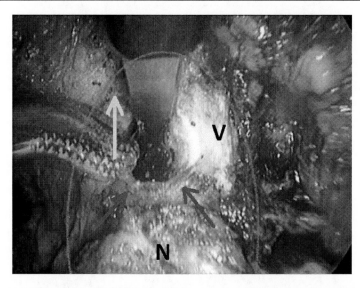

Figure 3. Resection of the posterior vaginal fornix (V) for an endometriotic nodule (N) at the rectovaginal septum. The green circle indicates the area to be resected. Red arrows indicate the presence of endometriotic glands in the vaginal wall. Yellow arrow indicates the extension of resection margin for complete removal of the disease.

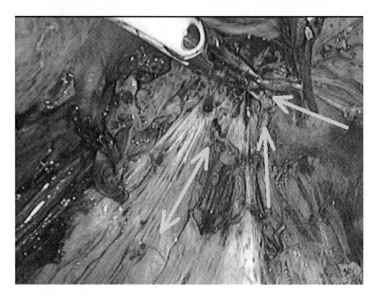

Figure 4. Retrocervical endometriotic lesion. The "arrows" (arrows in yellow) indicate the areas where coagulation-resection of tissue should occur.

However, the application of these principles is complex. In particular, the identification of boundaries between normal and diseased tissue is not always easy. The presence of black spots in the area of resection means that there is presence of micro-cysts of endometriosis, which indicates that the area of resection should be extended (Figure 3). When identification of boundaries are difficult, it is useful to read the monitor to look for the presence of arrows that indicate where to place the next incision (Figure 4). The identification of fatty tissue or normal muscle tissue means that the resection is complete. Conversely, unhealthy or fibrous tissue is suspected when there is a whitish appearance and reduced tendency to bleed. This notion of interpretation is more difficult in the deep part of the utero-sacral ligament. When the section is performed in a healthy tissue, one can realize that the sectioning of 1 or 2mm allows for the mobilization of 5, 10 or even 20mm of the retracted organ, confirming that the healthy tissue was released and became more mobile (Figure 5).

The identification of these limits requires perfect vision, which is only possible with strict hemostasis. However, hemostasis should not always be preventive. If tissue bleeds, it is usually a sign that is free of endometriosis. One should also be aware that the coagulation of blood vessels can produce images that appear similar those obtained in the periphery of the lesion of endometriosis.

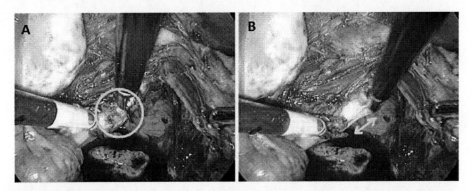

Figure 5. The yellow circle indicates the area to be sectioned and the yellow arrow indicates the mobility of the tissue obtained after resection.

Surgical Tactics

Adhesiolysis and Treatment of Endometriomas

The surgery begins with the release of adhesions that may exist between the posterior wall of the uterus, the adnexa, and the gastrointestinal tract (Figure 6).

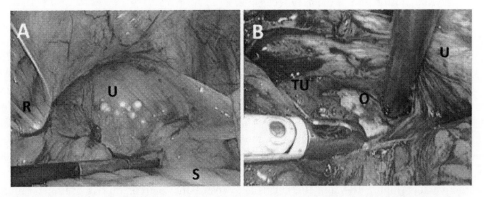

Figure 6. (A) Adhesion of the posterior uterine wall (U) to the left round ligament (R) and the fat of the sigmoid colon (S). (B) Adhesion of the left ovary (O) and tube (TU) to the posterior uterine wall (U).

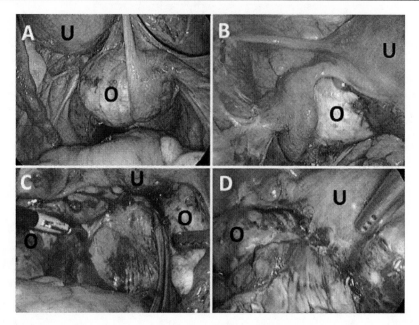

Figure 7. (A) Endometrioma of the right ovary (O) attached to the right utero-sacral ligament. (B) Endometrioma of left ovary (O) attached to the posterior uterine wall (U) and the pouch of Douglas. (C) Bilateral endometriomas attached to the pelvic sidewalls. (D) Endometrioma of left ovary (O) attached to the fat of the sigmoid colon, with total obliteration of the posterior cul-de-sac.

In the presence of ovarian endometriomas, they must be treated before the endometriotic nodule itself. Normally the ovaries containing endometriomas are adhered to the peritoneum of the ovarian fossa beneath which is the path of the ureter or to the ipsilateral utero-sacral ligament (Figures 7). In some instances there may be adhesions between the posterior uterine wall and anterior rectal wall. The lesions of superficial ovarian endometriosis can be treated by simple bipolar cauterization. The cystic endometriomas can be treated in two ways:

- Ovarian cystectomy;
- Draining the endometrioma associated with coagulation or laser vaporization, without resection of the pseudocapsule.

Mobilization of the Sigmoid Colon and Identification of the Ureter

The sigmoid colon should be mobilized at the level of the superior aperture of the pelvis in the left side. This allows identification of the ureter medial to the infundibulopelvic ligament beneath the lesions of ovarian endometriosis (Figure 8). As the ureter is dissected, the pneumoperitoneum viewed through the translucent serosa appears to have a bluish color, which indicates that the underlying ureter is no longer adherent to the peritoneum. The ureteral dissection guides the resection of the endometriotic lesion. The ureter should be left out in cases where the area of resection does not include the broad ligament (Figure 9). In the case of large lesions (more than 2 cm) the ureter is completely released up to the level of the uterine vessels (Figure 10A and 10B). This is to ensure that there is no risk of ureteral injury during the final resection. When the entire broad ligament is involved due to associated lesions, one must dissect all aspects of the ureter (Figure 10C to 10F).

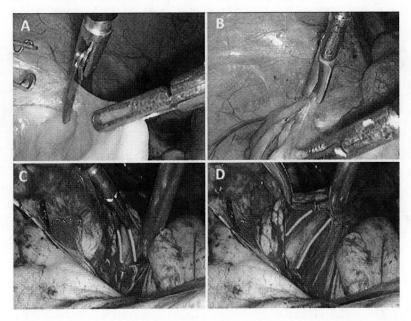

Figure 8. (A and B) Mobilization of the sigmoid colon to identify the ureter medial to the infundibulopelvic ligament.

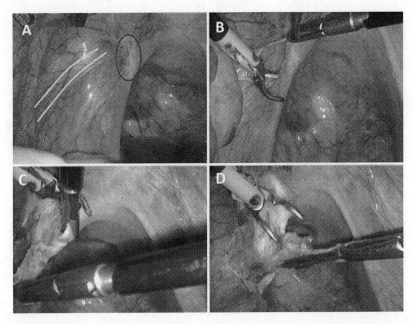

Figure 9. Endometriotic lesion (blue circle) involving only the left utero-sacral ligament (in green), with ureteral path away from the lesion (yellow lines).

When resection involves only the utero-sacral ligament, dissection of the lateral aspect of the ureter is not necessary (Figure 9).

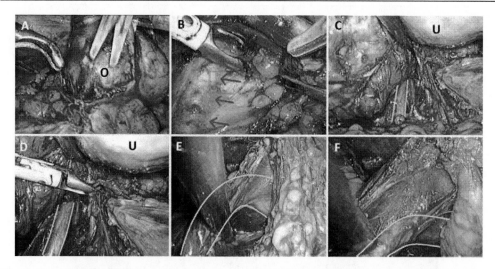

Figure 10. (A) Left ovarian endometrioma (O) attached to the pelvic sidewall and the posterior aspect of the uterus (U). (B) Starting the dissection at the level of the iliac vessels (the blue arrows indicate the left external iliac artery). (C and D) Dissection of the lateral and the medial aspects of the ureter (yellow lines). (E and F) Dissection of the anterior aspect of the ureter (yellow lines).

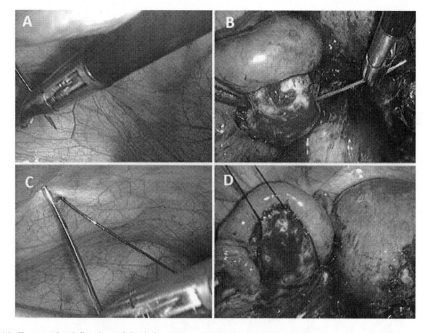

Figure 11. Transparietal fixation of the left ovary to improve exposure.

During this phase of ureteral dissection, ovarian suspension is very useful because it liberates a surgical instrument for other maneuvers. The suspension can be accomplished by the use of a straight needle, which can suture the ovary and attach it to the anterior abdominal wall after it is released from the broad ligament (Figure 11).

Transection of the Utero-Sacral Ligament and
Identification of the Pararectal Space

After identifying the ureter posterior-lateral to the lesion, the utero-sacral ligament is pulled medially with an atraumatic grasping forceps, scissors are positioned in the midline trocar and the bipolar forceps are positioned in the trocar on the same side of the ligament being treated. The cleavage planes are easily identified by the presence of bubbles arising from CO_2 entering the loose connective tissue and the fatty tissue. Divergent traction facilitates penetration of CO_2 into the tissues (Figure 12). After sectioning the posterior-lateral border of the nodule on the utero-sacral ligament, the para-rectal fossa is identified. At this level, resection should not be systematic but guided by the extent of the lesion. The need for extensive resection of the two utero-sacral ligaments is rare, thus limiting the frequency of postoperative voiding complications.

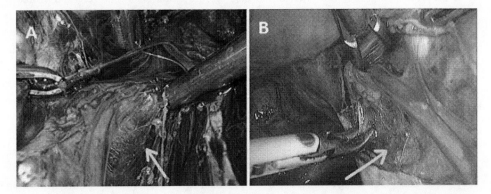

Figure 12. (A) Dissection medial to the left ureter (green lines) to identify the para-rectal fossa driven by bubbles (yellow arrows) that indicate the path to be followed. (B) The same dissection in the right side.

Identification of the Posterior Fornix of the Vagina

Once the para-rectal fossa is identified, dissection is continued anteriorly to define the lateral and distal limits of the nodule. The aim here is to find the disease-free vaginal fornix at the rectovaginal septum. It is important that the lateral limit of the resection is far away from the ureter, which should be located laterally. The risk of ureteral injury must not exist during vaginal resection. There must also be a margin of safety to allow for bipolar hemostasis of any eventual bleeding vessel without risk of thermal injury to adjacent vital structures. To ensure that the dissection is sufficient, the surgeon performs a vaginal palpation with his left hand and manipulates a laparoscopic forceps with the right hand in contact with the vagina in an attempt to discern for a soft and clinically normal vaginal distal to the endometriotic nodule at the posterior vaginal fornix.

Dissection of the Contralateral Border of the Nodule and
Separation of the Nodule from the Anterior Rectal Wall

The next step is to identify and dissect out the other side of the nodule. This may lie outside the other utero-sacral ligament or within the pouch of Douglas, internally to the contralateral utero-sacral ligament. The goal here is to identify the healthy vagina below and outside the nodule that will be resected. Two surgical approaches can be used:

- Recto-vaginal dissection and resection of the nodule: traditionally, gynecologists separate the posterior surface of the nodule from the anterior rectal wall. It is important to remember that the lower this dissection, the more anterior must be the application of the scissors in order to avoid rectal injury. Retraction caused by the endometriotic nodule displaces the involved rectum; therefore the axis of dissection is not always the same. The axis of dissection is directed anteriorly in the lowest part of the dissection. The goal is to continue the release of the nodule from the anterior rectal wall to identify the healthy vagina distal to the nodule. After the release of the posterior surface of the nodule from the rectal wall (lower and distal limits), it must be released from the posterior surface of the uterus, the base of the broad ligament and the vagina. The vaginal resection can be performed using scissors or a fine monopolar tip in pure cut mode.
- Reverse technique: the anterior surface of the nodule is first released from the posterior surface of the uterus and vagina (Figure 13). The mobility obtained after the release of the anterior aspect of the nodule allows for better exposure of it during dissection of the most difficult area to be treated, which is in contact with or near the rectum. When the nodule infiltrates the vagina, it is opened at the superior aspect and then laterally, in each side of the rectum, towards the disease-free zones that have already been dissected at the distal portion and around the nodule. The distal section is held in the disease-free rectovaginal plane, distal to the vaginal nodule (Figure 14). Then, the vagina is sutured and the nodule is pulled with a grasper to expose its posterior surface adhered to the anterior rectal wall (Figure 15). This approach though harder to conceive, seems to simplify and make the surgery more feasible. This bears out a basic surgical principle that says that exposure is the key to any surgery, which means that more difficult steps of the procedure must be executed with an even better exposure. However, to gynecologists this approach seems less logical because the more distressing step of the procedure (dissection of the nodule from the rectum) is the last to be performed.

Vaginal Suture Repair

The vaginal closure can be performed vaginally or laparoscopically. Performance of this step vaginally limits the amount of suture material that remains in the peritoneal cavity, reducing the risk of postoperative adhesions. Laparoscopic intra- or extracorporeal suturing is performed only for small vaginal openings and for patients who have a very narrow vagina.

Final Checklist

The intervention must end with a checklist that includes:

- Methylene blue test for assessment of tubal patency;
- Verification of hemostasis with and without uterine anteversion;
- Check the integrity of the rectum: 100ml of air injection into the rectum after placing 100ml of ringer lactate in the pelvis;
- Verification of peristalsis and color of the ureter (no blue or white zones);

- In the event of bleeding or visceral injury, it must be fixed immediately and completely; secondary treatment of complications is always infinitely more difficult and stressful than immediate treatment.

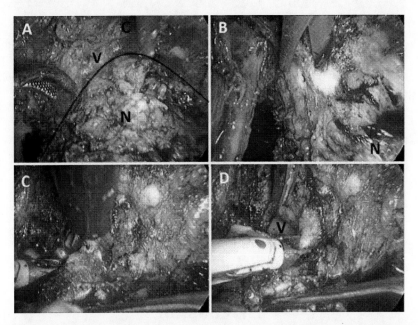

Figure 13. Separation of the endometriotic nodule (N) from the retrocervical area (C) and the posterior fornix of the vagina (V).

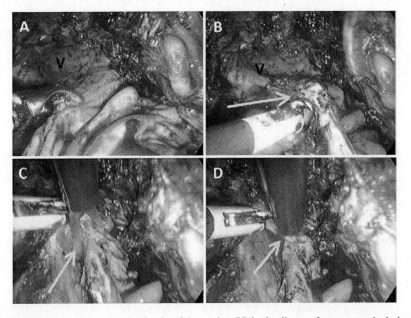

Figure 14. Distal section of the posterior fornix of the vagina (V) in the disease-free rectovaginal plane (yellow arrows).

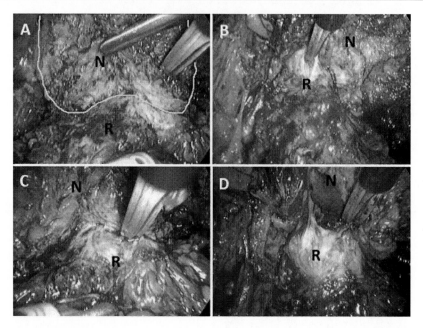

Figure 15. Separation of the endometriotic nodule (N; yellow line) from the anterior rectal wall (R).

Discussion

The effectiveness of surgical treatment for severe endometriosis in relieving pain symptoms was demonstrated in a prospective randomized study by Abbott et al. [20]. Other studies have confirmed the efficacy of surgery for treat deep infiltrating disease [16,49-51] but only few papers exist, that expresses in detail the technical methodology or approach to the lesion. In particular, the precise resection of gastrointestinal, vaginal opening and segmental ureteral resection are not fully described in the literature. There are some issues to be discussed at the end of this chapter such as:

- What is the significance of ovarian endometriomas and which is the current treatment of choice?
- Is it necessary to open the vagina for the resection of deep nodules of endometriosis?
- Should bowel resection be performed routinely? If not, when is it indicated?
- Should the ureter be treated by means of a ureteral resection?
- What is the role of reoperation in cases of recurrent deep endometriosis?

Ovarian Endometriosis

The presence of an ovarian endometrioma should normally cause the gynecologist to pay attention to the fact that there may be concomitant lesions of deep endometriosis. In 1999, Redwine [52] noted that superficial or deep ovarian endometriosis is a marker for the presence of extensive pelvic and intestinal disease. Surgeons diagnosing and treating only ovarian endometriosis may be underdiagnosing and undertreating their patients. Banerjee et al. [53] prospectively evaluated 295 women with histological confirmed diagnosis of endometriosis. Of the total, 61 (21%) had ovarian endometrioma. A higher proportion of women with ovarian endometrioma showed endometriotic disease affecting the intestine compared with women without endometrioma (77 vs. 21%, p <0.001). A strong relationship was observed between the presence of endometrioma and obliteration of the cul-de-sac, recto-sigmoid disease and involvement of the sero-muscular layer of the intestine. The presence of an endometrioma significantly increased the probability of having disease in the rectum-sigmoid, with a positive likelihood ratio of 6.96 (95% CI 4.04 to 12). However, the absence of endometrioma did not rule out the presence of disease in the recto-sigmoid, with a negative likelihood ratio of 0.55 (95% CI 0.45 to 0.67). The study by Chapron et al. [54] included 500 women with deep infiltrating endometriosis. In women with associated ovarian endometrioma, deep lesions of endometriosis were more severe with higher rates of vaginal, intestinal, and ureteral lesions.

The guidelines of the ESHRE (European Society of Human Reproduction and Embryology) [55] recommend that superficial ovarian lesions can be coagulated or vaporized. The primary surgical indication of an endometrioma is to determine that it is not a malignant lesion. Small endometriomas (less than 3cm) can be aspirated, irrigated and inspected internally to seek intra-cystic lesions. The lining of the cyst may be coagulated or vaporized to destroy the cells. Endometriomas larger than 3 cm should be preferably completely removed [56]. Saleh and Tulandi [57] retrospectively evaluated 231 women with endometriomas treated by laparoscopy and found that the cumulative rate of reoperation was higher after fenestration and destruction of the inner layer of the cyst compared with cystectomy. The rates of reintervention at 18 and 49 months were respectively 6.1% and 23.6% after cystectomy and 21.9% and 57.8% after fenestration, aspiration and destruction of the inner wall of the cyst.

Hayasaka et al. [58] evaluated 173 women (minimum of 1 year of follow-up) in an attempt to identify risk factors for recurrence and re-recurrence of endometriomas after first and second laparoscopic excision. The overall rate of recurrence and re-recurrence were 45.1% and 45.5%, respectively. A high revised American Society for Reproductive Medicine score (1997) [59] was associated with an increased risk of recurrence. Only postoperative pregnancy was associated with a decreased risk of recurrence. Short periods of normal menstruation without pregnancy or GnRH analogues between the first surgery and primary recurrence were associated with higher rates of re-recurrence.

Resection of the Posterior Vaginal Fornix

In those patients with a palpable lesion on digital vaginal examination, surgery is only complete when resection of the posterior fornix of the vagina is performed. According to the literature, resection of the posterior vaginal fornix for the treatment of infiltrative lesions is required in 20% to 100% of cases [30,39,60,61]. Complete surgical resection of deep endometriosis with excision of adjacent tissue of the posterior vaginal fornix improves quality of life with persistence of long-term results in patients who are unresponsive to non-surgical treatment [50].

A study conducted in Clermont-Ferrand[33] showed that in women with recto-vaginal endometriotic nodules larger than 2cm in diameter, the distance between the vaginal epithelium and endometriotic glands was <1mm in 49.2% of cases, <2mm in 70% and <5mm in 98.4% of cases, which provides histological evidence that resection of the posterior vaginal fornix is necessary to completely remove rectovaginal endometriotic nodules of large volume. Every time the lesion is visible in the vaginal fornix, whether in the form of a bluish cyst or a pseudo-polypoid appearance, vaginal resection of the entire thickness of the vaginal wall is essential. If the lesion is not visible but palpation shows an infiltration of the vaginal mucosa, it is necessary to resect the posterior vaginal fornix to achieve full treatment.

Treatment of Rectal Lesions

For lesions infiltrating the muscular layer of the rectum three technical options are available:

- Shaving (skinning): the aim is to find a healthy plane with no more active endometriotic lesions (Figures 21A and B and 24) within the muscle layer of the rectum, This procedure can be performed more or less deeply with a corresponding greater or lesser risk of opening the rectal lumen. Donnez et al. [60] suggested that this resection should avoid the risk of bowel perforation almost at all cost. For others, the resection must be complete, accepting the risk of opening the rectal lumen in a certain number of patients, instead of performing a segmental bowel resection routinely for such lesions [62].
- Disk Resection: consist of the resection of the anterior rectal wall. Two techniques can be applied: (1) resection with scissors followed by suture repair of the rectum, or (2) resection performed with a trans-anal circular stapler [63]. Most authors who use these methods state that they can only be applied in cases of lesions of moderate size.
- Segmental resection of the rectum (Figures 21C-F): allows the establishment of healthy tissue margins [61,62]; however, there is an increased short and long-term morbidity. For some, this procedure should be routine whenever there is muscular infiltration [61,64]. One of the important arguments in favor of this procedure is the certainty of complete treatment, since Remorgida showed that on histological examination of a bowel resection after rectal shaving, endometriotic lesions were found in a high percentage of cases [65].

All authors agree to perform a bowel resection when there is intestinal stenosis of more than 50% or cyclic rectal bleeding [66, 34]. All three approaches have inherent complications. In 2005, Mohr et al [35] described 187 women treated laparoscopically for intestinal endometriosis. The complete pain relief in the immediate postoperative period was significantly greater with segmental bowel resection compared with shaving alone (92 vs. 80%, respectively, p <0.04). Rectal shaving, the less invasive procedure, was associated with a higher rate of pregnancy and a lower complication rate: 6% compared with 23% for the disc resection (p <0.007) and 38% with bowel resection (p <0.001). In the experience of Clermont-Ferrand [30], the rate of major postoperative complications in women undergoing treatment for severe endometriosis that required some intestinal procedure was 9.3%. The postoperative complications occurred in 6.7% of women who underwent rectal shaving and 24% of women who underwent segmental bowel resection. In a prospective analysis of 500 cases of deep nodules of endometriosis treated by rectal shaving [67], major complications included seven cases of rectal perforation (1.4%), 4 cases of ureteral injury (0.8%), bleeding exceeding 300ml in one case (0.2%) and urinary retention in 4 cases (0.8%). Of the 388 women who wished to become pregnant, 221 (57%) became pregnant spontaneously and 107 through *in vitro* fertilization. In total, 328 women conceived (84%). The recurrence rate was 8% which was significantly lower ($p<0.05$) in women who became pregnant (3.6%) than in women who did not (15%). In the group of women who failed to conceive or who did not desire to become pregnant, the rate of severe pelvic pain recurrence was 16 to 20%.

Everything would have been simpler if the opening of the vagina were not so often necessary. Dehiscence of a rectal suture or a colorectal anastomosis in the presence of concomitant vaginal suture carries the risk of a very unpleasant and difficult to treat complication: recto-vaginal fistula. Most women with deep lesions affecting the bowel were of childbearing age and wished to become pregnant. Thus, postoperative intestinal complications can severely damage the reproductive future of these patients [68]. A prospective study with intention to treat is needed to elucidate the best technique and the precise indication for intestinal resection in cases of severe endometriosis.

A systematic review by De Cicco et al [69] of segmental bowel resection for endometriosis included 34 published articles and 1889 patients. The indications for resection were variable and rarely described accurately. The duration of surgery varied widely, and endometriosis was not confirmed in all cases in the pathologic examination. Recurrence of pain was reported in 45 of 189 women. Recurrence requiring reintervention occurred in 61 of 314 women. The recurrence of endometriosis was reported in 37 of 267 women. The authors concluded after the systematic review that the observed indication for performing segmental intestinal resection was poorly documented and that the data did not allow analysis of indications and results according to the location or the diameter of the endometriotic nodule.

An important situation arises in a woman who desires pregnancy but has a confirmed rectal endometriotic lesion is the presence of concomitant adenomyosis. The combined excision of pelvic endometriosis with bowel resection significantly improves chronic pelvic pain, dyspareunia and gastrointestinal symptoms; however, the presence of uterine adenomyosis can give rise to persistent dysmenorrhea [70]. In such cases we must consider whether or not treatment with radical resection with possible postoperative complications that may impair fertility is the best treatment option.

Treatment of the Ureter

Ureteral involvement is a serious complication that should be suspected in all cases of deep infiltrating endometriosis. Isolation and retroperitoneal laparoscopic inspection of both ureters help to diagnose silent ureteral involvement. Conservative laparoscopic surgery provides a safe and feasible modality for the management of ureteral endometriosis [71]. The study by Seracchioli et al. [71] included 30 women with endometriosis with ureteral involvement which was diagnosed by laparoscopy and confirmed by histology. Ureteral involvement was suspected preoperatively in only 40% of patients. The involvement of the left ureter occurred in 46.7%, right side in 26.7% and bilateral in 26.7%. There was associated endometriosis of the ipsilateral utero-sacral ligament in 100% of cases, the bladder in 50%, the rectovaginal septum in 80%, the ovaries in 53.3% and the intestine in 36.7%. Donnez et al. [72] demonstrated a high prevalence (11.2%) of ureteral stenosis in women with rectovaginal endometriotic nodule ≥3cm in diameter.

Patients with endometriosis and moderate to severe ureteral dilatation may require concomitant procedures for resection of endometriosis, including ureterolysis, uretero-ureterostomy, ureterocystoneostomy, or nephrectomy [37,73]. In instances where the ureter is released by means of a simple ureterolysis, and there is no modification of the caliber of the ureter or no dilation of the urinary tract proximal to the operated area, no additional action is required. On the other hand, if after ureterolysis there exists a permanent stenosis of the ureter or discovery of a cystic lesion in the wall of the ureter, ureteral segmental resection is required. The question of whether there should be a systematic reimplantation or an end-to-end anastomosis after ureteral resection, depends primarily on technical considerations and in particular the extent of the resected area. In the event that there is a dilation of the urinary tract, the indications for ureteral resection should be extended even when the ureterolysis appears to have occurred in good conditions.

Indications for Reintervention

The best available evidence on the role of reoperation for the treatment of symptomatic recurrent endometriosis was revised to define the results of conservative repetitive surgery, the effects of pelvic denervation procedures and postoperative clinical treatments, and the long-term results of definitive surgery. Based on the limited information available, the long-term results appear to be suboptimal, with a cumulative probability of recurrence of pain between 20 and 40%, and the need for an additional surgical procedure between 15 and 20%. The results of hysterectomy for pain associated with endometriosis in a medium-term follow-up looked good. However, approximately 15% of patients had persistent symptoms and 3 to 5% had worsening of pain. The performance of concomitant bilateral oophorectomy resulted in a sixfold reduction of the risk of reoperation for recurrent pelvic pain. However, at least one gonad should ideally be preserved in young women, especially in those with objections to the use of estrogen-progestin replacement. The risk of recurrence of endometriosis during hormone replacement therapy seems to be marginal when combined preparations or tibolone are used; unopposed estrogen treatments should be avoided [74].

References

[1]   Darai E, Thomassin I, Barranger E, Detchev R, Cortez A, Houry S, Bazot M. Feasibility and clinical outcome of laparoscopic colorectal resection for endometriosis. *Am. J. Obstet. Gynecol.* 2005;192(2):394-400.

[2]   Pritts EA, Taylor RN. An evidence-based evaluation of endometriosis-associated infertility. *Endocrinol. Metab. Clin. North Am.* 2003;32(3):653-67.

[3]   Koninckx PR, Martin D. Treatment of deeply infiltrating endometriosis. *Curr. Opin. Obstet. Gynecol.* 1994;6(3):231-41.

[4]   Nisolle M, Donnez J. Peritoneal endometriosis, ovarian endometriosis, and adenomyotic nodules of the rectovaginal septum are three different entities. *Fertil. Steril.* 1997;68(4):585-96.

[5]   Eskenazi B, Warner ML. Epidemiology of endometriosis. *Obstet. Gynecol. Clin. North Am.* 1997;24(2):235-58.

[6]   Carter JE. Combined hysteroscopic and laparoscopic findings in patients with chronic pelvic pain. *J. Am. Assoc. Gynecol. Laparosc.* 1994;2(1):43-7.

[7]   Laufer MR, Goitein L, Bush M, Cramer DW, Emans SJ. Prevalence of endometriosis in adolescent girls with chronic pelvic pain not responding to conventional therapy. *J. Pediatr. Adolesc. Gynecol.* 1997;10(4):199-202.

[8]   Strathy JH, Molgaard CA, Coulam CB, Melton LJ 3rd. Endometriosis and infertility: a laparoscopic study of endometriosis among fertile and infertile women. *Fertil. Steril.* 1982;38(6):667-72.

[9]   Mahmood TA, Templeton A. Prevalence and genesis of endometriosis. *Hum. Reprod.* 1991;6(4):544-9.

[10]   Kondo W, Ferriani RA, Petta CA, Abrão MS, Amaral VF. Endometriose e infertilidade: causa ou conseqüência? *JBRA - Jornal Brasileiro de Reprodução Assistida.* 2009;13(2):33-8.

[11]   Catenacci M, Sastry S, Falcone T. Laparoscopic surgery for endometriosis. *Clin. Obstet. Gynecol.* 2009;52(3):351-61.

[12]   Fauconnier A, Chapron C. Endometriosis and pelvic pain: epidemiological evidence of the relationship and implications. *Hum. Reprod. Update.* 2005;11(6):595-606.

[13]   Kwok A, Lam A, Ford R. Deeply infiltrating endometriosis: implications, diagnosis, and management. *Obstet. Gynecol. Surv.* 2001;56(3):168-77.

[14]   Cornillie FJ, Oosterlynck D, Lauweryns JM, Koninckx PR. Deeply infiltrating pelvic endometriosis: histology and clinical significance. *Fertil. Steril.* 1990;53(6):978-83.

[15]   Ripps BA, Martin DC. Correlation of focal pelvic tenderness with implant dimension and stage of endometriosis. *J. Reprod. Med.* 1992;37(7):620-4.

[16]   Anaf V, Simon P, El Nakadi I, Fayt I, Simonart T, Buxant F, Noel JC. Hyperalgesia, nerve infiltration and nerve growth factor expression in deep adenomyotic nodules, peritoneal and ovarian endometriosis. *Hum. Reprod.* 2002;17(7):1895-900.

[17]   Tamburro S, Canis M, Albuisson E, Dechelotte P, Darcha C, Mage G. Expression of transforming growth factor beta1 in nerve fibers is related to dysmenorrhea and laparoscopic appearance of endometriotic implants. *Fertil. Steril.* 2003;80(5):1131-6.

[18]   Anaf V, Simon P, El Nakadi I, Fayt I, Buxant F, Simonart T, Peny MO, Noel JC. Relationship between endometriotic foci and nerves in rectovaginal endometriotic nodules. *Hum. Reprod.* 2000;15(8):1744-50.

[19]   Sutton CJ, Ewen SP, Whitelaw N, Haines P. Prospective, randomized, double-blind, controlled trial of laser laparoscopy in the treatment of pelvic pain associated with minimal, mild, and moderate endometriosis. *Fertil. Steril.* 1994;62(4):696-700.

[20]   Abbott J, Hawe J, Hunter D, Holmes M, Finn P, Garry R. Laparoscopic excision of endometriosis: a randomized, placebo-controlled trial. *Fertil. Steril.* 2004;82(4):878-84.

[21]   Chapron C, Fauconnier A, Vieira M, Barakat H, Dousset B, Pansini V, Vacher-Lavenu MC, Dubuisson JB. Anatomical distribution of deeply infiltrating endometriosis:

surgical implications and proposition for a classification. *Hum. Reprod.* 2003;18(1):157-61.

[22] Vercellini P, Trespidi L, De Giorgi O, Cortesi I, Parazzini F, Crosignani PG. Endometriosis and pelvic pain: relation to disease stage and localization. *Fertil. Steril.* 1996;65(2):299-304.

[23] Porpora MG, Koninckx PR, Piazze J, Natili M, Colagrande S, Cosmi EV. Correlation between endometriosis and pelvic pain. *J. Am. Assoc. Gynecol. Laparosc.* 1999;6(4):429-34.

[24] Gruppo Italiano per lo Studio dell'Endometriosi. Relationship between stage, site and morphological characteristics of pelvic endometriosis and pain. *Hum. Reprod.* 2001;16(12):2668-71.

[25] Chapron C, Barakat H, Fritel X, Dubuisson JB, Bréart G, Fauconnier A. Presurgical diagnosis of posterior deep infiltrating endometriosis based on a standardized questionnaire. *Hum. Reprod.* 2005;20(2):507-13.

[26] Fauconnier A, Chapron C, Dubuisson JB, Vieira M, Dousset B, Bréart G. Relation between pain symptoms and the anatomic location of deep infiltrating endometriosis. *Fertil. Steril.* 2002;78(4):719-26.

[27] Redwine DB. Laparoscopic en bloc resection for treatment of the obliterated cul-de-sac in endometriosis. *J. Reprod. Med.* 1992;37(8):695-8.

[28] Garry R, Clayton R, Hawe J. The effect of endometriosis and its radical laparoscopic excision on quality of life indicators. *BJOG.* 2000;107(1):44-54.

[29] Kondo W, Bourdel N, Jardon K, Tamburro S, Cavoli D, Matsuzaki S, Botchorishvili R, Rabischong B, Pouly JL, Mage G, Canis M. Comparison between standard and reverse laparoscopic techniques for rectovaginal endometriosis. *Surg. Endosc.* 2011; *in press.*

[30] Kondo W, Bourdel N, Tamburro S, Cavoli D, Jardon K, Rabischong B, Botchorishvili R, Pouly J, Mage G, Canis M. Complications after surgery for deeply infiltrating pelvic endometriosis. *BJOG.* 2011;118(3):292-8.

[31] Chapron C, Dubuisson JB, Fritel X, Fernandez B, Poncelet C, Béguin S, Pinelli L. Operative management of deep endometriosis infiltrating the uterosacral ligaments. *J. Am. Assoc. Gynecol. Laparosc.* 1999;6(1):31-7.

[32] Donnez J, Nisolle M. Advanced laparoscopic surgery for the removal of rectovaginal septum endometriotic or adenomyotic nodules. *Baillieres Clin. Obstet. Gynaecol.* 1995;9(4):769-74.

[33] Matsuzaki S, Houlle C, Botchorishvili R, Pouly JL, Mage G, Canis M. Excision of the posterior vaginal fornix is necessary to ensure complete resection of rectovaginal endometriotic nodules of more than 2 cm in size. *Fertil. Steril.* 2009;91(4 Suppl):1314-5.

[34] Canis M, Botchorishvili R, Slim K, Pezet D, Pouly JL, Wattiez A, Pomel C, Masson FN, Mage G, Chipponi J, Bruhat MA. Bowel endometriosis. Eight cases of colorectal resection. *J. Gynecol. Obstet. Biol. Reprod.* (Paris). 1996;25(7):699-709.

[35] Mohr C, Nezhat FR, Nezhat CH, Seidman DS, Nezhat CR. Fertility considerations in laparoscopic treatment of infiltrative bowel endometriosis. *JSLS.* 2005;9(1):16-24.

[36] Chapron C, Dubuisson JB. Laparoscopic management of bladder endometriosis. *Acta Obstet. Gynecol. Scand.* 1999;78(10):887-90.

[37] Ghezzi F, Cromi A, Bergamini V, Bolis P. Management of ureteral endometriosis: areas of controversy. *Curr. Opin. Obstet. Gynecol.* 2007;19(4):319-24.

[38] Canis M. Endometriosis is a simple disease! *J. Gynecol. Obstet. Biol. Reprod.* (Paris). 2007;36(2):106-7.

[39] Koninckx PR, Timmermans B, Meuleman C, Penninckx F. Complications of CO2-laser endoscopic excision of deep endometriosis. *Hum. Reprod.* 1996;11(10):2263-8.

[40] Varol N, Maher P, Healey M, Woods R, Wood C, Hill D, Lolatgis N, Tsaltas J. Rectal surgery for endometriosis - should we be aggressive? *J. Am. Assoc. Gynecol. Laparosc.* 2003;10(2):182-9.

[41] Golfier F, Sabra M. Surgical management of endometriosis. *J. Gynecol. Obstet. Biol. Reprod.* (Paris). 2007;36(2):162-72.

[42] Panel P, Renouvel F. Management of endometriosis: clinical and biological assessment. *J. Gynecol. Obstet. Biol. Reprod.* (Paris). 2007;36(2):119-28.

[43] Mihalyi A, Gevaert O, Kyama CM, Simsa P, Pochet N, De Smet F, De Moor B, Meuleman C, Billen J, Blanckaert N, Vodolazkaia A, Fulop V, D'Hooghe TM. Non-invasive diagnosis of endometriosis based on a combined analysis of six plasma biomarkers. *Hum. Reprod.* 2010;25(3):654-64.

[44] Kafali H, Artuc H, Demir N. Use of CA125 fluctuation during the menstrual cycle as a tool in the clinical diagnosis of endometriosis; a preliminary report. *Eur. J. Obstet. Gynecol. Reprod. Biol.* 2004;116(1):85-8.

[45] Abrao MS, Gonçalves MO, Dias JA Jr, Podgaec S, Chamie LP, Blasbalg R. Comparison between clinical examination, transvaginal sonography and magnetic resonance imaging for the diagnosis of deep endometriosis. *Hum. Reprod.* 2007;22(12):3092-7.

[46] Bazot M, Lafont C, Rouzier R, Roseau G, Thomassin-Naggara I, Daraï E. Diagnostic accuracy of physical examination, transvaginal sonography, rectal endoscopic sonography, and magnetic resonance imaging to diagnose deep infiltrating endometriosis. *Fertil. Steril.* 2009;92(6):1825-33.

[47] Takeuchi H, Kuwatsuru R, Kitade M, Sakurai A, Kikuchi I, Shimanuki H, Kinoshita K. A novel technique using magnetic resonance imaging jelly for evaluation of rectovaginal endometriosis. *Fertil. Steril.* 2005;83(2):442-7.

[48] Chassang M, Novellas S, Bloch-Marcotte C, Delotte J, Toullalan O, Bongain A, Chevallier P. Utility of vaginal and rectal contrast medium in MRI for the detection of deep pelvic endometriosis. *Eur. Radiol.* 2010;20(4):1003-10.

[49] Chopin N, Vieira M, Borghese B, Foulot H, Dousset B, Coste J, Mignon A, Fauconnier A, Chapron C. Operative management of deeply infiltrating endometriosis: results on pelvic pain symptoms according to a surgical classification. *J. Minim. Invasive Gynecol.* 2005;12(2):106-12.

[50] Angioni S, Peiretti M, Zirone M, Palomba M, Mais V, Gomel V, Melis GB. Laparoscopic excision of posterior vaginal fornix in the treatment of patients with deep endometriosis without rectum involvement: surgical treatment and long-term follow-up. *Hum. Reprod.* 2006;21(6):1629-34.

[51] Dubernard G, Rouzier R, David-Montefiore E, Bazot M, Darai E. Use of the SF-36 questionnaire to predict quality-of-life improvement after laparoscopic colorectal resection for endometriosis. *Hum. Reprod.* 2008;23(4):846-51.

[52] Redwine DB. Ovarian endometriosis: a marker for more extensive pelvic and intestinal disease. *Fertil. Steril.* 1999;72(2):310-5.

[53] Banerjee SK, Ballard KD, Wright JT. Endometriomas as a marker of disease severity. *J. Minim. Invasive Gynecol.* 2008;15(5):538-40.

[54] Chapron C, Pietin-Vialle C, Borghese B, Davy C, Foulot H, Chopin N. Associated ovarian endometrioma is a marker for greater severity of deeply infiltrating endometriosis. *Fertil. Steril.* 2009;92(2):453-7.

[55] Kennedy S, Bergqvist A, Chapron C, D'Hooghe T, Dunselman G, Greb R, Hummelshoj L, Prentice A, Saridogan E; ESHRE Special Interest Group for Endometriosis and Endometrium Guideline Development Group. ESHRE guideline for the diagnosis and treatment of endometriosis. *Hum. Reprod.* 2005;20(10):2698-704.

[56] Chapron C, Vercellini P, Barakat H, Vieira M, Dubuisson JB. Management of ovarian endometriomas. *Hum. Reprod. Update.* 2002;8(6):591-7.

[57] Saleh A, Tulandi T. Reoperation after laparoscopic treatment of ovarian endometriomas by excision and by fenestration. *Fertil. Steril.* 1999;72(2):322-4.

[58] Hayasaka S, Ugajin T, Fujii O, Nabeshima H, Utsunomiya H, Yokomizo R, Yuki H, Terada Y, Murakami T, Yaegashi N. Risk factors for recurrence and re-recurrence of ovarian endometriomas after laparoscopic excision. *J. Obstet. Gynaecol. Res.* 2010; *in press.*

[59] American Society for Reproductive Medicine. Revised American Society for Reproductive Medicine classification of endometriosis: 1996. *Fertil. Steril.* 1997;67(5):817-21.

[60] Donnez J, Nisolle M, Gillerot S, Smets M, Bassil S, Casanas-Roux F. Rectovaginal septum adenomyotic nodules: a series of 500 cases. *Br. J. Obstet. Gynaecol.* 1997;104(9):1014-8.

[61] Darai E, Ackerman G, Bazot M, Rouzier R, Dubernard G. Laparoscopic segmental colorectal resection for endometriosis: limits and complications. *Surg. Endosc.* 2007;21(9):1572-7.

[62] Leconte M, Chapron C, Dousset B. Surgical treatment of rectal endometriosis. *J. Chir.* (Paris). 2007;144(1):5-10.

[63] Woods RJ, Heriot AG, Chen FC. Anterior rectal wall excision for endometriosis using the circular stapler. *ANZ J. Surg.* 2003;73(8):647-8.

[64] Keckstein J, Wiesinger H. Deep endometriosis, including intestinal involvement--the interdisciplinary approach. *Minim. Invasive Ther. Allied Technol.* 2005;14(3):160-6.

[65] Remorgida V, Ragni N, Ferrero S, Anserini P, Torelli P, Fulcheri E. How complete is full thickness disc resection of bowel endometriotic lesions? A prospective surgical and histological study. *Hum. Reprod.* 2005;20(8):2317-20.

[66] Abrão MS, Podgaec S, Dias JA Jr, Averbach M, Silva LF, Marino de Carvalho F. Endometriosis lesions that compromise the rectum deeper than the inner muscularis layer have more than 40% of the circumference of the rectum affected by the disease. *J. Minim. Invasive Gynecol.* 2008;15(3):280-5.

[67] Donnez J, Squifflet J. Complications, pregnancy and recurrence in a prospective series of 500 patients operated on by the shaving technique for deep rectovaginal endometriotic nodules. *Hum. Reprod.* 2010;25(8):1949-58.

[68] Kondo W, Daraï E, Yazbeck C, Panel P, Tamburro S, Dubuisson J, Jardon K, Mage G, Madelenat P, Canis M. Do patients manage to achieve pregnancy after a major complication of deeply infiltrating endometriosis resection? *Eur. J. Obstet. Gynecol. Reprod. Biol.* 2011;154(2):196-9.

[69] De Cicco C, Corona R, Schonman R, Mailova K, Ussia A, Koninckx P. Bowel resection for deep endometriosis: a systematic review. *BJOG*. 2011;118(3):285-91.

[70] Ferrero S, Camerini G, Menada MV, Biscaldi E, Ragni N, Remorgida V. Uterine adenomyosis in persistence of dysmenorrhea after surgical excision of pelvic endometriosis and colorectal resection. *J. Reprod. Med.* 2009;54(6):366-72.

[71] Seracchioli R, Mabrouk M, Manuzzi L, Guerrini M, Villa G, Montanari G, et al. Importance of retroperitoneal ureteric evaluation in cases of deep infiltrating endometriosis. *J. Minim. Invasive Gynecol.* 2008;15(4):435-9.

[72] Donnez J, Nisolle M, Squifflet J. Ureteral endometriosis: a complication of rectovaginal endometriotic (adenomyotic) nodules. *Fertil. Steril.* 2002;77(1):32-7.

[73] Mereu L, Gagliardi ML, Clarizia R, Mainardi P, Landi S, Minelli L. Laparoscopic management of ureteral endometriosis in case of moderate-severe hydroureteronephrosis. *Fertil. Steril.* 2010;93(1):46-51.

[74] Vercellini P, Barbara G, Abbiati A, Somigliana E, Viganò P, Fedele L. Repetitive surgery for recurrent symptomatic endometriosis: what to do? *Eur. J. Obstet. Gynecol. Reprod. Biol.* 2009;146(1):15-21.

In: Laparoscopy: New Developments, Procedures and Risks   ISBN: 978-1-61470-747-9
Editor: Hana Terzic, pp. 141-164   © 2012 Nova Science Publishers, Inc.

Chapter VI

Laparoscopic Trainers and Surgical Virtual Simulators in Laparoscopic Learning Curve

Andrea Tinelli[*1]*, Lucio De Paolis*[2]*,*
Giovanni Aloisio[3]*, Giorgio De Nunzio*[4]*, Mario Bochicchio*[5]*,*
Ivan De Mitri [6] *and Antonio Malvasi*[7]

[1] Department of Obstetrics and Gynecology, Vito Fazzi Hospital, Lecce, Italy.
[2] Department of Innovation Engineering, University of Salento, Lecce, Italy.
[3] Information Processing Systems, Department of Innovation Engineering,
University of Salento, Lecce, Italy.
[4] Department of Materials Science, University of Salento, and INFN, Lecce, Italy.
[5] SET-Lab, Department of Innovation Engineering, University of Lecce, Italy.
[6] Department of Physics, University of Salento, and INFN, Lecce, Italy.
[7] Department of Obstetrics and Gynaecology, Santa Maria Hospital, Bari, Italy.

Abstract

This chapter fouses on the utilization of laparoscopic trainers and surgical virtual simulators, who provide deliberate practice, training, and assessment in a safe environment. Simulators range from simple task trainers to high-fidelity mock operating rooms, from organic to inorganic models. With the advent of laparoscopic surgery technical challenges raised, as altered depth perception, reduced tactile feedback, and the fulcrum effect. Thus surgical operations required a sophisticated level of practice, more than in open surgery. The laparoscopic box trainer was an early spark in the proliferation of depth and breadth in surgical skills training, now driven by forces including work-hour

* Dr. Andrea Tinelli, MD, Department of Obstetrics and Gynecology, Division of Experimental Endoscopic Surgery, Imaging, and Minimally Invasive Therapy and Technology., Vito Fazzi Hospital, Piazza Muratore, 73100 Lecce, Italy, Tel.: +39/339/2074078, Fax: +39/0832/661511, E-mail: andreatinelli@gmail.com

restrictions, patient safety concerns, financial cost of training, and emerging technology. Another help in surgical skills come from virtual reality, a computer simulation that enables users to perform operations on the system and shows effects in real time. Computerized simulators allow instant score reporting, feedback, and automated tutoring. Instruments' expensive cost is a major downside, but they really help young and skilled surgeons to trainee their daily work.

Introduction

The practical problems faced in abdominal surgery are the difficult management of hospital structures, the insufficient paramedical training and the insufficient hygiene, the lack of appropriate medication and the overcrowding of the wards by patients' relatives who are in charge of food supply to the patient; these problems are the direct cause of a high infection rate, hence longer hospital stay and unnecessary drainage of the already depleted means of care.

To overpass these problems, the industries, some years ago, discovered Minimally Invasive Surgery (MIS), such as surgical endoscopy and laparoscopy.

Usually, the advantages of laparoscopic surgery are: reduced infection risk thanks to the absence of large incisions, reduced patient immobilization, hence shorter hospital stay for the patient and his relatives, which is of the utmost importance in a system where social coverage does not exist, and a readily available diagnostic tool, advantageously replacing more expensive equipment as Computer Tomography scan and Magnetic Resonance. Laparoscopic simulators could already reproduce a female abdominal wall with the classical trocar position for a gynaecological laparoscopy (Figure 1).

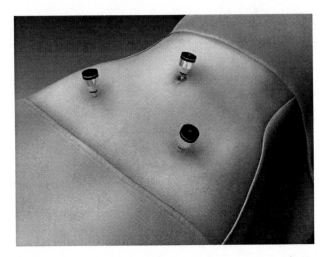

Figure 1. A simulated female abdominal wall with the trocar position for a gynaecological laparoscopy.

Nevertheless, actually, the theoretical disadvantages of laparoscopy are: the relative technical sophistication of the technique (maintenance problems) and the expensive cost of the equipment.

The only weak link in the chain are the relatively sophisticated insufflator and video camera, which constitute the only and absolute priority in the laparoscopic surgeon armamentarium; taking care of these instruments however is less time consuming for a surgeon than the alternatives (supervising administration, nursing care and long stays).

The practical application areas of laparoscopy are: abdominal emergencies (in case of traumatic acute abdomen, laparoscopy permits a quick diagnosis of visceral damage), second look (easily performed in patients with a rapidly degrading condition), infection diagnosis and treatment (in the case of peritonitis, laparoscopy can determine or confirm the source of the infection as well as its localization).

Pathology treatment can then be undertaken either laparoscopically (e.g. in appendicitis, ectopic pregnancy, perforated ulcer) or conventionally, but via a well-defined incision, right across from the target organ as diagnosed laparoscopically.

Laparoscopy is useful in functional gastric surgery (Figure 2): ulcer disease, cholecystectomy and gastro-oesophageal reflux can thus be cured at low cost (as compared with a lifelong drug treatment in a poorly complying population); also, the surgical procedure (application of the fundus, vagotomy) is relatively benign since no organectomy or organotomy is performed.

The morbidity of the open procedure lies in the way of access (long laparotomy incision, long retraction), which is much more advantageous in the laparoscopic procedure and the surgical treatment of infectious and parasitic disease (echinococcal cyst, deeply located abscesses) is corrected by laparoscopy.

In so many Gynecologic and Obstetric Departments, doctors contemporarily utilized traditional surgery and minimally invasive surgery, although in rapid changeover of the relationship in favour of endoscopy; it has been interesting to note that, during the post-operative period, patients often wonder and ask a series of embarrassing questions regarding the significant difference between the two post-operative recoveries.

In fact, patients who have undergone a traditional intervention start to eat on the second or third post-operative day, while those operated with minimally invasive techniques have already been, or are about to be, discharged.

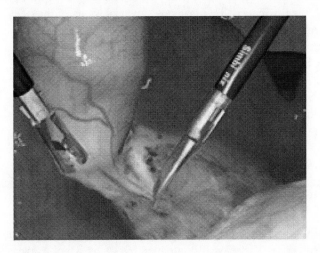

Figure 2. A simulated cholecystectomy.

Finally, by these key points, the minimally invasive surgery presents, on the contrary, the following advantages: less pain, earlier mobilization, the possibility of eating immediately, earlier autonomy, not using analgesics reduces the general lethargic effect of surgery and, particularly, the consequences on the intestine, general feeling of well-being leads the patient to desire to return soon to normal standards of life. The abdominal accesses for the passage of laparoscopic tools are incisions smaller than 1 centimetre (1 suture is sufficient) and they may reach 5 in the most difficult and serious cases. Once healed, these small wounds are almost invisible and, therefore, visible scarring is avoided, reduced trauma to the abdominal wall and neighbouring tissues reduces long-term sequelae (adhesions, cicatritial sclerosis, etc.), the hospitalization period is significantly less, varying between one day in day-hospital and a maximum of 3 days for the most serious cases, normal activity can be resumed after 1-2 weeks.

The Simulation in MIS

In recent years the latest technological developments in medical imaging acquisition and computer systems have permitted physicians to perform more sophisticated as well as less invasive treatments of patients.

One trend in surgery is the transition from open procedures to minimally invasive laparoscopic interventions, where visual feedback to the surgeon is only available through the laparoscope camera and direct palpation of organs is not possible.

In traditional open surgery, surgeons often have to cut through many layers of healthy tissue to reach the target of interest, thereby inflicting significant damage on the tissue. This is very traumatic for the patient.

In the last 15 years the MIS, such as laparoscopy or endoscopy, has become very important and the research in this field is ever more widely accepted because these techniques provide surgeons with less invasive means of reaching the patient's internal anatomy and allow entire procedures to be performed with only minimal trauma to the patient [1].

The diseased area is reached by means of small incisions in the body, called ports, and specific instruments are used to gain access to the operation area. The surgical instruments are inserted through the ports using trocars and a camera is also inserted. During the operation a monitor shows what is happening inside the body. This is very different to what happens in open surgery, where there is full visual and touch access to the organ.

The idea of MIS is to reduce the trauma for the patient by minimizing the incisions and the tissue retraction. Since the incision is kept as small as possible, the surgeon does not have direct vision and is thus guided by camera images. As a promising technique, the practice of MIS is becoming more and more widespread and is being adopted as an alternative to the classical procedure.

The advantages of the use of this surgical method are evident for the patients because the possible trauma is reduced, the postoperative recovery is nearly always faster and scarring is reduced.

Despite the improvement in outcomes, these techniques have their limitations and come at a cost to the surgeons. The view of the patient's organs is not as clear and the ability to manipulate the instruments is diminished in comparison with traditional open surgery. The indirect access to the operation area causes restricted vision, difficulty in hand-eye coordination, limited mobility in handling instruments and two-dimensional imagery with a lack of detailed information and a limited field of view during the whole operation. In particular, the lack of depth in perception and the difficulty in estimating the distance of the specific structures in laparoscopic surgery can impose limits on delicate dissection or suturing.

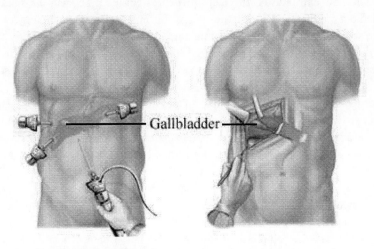

Figure 3. Cholecystectomy in laparoscopic and open surgery.

This situation, where eye-hand co-ordination is not based on direct vision, but more predominantly on image guidance via endoscopes (Figure 3), requires a different approach to conventional surgical procedures. On the other hand, the quality of medical images and the speed with which they can be obtained, the increasing ability to produce 3-dimensional models and the advanced developments in Virtual Reality technology make it possible to localize the pathology accurately, to see the anatomic relationships like never before and to practice new methods such as surgical navigation or image-guided surgery.

The outcome of a surgical procedure is closely related to the skills of the surgeon; these skills are being developed by means of the previous training on animals, cadavers, and patients. In many countries, due to ethical reasons, some methods are becoming increasingly unpopular and new and alternative ways of performing surgical training are required for the surgeons to remain at a high level of technical skills and for surgical trainees to reach such a high level. Although learning by apprenticeship in the operating room (OR) under the supervision of experienced mentors has benefits, it has major disadvantages as well because there are potential risks to the patient.

Given that a large part of the difficulties involved in MIS are related to perceptual disadvantages, many research groups are now focusing on the development of surgical assistance systems, motivated by the benefits MIS can bring to patients. Advances in technology are making it more and more possible to develop systems that can help surgeons to perform training in a realistic environment and without risks for the patient.

For more than a decade, advancing computer technologies have allowed incorporation of Virtual Reality (VR) into surgical training. This has become especially important in training for laparoscopic procedures where a valid VR-assisted surgery simulator could minimize the steep learning curve associated with many of these complex procedures and thus enable better outcomes.

The training on virtual patients met the growing need for training in MIS; many minimally invasive procedures need to be learned by repetition. Virtual simulators provide a new method for apprenticeship which can reduce the length of training repeating procedures as many times as needed, without the need for supervision and without hurting the patient.

In addition, new and unusual surgical procedures can be practiced, the same procedure can be carried out on different case studies that differ in terms of the pathology or anatomical structure and some complications can be simulated in a safe manner.

Many research groups have recognized the potential of virtual environments and developed surgical applications focused on real-time methods for simulating the physical behaviour of deformable tissue.

A surgery simulator requires modelling of deformations, cutting in tissue, and also the ability to calculate a force feedback sensation. The most critical issues in designing surgical simulators are accuracy - the simulator should generate visual and haptic sensations very close to reality - and efficiency - deformations must be rendered in real-time. Accuracy and efficiency are two opposite requirements; in fact, increased accuracy implies higher computational time and vice versa. So, it is necessary to find a trade-off according to the application. However, substantial differences between the real and the virtual deformations may lead to a wrong learning of the procedure [2].

Another major research emphasis in surgical simulation has been in the development of realistic haptic devices; haptic sensation is important in the performance of many surgical skills and in the learning of surgical procedures in laparoscopy, endoscopy, catheter navigation and epidural anesthesia.

Because of the growing acceptance of simulators for surgical training and the promoting choice of these systems over animal and cadaver use, the market for virtual reality surgical systems is estimated to increase due to their acquisition by medical centres and teaching hospitals.

The utilisation of surgical computer simulations allows repeatedly exploring the structures of interest and viewing them from almost any perspective. This is obviously impossible with real patients, and is economically infeasible with cadavers that, in any case, have already lost many of the important characteristics of live tissue. Animal experiments are expensive, and of course the anatomy is different.

The advantage is that it provides safe controlled medical environment to practise and to plan surgical procedures reducing the costs of education; different scenarios can be built in the simulator to provide a wide experience that can be repeated as needed. Training can be done anytime and anywhere the equipment is available. Training systems make possible the reduction of operative risks associated with the use of new techniques, reducing surgical mortality.

However, the big challenge is to simulate with sufficient fidelity so as to minimise the difference between performing the surgical operation with the simulator and on real patients. Since all of the human organs are not rigid, their shape can change during the interaction. For this reason the realism of the deformation is very important in surgery simulation. Most of the existing training simulations are for applications, where there are no large deformations and mostly concern manipulation of hard objects. For other applications, deformable models are required to build realistic and efficient simulations. For this reason it is necessary the use of force feedback, modelling of soft tissue and real-time response to user's action [3].

Visual realism and real-time interactions are essential in surgery simulation. Real-time interaction requires that each action of the user generate an instantaneous response in the virtual environment, whatever the complexity of its geometry.

The realism can be enhanced using a device that allows integrating the force feedback sensations in order to provide the surgeon with forces as close as possible to reality [4].

Sometimes it is very important to have images obtained from the actual patient, since life-critical decisions are based on the presentation of patient data.

Requirements of a Virtual Surgical Simulator

In order to transfer surgical skills it is necessary to provide a realistic interactive environment that reflects real life procedures. The simulated model needs to be a flexible representation of the system that can be interactively manipulated by the user.

The increasing computational power, as well as the achievements in the field of interactive computer graphics, Virtual Reality and robotics technologies and the advanced medical image acquisition methods, have already led to the rapid development of sophisticated surgical simulators. These systems incorporate realistic graphics and the sense of touch and offer an interesting way to provide adequate training without any risks for the patient.

The utilisation of surgical training devices combined with a computer simulation allows avoiding the problems of in vivo practice or the use of animal models. The advantage of using a virtual reality simulator is that it provides a safe controlled medical environment to practise and to prepare procedures; different scenarios can be build in the simulator to provide a wide experience that can be repeated as needed.

Ideal surgical simulations and training systems demand:

- realistic virtual environments;
- physical modelling of deformable tissues;
- real-time tissue-tool interactions;
- force feedback provided to the operator;
- visual feedback;
- integration of all components in a real-time system.

For this reason, a realistic simulation combines a visualization system, where a representation of the real environment is reproduced, and a haptic device that provides a force feedback to the user during the interaction in the virtual environment.

The haptic sensation could be an essential component of the procedure. The information flow forms a closed loop: the motion of the medical instruments is reproduced in the virtual environment, contact forces are computed and the loop is closed by generating these forces on the surgeon's hand by means of the haptic interface.

The realism of the interactions can be enhanced using specific haptic interfaces that provide force feedback sensations as close as possible to reality, but also computations performed in real-time are required. Only by obtaining a realistic representation of the anatomy, a fair force feedback and real-time tissue-tools interaction the training experience can be considered useful and provide a rapid learning curve.

To obtain a realistic simulation the main difficulty is related to the real-time constraint that imposes a very high frequency in force computing. The realism of the sensation of force is highly dependent on the physical realism of the model. The modelling of the virtual environment involves a geometrical description of the organs, their behaviour and their interactions with the medical instruments. In many surgical procedures the organs are soft tissues, their shape may change during operation; for this reason physical modelling of the organs is necessary to render their behaviour under the influence of surgeon's instruments.

Physical modelling gives the constitutive equations that describe the mechanical properties of the real body. The two main constraints for the modelling of soft tissues are deformation accuracy and computational time. For surgery procedure training, computational time is more important than the accuracy of deformation in order to achieve smooth user interaction. The desired realism of the physical models must be balanced against the need for speed.

The real-time deformation of soft tissue is an important constraint for medical simulators. Delay between user action and environment reaction disturbs the perception of correct interaction in the virtual environment and reduces the immersion sensation.

There are several causes contributing to latency: communication between the haptic interface and the virtual environment, computation time for collision detection, force feedback and deformation; the total latency is not the sum of those delays because many elements are asynchronous. The latency depends greatly on the hardware used and it is important to reduce it to its minimum value.

The ability of the operator to learn from a computer-simulated system is directly connected to the bandwidth of the system; an acceptable bandwidth for visual feedback is in the range of 20-60 Hz, while an acceptable bandwidth for haptic feedback is in the range of 500-1000 Hz [5].

To build a surgical simulator it is necessary to model the anatomy of the organs in an accurate and realistic way. The modelling of the virtual environment involves geometrical description of the virtual objects, their behaviour and their interactions in the virtual environment.

An interactive environment should be able to get the result of the manipulation like a visual-kinaesthetic interaction, very similar to the eye-hand coordination required in the real situation. Moreover, the haptic device has to be able to reproduce, without distortion, the sensations associated with the interaction in the virtual environment; the workspace has not to be reduced by mechanical constraints.

The modelling of the simulation environment is very important to achieve a highly realistic simulation of human soft tissue behaviour under the effect of external stimulations. This leads to a system of deformable objects with specified geometrical shape and natural physical/mechanical behaviour. A realistic simulation of the interaction requires the following topics:

- geometrical modelling: a description of the geometric shapes of organs, tissues and vessels and their graphical representation;
- physical modelling: an imitation of the behaviour of soft tissues;

- model interactions: an interactive manipulation of deformable objects using the simulated instruments.

The interactions can be divided into collision detection (check for space sections simultaneously used by two objects), collision response (calculation of the forces in order to provide a force feedback) and interaction management (evaluation and handling of the different interactions).

Building a surgical simulator in an accurate and realistic way includes activities such as real-time rendering of dynamic models, real-time collision detection among objects, real-time physical modelling, force computation and interaction using a haptic interface.

The use of a haptic device, which is able to return to the user's hand a realistic force feedback, is very important because the force and the visual feedback sensations at the same time enhance the user performance.

Specific haptic devices have been designed for the different surgical procedures.

The user interacts with the simulator (Figure 4) using the haptic interface and the data acquired from the haptic device sensors are used both to graphically represent the surgical tools and their positions in the virtual environment, and to determine possible collisions between the virtual objects. Movements of the haptic device lead to changes in the virtual scene.

Collisions between virtual objects produce both forces, which have to be replicated on the user's hand by means of the haptic interface, and virtual organs deformations, which have to be rendered by the visual interface.

In order to obtain a realistic simulation, real-time interactivity is the most critical issue. The movements of the surgical tools have to produce without delay the corresponding virtual instrument motions; delays between the user action and the environment reaction reduce the immersion sensation.

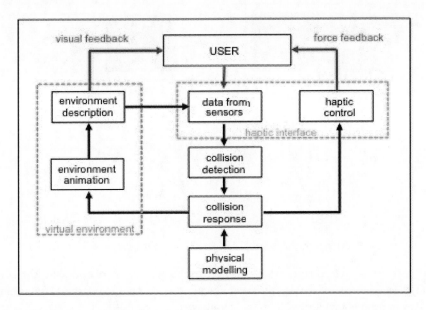

Figure 4. A schema of a generic virtual surgical simulator.

Building of the Virtual Environment

In order to provide a meaningful educational experience, a surgical training simulation must depict the relevant anatomy accurately; unrealistic anatomic models could confuse or even misinform trainers as to what they might encounter in the operating room.

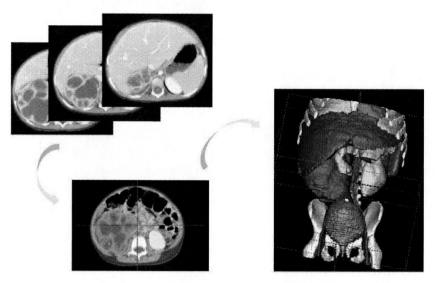

Figure 5. Building of the Virtual model of the organs (AVR Lab, Salento University, Italy).

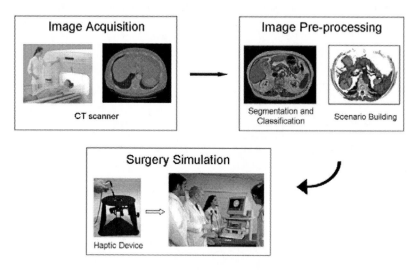

Figure 6. Integration of a virtual environment built from real patient images.

The use of digital images for medical diagnosis has increased considerably and, depending on simulation needs, the anatomical images can be derived from magnetic resonances or from computerized tomography images.

To build a virtual environment from the real patients' images, the geometric models of the human organs have been reconstructed using data acquired by a medical scanner; data are processed to distinguish the anatomical structures and to associate different chromatic scales to the organs.

The segmentation and classification phases are carried out in order to obtain information about the size and the shape of the human organs.

The visual and haptic feedbacks and the interaction management, working in conjunction, are able to produce a realistic impression that the surgeon is interacting with a real tissue [6] (Figures 5 and 6).

Collision Detection and Response Algorithms

Physical modelling has the task of determining the dynamic behaviour of virtual objects in order to add realism to the simulation. Simulations based on physical modelling depend highly on the physical interaction between objects in a scene.

Collision detection involves the automatic detection of an interaction of two objects and of the location where this interaction takes place. At the moment of impact, the simulation produces a collision response that generates a haptic feedback to the user.

Collision detection is considered as the major computational bottleneck of physically-based animation systems. The problem is still more difficult to solve when the simulated objects deform over time [7,8].

Generally, detecting a collision between two objects basically consists in testing if the volume of the first one intersects the second one. In surgical applications it is necessary to perform dynamic collision detection by testing for a precise intersection between the surgical tool extremity and the triangle mesh that models the organs; this computation is performed at each time step.

A general description of collision detection and response algorithms in surgical simulators is reported hereafter. At each time step, it is necessary to check if there is an intersection between the actual position of the surgical instrument and each triangle mesh that models a short area of the organ; if there is a collision the algorithm:

- will find the exact intersection point between a triangle and the segment obtained from the previous and actual positions of the surgical tool;
- will compute the incidence angle between this segment and the plane that include the triangle;
- will compute the force proportional to the penetration distance (between the actual position of the tool and the contact point in the triangle).

Deformable Tissue Models

Physical modelling has the task of determining the dynamic behaviour of virtual objects in order to add realism to the simulation.

The idea is to define a model that computes the tissue displacement with time; the displacement is used to calculate the response of the tissue to the surgical tool external stimuli.

Information about surgical tool displacements and tissue responses are also used to graphically model the artery wall and virtual surgical instrument deformations generated in consequence of their contact.

To obtain a correct representation of soft–tissue deformability it is necessary to compare the computed soft-tissue model with the actually deformed tissue. For this reason it is necessary to have a qualitative knowledge of the biomechanical behaviour of soft tissue.

Research in biomechanics has shown that a realistic model for soft tissues is a visco-elastic non-linear model; this model has high computational complexity. Biomechanics has proposed complex mathematical models for representing the deformation of soft tissue and computer graphics has developed many algorithms for the real-time computation of deformable objects.

A reasonable approximation for soft tissue deformations can be obtained using linear elasticity theory. The physical behavior of a soft tissue model may be considered linear-elastic if the applied displacement remains small (less than 10% of typical object size) [9].

These models (e.g. mass-spring models) have frequently been used because they are very easy to implement and they yield reasonable speeds.

Mass-Spring Model (the nodes of the mesh connected by springs and dampers) and Finite Element Method (organs divided into surface or volumetric elements, calculation of the proprieties of each element and assemblage of all finite elements) are the most used methods to compute the deformation of the organs under the applied forces.

Mass-spring model is a physically based technique and consists of a set of nodes linked by springs; mass and damping are assigned to the nodes. Springs exert forces on neighbouring points and the spring behaviour is governed by a deformation law (typically Hooke's law). The amount of stiffness of the springs can be derived from the intensity of voxels in a CT-scan image; in this way the stiffness is proportional to tissue density and therefore to the Hounsfield units.

A mass-spring method does not require continuous parameterization and can be used to model cutting or suturing simply by removing or adding connections between vertices.

The behaviour of a mass-spring mesh depends heavily on its topological and geometric configuration. In addition, configurations with large forces (e.g. nearly-rigid objects) lead to stiff differential equations with poor numerical stability, requiring small time-steps of the integration. Nevertheless a mass-spring model is an easily understandable concept, which is simple to implement and has low computational demands.

Therefore, mass-spring models are used in a wide range of computer graphics and VR applications, e.g. in the animation of facial expressions, the simulation of cloth or the modelling of inner organs, including visco-elastic tissues encountered in surgery. Several improvements to spring models have been proposed, specifically with regard to their dynamical behaviour.

A brain model was built using the mass-spring method and composed from about 27.000 nodes (Figure 7); together with the external layer of springs, two other layers have been modelled and connected to the corresponding points of the tier immediately above by means of springs and dampers.

Figure 7. A brain model built using the mass-spring method (Salento University, Italy and Karlsruhe University, Germany).

Several research groups have been involved in the modelling of virtual organs using the mass-spring method.

Cover et al. [10] were the first to present a real time model for gall bladder surgery simulation.

Kühnapfel et al. [11] used a mass-spring model to simulate a realistic interaction between surgical tools and organs in KISMET system, a virtual reality training system for minimally invasive surgery. Virtual organ geometry is modelled as elastic body and the control points of the object surface form, together with additional internal nodes, an elastic 3D-mesh of virtual mass points, which are interconnected by virtual springs with damping elements.

Gibson [12] proposed a "ChainMail" model, where volume elements are linked to their nearest neighbours. Each node must satisfy a given maximum and minimum distance constraint to its adjacent nodes. When an element is moved and one of its constraints is violated, a displacement of the respective neighbouring element takes place. In this way small displacements of a selected point in a relatively slack system result only in local deformations of the system, while displacements in a system that is already stretched or compressed to its limit cause the whole system to move.

Another model used for soft tissues is the Finite Element Method (FEM) that uses basic element (triangles, quadrilaterals, tetrahedral, etc) in order to describe the object's shape. Simple interpolation functions within these elements make the problem numerically tractable; appropriate boundary conditions guarantee a physically correct solution.

One major advantage of FEM is the scalability of the solution method because with the same mesh structure it is possible to increase or decrease the precision and complexity of the model allowing to have an advanced model or a less advanced but faster model.

The use of FEM in computer graphics has been limited because of the computational requirements; in particular it is difficult to apply FEM in real-time systems. Several modifications and simplifications have been introduced to reduce computational time. In particular, only valid for small displacements, linear elasticity has often been used as a trade-off between biomedical realism and real-time computation.

Several research groups have been involved in the modelling of virtual organs using the FEM method.

Bro-Nielsen et al. [13] use a different approach to achieve real-time performance for application of 3D solid volumetric FEM. This improvement, called "Condensation", allows compressing the linear matrix system resulting from the volumetric FE model to a system with the same complexity as a FE surface model of the same object. The cutting or suturing procedures require a redefinition of the finite element model and, for this reason, they can not be used since the calculation cost is too high.

Cotin et al [14] propose a new method, called "tensor-mass model", that is as simple to implement and as efficient as spring-mass models, but it is based on continuum mechanics and linear elasticity theory. In this method the stiffness matrix only depends on the material characteristics within a tetrahedron and, for this reason, it is possible to simulate cutting and tearing of soft tissue. A limited number of elements (around one thousand) is allowed for real-time situation.

Moreover in [15] it is proposed a "hybrid elastic method" enabling to cut and deform large anatomical structures. A simulation of a hepatectomy has been chosen to demonstrate the approach efficiency.

Simulators for Surgical Training

Technical skills in the field of surgery have been taught using the apprenticeship model for the last 100 years.

The advent and popularization of minimally invasive surgery brought about the use of simulation as a training tool; videoendoscopic techniques are especially suited for simulation because the field of view is limited, peripheral vision is not possible and the operative field is represented in two dimensions on a video monitor (Figure 8).

The Minimal Invasive Surgery techniques are complex procedures and difficult to master. Surgical educators have highlighted in numerous editorials that minimally invasive technique is difficult to learn using the conventional apprenticeship concept, as the specific psychomotor skills cannot be acquired by observation and assistance alone. Several reports of serious complications attributable to technical errors have demonstrated the need for more efficient and intensive training and assessment before surgeons are allowed to perform laparoscopic procedures on patients [17].

Traditional learning methods, assuming the importance of the force feedback, use real surgical instruments with plastic models for training; due to the incisions, these models become soon unusable.

Virtual Reality simulation has the potential to play a key role in the training process. Developments in computer technology and haptic interfaces allow creating specific simulations of minimally invasive surgical procedures and makes possible to practice training on new and difficult procedures avoiding risks for the patients. Virtual simulators can allow repeated practice of basic tasks and complete surgical procedures before performing the same procedures on patients in the operating room.

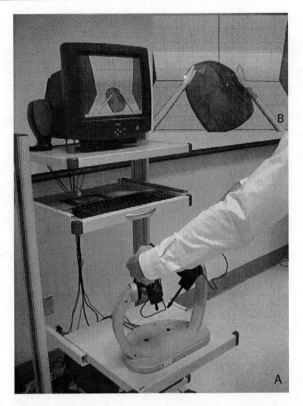

Figure 8. MIST-VR system.

The virtual procedure repetition brings several advantages, including anticipation of complications, better selection of tools and techniques to be used, and reduction of procedure time; the trainee learns to handle the surgical instruments and to recognize the pathologies [16].

Furthermore, the mentoring surgeon has a limited ability to direct the operation; indeed, unlike open procedures, where the mentor may employ verbal and manual direction from the opposite side of the operating table, in videoendoscopic surgery verbal direction is the only basis for instruction and there is an increased reliance on the technical skills of the trainee.

To achieve these basic skills, training in simulated operative environments has become increasingly common despite little evidence regarding the efficacy of these techniques.

Simulation may be divided into four main categories: skill stations, synthetic material, animal models and virtual environments.

Skill stations have been designed to train on specific functions with laparoscopic instruments in a two-dimensional environment; the skills practiced in such simulators usually represent a component of a more complex procedure performed in the operating room.

Synthetic material simulation uses man-made material to approximate tissues and anatomic relationships found clinically.

Animal model simulation is based on finding an animal model similar to human anatomy for the respective surgical procedure; this approach was used widely with the introduction of laparoscopic cholecystectomy.

Virtual environments vary in complexity from simple skill station tasks to anatomical recreations of common operative fields complete with realistic tissue deformation and force feedback.

Each of these simulation models has differing attributes as a training tool.

Skill stations are inexpensive; they are easy to use, but at best, they only train the student in one limited aspect of the operation.

Animals may provide an excellent model, but ethical and cost considerations require that they be used at a more advanced stage of the learning process.

Synthetic material is robust, relatively inexpensive, may be similar to the operative environment and avoids ethical considerations.

Virtual environments are free of these ethical considerations, but tend to be expensive.

Prior studies assessing the clinical impact of simulation training have been complicated because these skills were incorporated into a broader educational program in individuals of varying experience.

Thus, objective improvement in the trainee's ability to perform a clinical skill after training on simulation has not been clearly demonstrated.

Virtual Reality Training Systems

A new and very promising technology is the use of computers and robots in medical education and training and usually consists of a computer, a force-feedback device and a display system.

The user interacts with the training system via an input device that resembles the handles of instruments as they are used in real patient treatment. A specialized medical simulation software is fed with digital models of a real patient's anatomy derived from CT or MR data: the computer also receives the position of the virtual instruments, pretended by the current position of the handles while they are manipulated as they would be during a real procedure. The software simulates physics such as gravity and behaviour of fluids as well as the optical appearance such as shadows and glossiness of a virtual scenario. A realistic visual impression is mostly achieved by using specialized software that runs for performance reasons on the processor of high-end graphic cards instead of the main unit processor.

The force feedback, or haptic feedback, introduces the physical sensation into the virtual environment by means of advanced human-machine interfaces (haptic interface) that consist of one or more handles that resemble to the tool-holders of real procedure and are able to replicate the user's movements in the virtual environment and to reproduce the sensations associated with the interactions in the virtual environment. In other words, the user feels the forces generated in the virtual environment in response to the forces that he applies.

If the computation of the force feedback is fast enough, the user gets the illusion of touching the organs and the user can train basic tasks as well as complex surgical procedures under very realistic conditions.

The value of Virtual Reality computer simulators has been assessed in a consensus document, indicating that several systems can be considered valid tools for assessment of technical skills [18]. Such systems give us for the first time the unique possibility to quantify surgical performance and provide an objective and unbiased assessment of technical skills

[19]. The assessment can serve as an excellent tool to monitor progress during the training period, provide structured feedback, and, finally, ensure that the objectives of the training program have been met [18].

The first commercially successful surgical simulator was the MIST-VR (Minimally Invasive Surgery Trainer–VR) of Mentice Inc, which combined a mechanical trainer with an abstract graphic image. The skills and tasks included for training were the most fundamental—pick and place, transfer, etc [19].

The Swedish Mentice Corporation is a supplier of several virtual reality based applications with special attention to the minimally invasive surgery and the endovascular interventions [20].

The modern Procedicus MIST is an endoscopic simulator divided into several modules providing a vehicle for acquiring basic skills and a framework for enhancing clinical knowledge and cognitive skills. Trainees are guided through a series of exercises of progressive complexity, enabling them to develop the skills essential for good clinical practice. The Procedicus MIST system enables to practice basic skills, atrialfibrillation, arthroscopy for shoulder and knee and nephrectomy. The system measures performance by time to task completion, number of errors, and overall exercise efficiency [21].

Procedicus MIST system is the first virtual reality system that is validated for the automatic objective assessment of surgical skills: it sets a benchmark for all subsequent systems [21].

The Select-IT VEST Systems AG Company has developed, in collaboration with the Forschungszentrum Karlsruhe, Institut für Angewandte Informatik, the Virtual Endoscopic Surgery Training (VEST) system VSOne (Figure 9), a virtual reality simulator for minimal invasive surgery that is commercially available. The simulator allows users to practice surgical procedures using three haptic devices as mock-up endoscopic instruments and provides laparoscopic cholecystectomy and gynaecology scenario [22].

LapSim System (Surgical Science Ltd, Sweden) utilizes advanced 3D technology, including interactive live video, to provide the student with a realistic virtual working environment [23].

LapSim System (Figure 10) allows the trainee to learn and practice a range of basic skills that are essential to any surgeon. Practice sessions can vary in graphic complexity as well as in the level of difficulty and exercises as basic navigation, grasping, cutting and advanced suturing can be carried out [4].

The simulated tissue in LapSim Dissection reacts realistically to the user's manipulations, and dissection may be carried out using different instruments, each interacting with the simulated tissue in a realistic way.

The Simbionix LAP Mentor is multi-disciplinary laparoscopy surgery simulator that enables simultaneous hands-on practice for a single trainee or a team. The system offers training opportunities to new and experienced surgeons to performing complete laparoscopic surgical procedures. The new second generation LAP Mentor II Simulator features an advanced, ergonomic design that is both portable and user-friendly. The simulator handles on this sleek system are completely extractable for easy switching to suturing handles.

In addition, the improved haptic interface on the new LAP Mentor II (Figure 11) offers enhanced tactile feedback, performance and reliability.

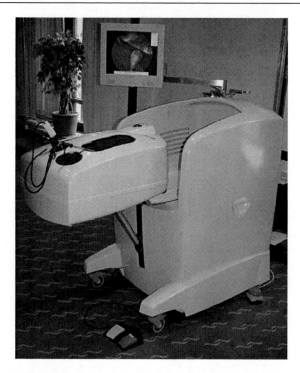

Figure 9. VEST system VSOne.

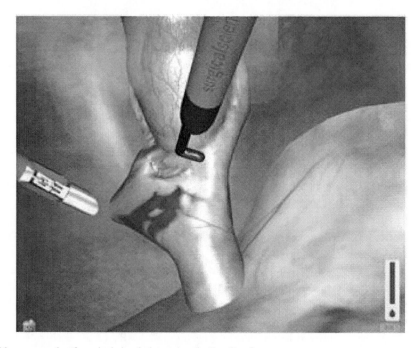

Figure 10. an example of surgical simulation using the LapSim System.

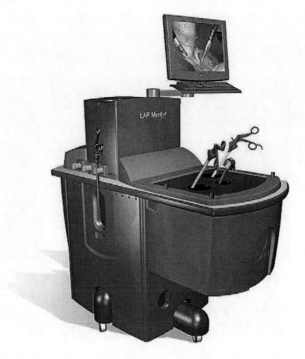

Figure 11. Simbionix LAP Mentor II.

There is also a portable solution, the LAP Mentor Express, that is a "personal trainer" for integrated training and practice of basic laparoscopic skills and laparoscopic procedures for use in clinics, smaller courses and local meetings [25].

Female Surgical Pelvic Trainer

Although great enthusiasm exists for developing skills in laparoscopic gynaecology in the scientific surgical world, training opportunities are limited; this is primarily due to a lack of approved gynaecology/laparoscopy fellowships, as exist in the surgical school.

It is an unfortunate fact that many interested gynaecologists do not progress beyond the initial courses stage and indeed a number of gynaecologists who have attended animal laboratory training as well have not proceeded to regular pelvic laparoscopic practice.

It was therefore thought prudent to create a fluid "mini" fellowship, enabling supervised training so that interested gynaecologists could become comfortable and competent with laparoscopy.

Female pelvic surgical approach is a critical procedure that needs to be taught away from the patient; a clinical female pelvic trainer presents a possible accurate anatomical and tactile representation of the female pelvis for an endoscopical examination and a surgical diagnosis of pathologies and abnormalities.

A pelvic trainer can be used for many levels of training from undergraduate onwards as well as for young surgeons; it can be designed as a model trainer able to concentrate on essential anatomy and procedures. The pelvic trainer skills, usually, are: recognition of anatomy and appropriate landmarks, enscopic examination procedure, pre-operative procedure evaluation, pre-surgical instrumental planning and intra-abdominal surgical exercitation (Figure 12).

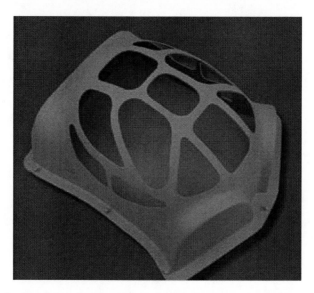

Figure 12. An example of a pelvic trainer for the gynaecological laparoscopy.

The pelvic trainer features are: interchangeable genital assemblies with different complications, realistic genital and abdominal assemblies, realistic abdominal wall, partial thighs aid anatomical orientation, removable abdominal fat pad to represent different thicknesses of abdominal tissue, realistic anus and lower bowel, freedom to present different training scenarios at appropriate levels, the surface of each foam component is washable using soap and water.

Accurate anatomical and tactile representation provides for extensive training at undergraduate level for both doctors and assistants and has many uses in surgical community care. The simplicity of the model enables the trainee to focus on essential anatomy and procedure. Different assemblies can be introduced according to the need of that training requirement; so, simulation for training videoendoscopic surgical skills has become increasingly important (Figure 13).

Video technology and computerized pelvic trainer are more widely accepted in surgical education because of advances in simulator technology; according to this progress, some medical teachers decline in formal study of human anatomy in graduate medical education.

Several factors are responsible for this change in curriculum including competing subject matter, redirection of teaching toward clinical sciences, and attrition in faculty university members; surgical educators have turned to anatomic models to teach various surgical procedures including pelvic and laparoscopic surgery.

Although these computer-assisted mannequins are highly realistic, institutions may be limited by their costs coupled with the concerns that the technology may rapidly be outdated.

The realistic anatomic model with modest physiologic responses allows for a cost-effective realistic model that may function as an alternative to animal or cadaver models; animal models are limited to institutions that have a veterinary facility on the premises.

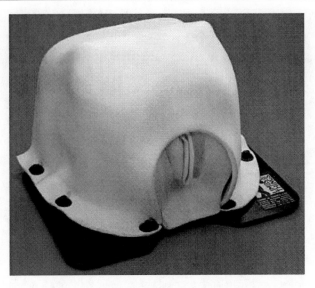

Figure 13. An example of a pelvic trainer for the study of female anatomy in gynaecological laparoscopy.

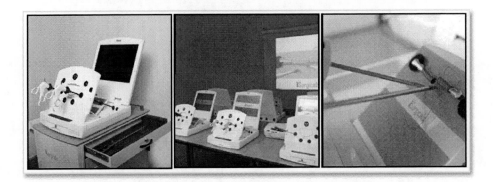

Figure 14. Video technology applied to laparoscopical trainer simulator.

Institutions with remote animal laboratories must either shuttle their students over long distances or restrict their courses offering to refresher courses that do not include the surgical skills station.

Simulation is routinely incorporated into programs designed to facilitate videoendoscopic technical skill training (Figure 14).

The impact of this training is difficult to discern because different types of simulation are often employed during the same course, and clinical performance after the course has not been assessed objectively.

Some of the earliest and most thorough analysis of simulation training showed significant correlation between the performance at three skill stations and the ability to perform a laparoscopic suturing exercise on pig intestine.

Similarly, a surgeon showed that surgical residents who were evaluated with skill stations before and after a 6-hour suturing course did improve their ability to perform at the skill stations (Figure 15).

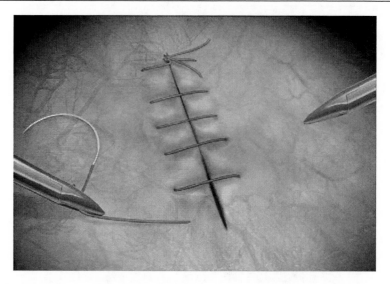

Figure 15. Video technology applied to laparoscopical trainer simulator during a suturing course.

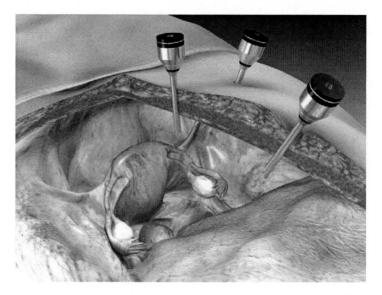

Figure 16. the virtual reproduction of the female pelvis in endoscopy.

More recently, an author showed through a series of seven simulators that concurrent repetition at multiple skill stations will improve the ability of the participant to perform each of the tasks.

In this study, performance at four of the seven tasks was also improved in a control group of participants who had no repetition between testing.

This study reveals two important points: repetition of a task will improve the ability to perform the task and some tasks require little repetition to see improvement (i.e. a very rapid learning curve).

Some companies, involved in endoscopic imaging, have already taken the option to donate such instruments to projects in the third world or to sponsor punctuate medical missions (Algeria, Vietnam, Rumania).

One of the most efficient teaching forms is the partnership between well experienced European laparoscopic departments, endoscopical industries and third-world university departments, with a clear hierarchic structure and a well defined teaching mission.

This partnership should be based on a man-to-man contact and implemented by cooperative aid structures providing financing and helping in obtaining the necessary permits from the involved embassy as well as non-governmental organizations and commercial firms.

As for now, teaching implies frequent travels for teachers and students.

Financing for travels and fellowships up to 1 year can be granted by organizations in the third-world country as well as in the western countries.

At the present, some industries have run an educational program specifically targeted at medical professionals in developing countries.

Disclosure of Interest

Authors certify that there is no actual or potential conflict of interest in relation to this article and they reveal any financial interests or connections, direct or indirect, or other situations that might raise the question of bias in the work reported or the conclusions, implications, or opinions stated – including pertinent commercial or other sources of funding for the individual author(s) or for the associated department(s) or organization(s), personal relationships, or direct academic competition.

References

[1]   Harrell AG, Heniford TB. Minimally Invasive Abdominal Surgery: Lux et Veritas Past, Present, and Future. *Am. J. Surg.* 2005, 190:239-243.

[2]   Gorman PJ, Meier AH, Kummel TM. Simulation and Virtual Reality in Surgical Education: real or unreal? *Arch. Surg.* 1999 Nov;134(11):1203-8.

[3]   Dawson SL, Cotin S, Meglan D, Shaffer DW, Ferrell MA. Designing a Computer-Based Simulator for Interventional Cardiology Training. *Catheter Cardiovasc. Interv.* 2000 Dec;51(4):522-7.

[4]   Zorcolo A, Gobbetti E, Pili P, Tuberi M. Catheter Insertion Simulation with Combined Visual and Haptic Feedback. Proc. First PHANToM Users Research Symposium (PURS'99), Heidelberg, Germany, 21-22 May, 1999.

[5]   Jackson B, Rosenberg L. Force Feedback and Medical Simulation. In: Interactive Technology and the New Paradigm for Health-Care, chapter 24, IOS Press 1995, pp.147-151.

[6]   Van den Bergen G. Collision Detection in Interactive 3D Environments. Elsevier Morgan Kaufmann Publishers, San Francisco, 2004.

[7]   Lombardo J, Cani MP, Neyret F. Real-time Collision Detection for Virtual Surgery. Proc. *Computer Animation* 1999, pp. 33-39.

[8] Watt A, Policarpo F. 3D Games: Real-time Rendering and Software Technology. Addison Wesley Publishing Company, 2001.

[9] Delingette H. Towards Realistic Soft Tissue Modeling in Medical Simulation. *Proceedings of the IEEE: Special Issue on Surgery Simulation* 1998; 86(3):512-523.

[10] Cover S, Ezquerra N, O'Brien J. Interactively Deformable Model for Surgery Simulation. *IEEE Computer Graphics and Applications*, 1993, pp. 68-75.

[11] Kühnapfel UG, Cakmak HK, Maass H. Endoscopic Surgery Training using Virtual Reality and Deformable Tissue Simulation. *Computer and Graphics* 2000; 24: 671-682.

[12] Gibson S. 3D ChainMail: a Fast Algorithm for Deforming Volumetric Objects. Proc. Symposium on Interactive 3D Graphics, 1997.

[13] Bro-Nielsen M, Cotin S. Real-Time Volumetric Deformable Models for Surgery Simulation using Finite Elements and Condensation. *Proceedings of Eurographics '96 – Computer Graphics Forum* 1996;15: 57-66.

[14] Cotin S, Delingette H, Ayache N. A Hybrid Elastic Model allowing Real-Time Cutting, Deformations and Force-Feedback for Surgery Training and Simulation. *Visual Computer Journal* 2000;16(8).

[15] Cotin S, Delingette H, Ayache N. Real-time Elastic Deformations of Soft Tissues for Surgery Simulation", *IEEE Transactions on Visualization and Computer Graphycs* 1999;5(1): 62-73.

[16] Satava RM. Cybersurgery: advanced technologies for surgical practice. Wiley-Liss, 1998.

[17] Grantcharov TP. Virtual reality simulation in training and assessment of laparoscopic skills. *Eur. Clinics Obstet. Gynaecol.* 2007; 2:197–200.

[18] Carter FJ, Schijven MP, Aggarwal, Grantcharov T, Francis NK, Hanna GB, Jakimowicz JJ. Work Group for Evaluation and Implementation of Simulators and Skills Training Programmes. Consensus guidelines for validation of virtual reality surgical simulators. *Surg. Endosc.* 2005;19:1523–1532.

[19] Wilson MS, Middlebrook A, Sutton C, Stone R, McCloy RF. MIST-VR: a virtual reality trainer for laparoscopic surgery assesses performance. *Ann. R. Coll Surg. Engl.* 1997;79(6): 403–404.

[20] Seymour NE, Gallagher AG, Roman SA, O'Brien MK, Bansal VK, Andersen DK, Satava RM. Virtual reality training improves operating room performance: results of a randomized, double-blinded study. *Ann. Surg.* 2002; 236:458–463.

[21] Satava R. M., Historical Review of Surgical Simulation—A Personal Perspective. *World J. Surg.* 2008;32:141–148.

[22] Procedicus MIST, Mentice Inc., http://www.mentice.com.

[23] VEST system VSOne, http://www-kismet.iai.fzk.de/KISMET/VestSystem.html.

[24] LapSim, Surgical Science Ltd, http://www.surgical-science.com.

[25] Lap Mentor, Simbionix, http://http://www.simbionix.com/LAP_Mentor.html.

In: Laparoscopy: New Developments, Procedures and Risks ISBN: 978-1-61470-747-9
Editor: Hana Terzic, pp. 165-183 © 2012 Nova Science Publishers, Inc.

Chapter VII

Laparoscopy in Colorectal Cancer

Ker-Kan Tan and Dean C. Koh [*]

Division of Colorectal Surgery, University Surgical Cluster,
National University Health System, Singapore.

Abstract

This chapter highlights the present role of laparoscopy in colorectal cancer. There exists strong evidence supporting the use of laparoscopic approaches in the surgical treatment of colon cancer. Several randomised controlled trials comparing open and laparoscopic resection for colon cancer have confirmed the numerous short term advantages including reduced post-operative wound pain, fewer wound and pulmonary related complications, shorter hospitalization and a quicker return of bowel function without compromising the oncologic outcome and overall survival.

Evidence for laparoscopic proctectomy is only now emerging from the results of ongoing trials. Laparoscopic resection for rectal cancer has not been met with the similar enthusiasm seen in colon cancer. This may be attributed to laparoscopic mesorectal excision being technically more challenging as evidenced by the high conversion rates reported in early studies. While these studies have demonstrated the similar short-term benefits seen in laparoscopic colectomy for colon cancers, trials are presently still being conducted to evaluate the long-term oncologic outcomes and survival. The COREAN trial has demonstrated similar short-term advantages whilst retaining the quality of oncological resection of laparoscopic proctectomy in mid and low rectal cancers. The outcomes of similar trials such as the ACOSOG Z6051 and the ALaCaRT will provide more concrete conclusions on the role of laparoscopic proctectomy for rectal cancer.

There is emerging consensus on the various technical approaches to laparoscopic colonic mobilization, vessel ligation and creation of anastomoses, all of which aim to achieve comparable oncologic resections with the traditional open techniques. Conventional laparoscopic and hand-assisted laparoscopic techniques have been compared and evaluated extensively.

[*] Corresponding author: Dean Chi-Siong Koh, Division of Colorectal Surgery, University Surgical Cluster 1E Kent Ridge Road, Singapore 119228, National University Health System, TEL: [65]-67724235, FAX: [65]-67778206, Email: dean_koh@nuhs.edu.sg

Following the successful adoption of robotic technology in radical prostatectomy, robotic assisted laparoscopic colorectal surgery has seen increasing interest in an attempt to overcome the limitations of standard laparoscopy. The new technology provides a stable platform with three-dimensional visualization, endowrist range of movements with better manoeuvrability in confined spaces, and motion scaling for better precision in dissection. These advantages are most evident when performing mesorectal excision in the deeper confines of the pelvis. Early studies have shown robotic assisted total mesorectal excision to be associated with lower rates of positive resection margins and conversion.

To achieve even better cosmetic outcomes, single port access surgery for colon cancer has begun to emerge with several case series reported in the literature. These procedures have been reported to be safe and feasible through a smaller incision without compromising the oncologic principles. Early surgeon-modified single incision devices have now been replaced by a number of commercially manufactured ones.

Expert laparoscopists have begun to expand the role of the minimally invasive approach in non-elective situations. Recent reviews have proven the safety and feasibility of performing emergency laparoscopic surgery in well selected patients with obstructed or perforated colorectal cancers. In addition, certain conditions such as anastomotic dehiscence, adhesive small bowel obstruction and even reversal of Hartmann's procedures following prior surgery for colorectal cancer can also be treated using the laparoscopic approach.

The field of laparoscopy in colorectal cancer continues to evolve and is likely to become an integral part in the management of colorectal cancer in the near future.

Introduction

Laparoscopy has revolutionised the practice of general surgery over the past three decades. When initially described in the early 1990s, laparoscopic surgery for malignant colorectal conditions was met with much skepticism with several questions raised regarding its adherence to oncologic principles [1-5]. Despite reported benefits such as reduced hospital stays, quicker recovery, less narcotic analgesia requirements and improved cosmesis, adoption of laparoscopic colorectal resection at that juncture remained only in the practices of selected institutions and in the context of clinical studies [5]. That was until the results of several large, randomised controlled trials comparing laparoscopic and open resection for colon cancer emerged at the start of the millennium.

Laparoscopic Versus Open Surgery for Colon Cancer

Four large, prospective, randomised controlled trials from North America and Europe have published their short-term results comparing laparoscopic to open colectomy for colon cancers (Table 1). The same groups subsequently published their long-term follow up data (Table 2). These included the Barcelona Trial, the Clinical Outcomes of Surgical Therapy (COST) Trial, the Conventional versus Laparoscopic-Assisted Surgery in Patients with

Colorectal Cancer (CLASSIC) Trial and the Colon Cancer Laparoscopic or Open Resection (COLOR) Trial [6-13].

Short Term Outcome

All four randomised trials confirmed the safety and feasibility of performing colectomy for colon cancer via the laparoscopic approach. The short-term complications, morbidity and mortality rates were found to be similar, although the Barcelona trial did report a lower rate of morbidity in the laparoscopic group which was statistically significant. The COLOR, CLASSIC and the Barcelona trials were able to demonstrate an earlier return of bowel function in the laparoscopic group. The shorter hospital stays that were seen in the laparoscopic group were achieved in exchange for a slightly longer operative duration.

Following the results of these trials, several large retrospective reviews have correspondingly reported their short-term results comparing laparoscopic to open colectomy for colon cancer. These reviews highlighted the shorter lengths of stay, lengthier operative times and lower rates of post-operative complications, such as wound infection/dehiscence, pneumonia and urinary tract infection in the laparoscopic group [14-17]. These have been postulated to be due to the smaller incisions and the corresponding reduced immunological response to a 'less traumatic' procedure [14-17].

Oncologic and Long-Term Outcome

One of the early concerns with laparoscopic colectomy for colon cancer was the lack of convincing data demonstrating comparable long-term oncologic outcomes of this new technique. This was further augmented by initial reports of increased rates of port-site recurrences [18-19].

Table 1. Randomised trials demonstrating short-term outcomes between laparoscopic (L) and open (O) colectomy in colon cancer

Trial	Study period (year)	No. of patients (L vs. O)	Operative time (L vs. O) (minutes)	Conversion	Hospital stay (L vs. O) (Days)	Morbidity (L vs. O) (%)	Mortality (L vs. O) (%)
Barcelona [6]	1993–1998	111: 108	142 vs. 118*	11%	5.2 vs. 7.9*	11 vs. 29*	1 vs. 3
COST [8]	1994–2001	435: 428	150 vs. 95*	21%	5 vs. 6*	21 vs. 20	<1 vs. 1
CLASSIC [10]	1996–2002	273: 140	180 vs. 135	25%	9 vs. 9	35 vs. 35	4 vs. 5
COLOR [12]	1997–2003	536: 546	145 vs. 115*	17%	8.2 vs. 9.3*	21 vs. 20	1 vs. 2

*: Statistically Significant.

The aforementioned four major trials then published their long-term results to address these issues. There were no statistical differences seen between the groups in terms of the rates of positive resection margins and number of lymph nodes harvested (Table 2) [7, 9, 11, 13]. There were also no notable differences between the disease-free survival and overall survival rates (Table 2). The adequacy of oncologic resection has been further supported by a recent meta-analysis which demonstrated similar long-term oncologic outcomes between the two groups [20]. In addition, the incidences of wound/port-site, local and systemic recurrences were also similar.

Table 2. Randomised trials demonstrating long-term outcomes between laparoscopic (L) and open (O) colectomy in colon cancer

Trial	Median follow up period	Mean/Median lymph nodes harvested (L vs. O)	Local recurrence (L vs. O)	Chemotherapy administered (L vs. O) (%)	Disease free survival (L vs. O) (Months)	Overall survival (L vs. O) (Months)
Barcelona (95 months) [7]	95 months	11.1 vs. 11.1	7.5% vs. 13.7%	-	-	64 vs. 51
COST (5 yr) [9]	7 years	12 vs. 12	2.3% vs. 2.6%	No difference	69.2 vs. 68.4	76.4 vs. 74.6
CLASSIC (5 yr) [11]	56.3 months	12 vs. 13.5	-	-	57.6 vs. 64.0	55.7 vs. 62.7
COLOR (5 yr) [13]	53 months	10 vs. 10	4.9% vs. 4.8%	10.3 vs. 10.5	66.5 vs. 67.9	73.8 vs. 74.2

*: Statistically Significant.

Hence, there is now strong evidence supporting the role of laparoscopic colectomy for colon cancer that is well accepted.

Laparoscopic Versus Open Surgery for Rectal Cancer

There are considerable technical difficulties involved in performing a total mesorectal excision (TME) laparoscopically and achieving clear margins, in particular the circumferential resection margin (CRM). Furthermore, the results of the CLASSIC trial have somewhat limited the widespread adoption of laparoscopic proctectomy in rectal cancer.

This trial was the only one of the four described multicentre randomised trials that included patients with rectal cancer [10]. It reported a considerable conversion rate of over 34% in the subset of patients who underwent laparoscopic proctectomy. Conversion, as a factor, was associated with more post-operative complications and a prolonged length of stay. The CRM positivity rate in patients who underwent proctectomy was also noted to be two times higher in the laparoscopic (12%) compared to the open (6%) group. However, it was also noted that the laparoscopic group was able to achieve a higher rate of complete TME. In the conclusion of that study, the authors urged caution in the routine practice of laparoscopic proctectomy in all patients with rectal cancers.

The long-term outcomes reported from the same group addressed the initial concerns of possibly higher local recurrence rates anticipated in the laparoscopic group. It demonstrated a similar rate of local recurrence between the two groups (Local recurrence: 7.6% in open vs. 9.4% in laparoscopic, $p = 0.740$). There were also no differences seen in the disease free (5-year disease free survival rates: 52.1% in open vs. 53.2% in laparoscopic, $p = 0.953$) and overall survival rates (5-year overall survival rates: 52.9% in open vs. 60.3% in laparoscopic, $p = 0.132$) [11].

Several other smaller randomised single-institution trials subsequently reaffirmed the safety, feasibility and short-term benefits of laparoscopic proctectomy for rectal cancer. There were also no significant differences in the long term outcomes seen in these reports (Table 3) [20-24]. All the studies were able to demonstrate lower rates of conversion and incidences of CRM positivity compared to that of the CLASSIC trial.

With increasing adoption of neoadjuvant chemoradiation therapy for patients with advanced mid and distal rectal cancers, the COREAN trial was performed to address if there were any differences between laparoscopic and open proctectomy in these patients. It was the first such multi-centred randomised controlled trial that was performed with 170 patients in each arm [25]. They were able to demonstrate a low conversion rate of 1.2% with expectedly longer operative times in the laparoscopic group. The incidence of CRM positivity, quality of TME and peri-operative morbidity and mortality rates were comparable in both groups. The laparoscopic group demonstrated an earlier return of bowel function and reduced narcotic analgesia usage.

Benefits and Challenges of Laparoscopic Proctectomy

In addition to the above mentioned benefits of laparoscopic colectomy, there are unique advantages conferred by the laparoscopic approach in the resection of rectal cancers [26-28]. Apart from the CLASSIC trial, another series from Greece was also able to highlight the higher rate of completeness of TME achieved using the laparoscopic approach [29]. One reason reported has been the better visualisation and the high-resolution image qualities obtained by the modern laparoscope. This is especially evident when performing sharp mesorectal excision within the confines of a deep and narrow pelvis [29-30]. In addition, the pneumoperitoneum facilitates dissection in between the loose areolar planes once the overlying pelvic peritoneum is incised [30]. Moreover, an abdominoperineal resection (APR) performed via the laparoscopic approach is particularly beneficial because there is no requirement for an extraction incision [31].

Nevertheless, laparoscopic proctectomy with a good quality, complete TME remains arguably one of the most technically challenging procedures to master in the field of colorectal surgery. One technical challenge lies in the difficulty in applying the laparoscopic staplers across the distal rectum for transection. The angles of articulation provided by the current staplers are still unable to reproduce the similar cross-stapling achievable using conventional open staplers [30]. This often results in multiple fires and overlapping cross-staple lines. These have been postulated to potentially increase the risks of tissue ischaemia and anastomotic leakage [30].

Table 3. Randomised trials comparing laparoscopic (L) and open (O) proctectomy for rectal cancer

Trial	Study period (year)	Cases	No. of patients (L vs. O)	Neoadjuvant therapy (L vs. O)	Operative time (L vs. O) (minutes)	Conversion	% positive CRM (L vs. O)	Hospital stay (L vs. O) (Days)	Morbidity (L vs. O) (%)	Mortality (L vs. O) (%)
CLASSIC [10]	1996–2002 (Multicentre)	AR and APR	253 : 128	-	180 vs. 135	34%	16 vs. 14	11 vs. 13	59 vs. 50	4 vs. 5
Zhou ZG [21]	2001 – 2002	Low AR	82 : 89	-	120 vs. 106	-	0 vs. 0	8.1 vs. 13*	6.1 vs. 12.4*	0 vs. 0
Braga M [22]	-	AR and APR	83 : 85	16.9 vs. 14.1	262 vs. 209*	7.2%	1.2 vs. 2.4	10.0 vs. 13.6*	28.9 vs. 40.0	1.2 vs. 1.2
Ng SS [23]	1994 – 2005	APR	51 : 48	0%	214 vs. 164*	9.8%	5.9 vs. 4.2	10.8 vs. 11.5	45.1 vs. 52.1	2.0 vs. 2.1
Lujan J [24]	2002 – 2007	AR and APR	101 : 103	72.3 vs. 74.8	194 vs. 173*	7.9%	4.0 vs. 2.9	8.2 vs. 9.9	33.7 vs. 33.0	1.9 vs. 2.9
COREAN [25]	2006 – 2009 (Multicentre)	AR and APR	170 : 170	100% vs. 100%	245 vs. 197*	1.2%	2.9 vs. 4.1	8 vs. 9	21.2 vs. 23.5	0 vs. 0

*: Statistically Significant,

Bladder and Sexual Function

Bladder and sexual dysfunctions are known complications of rectal surgery that are often under-reported. The CLASSIC trial demonstrated similar rates of bladder dysfunction in both open and laparoscopic groups but worse sexual function in the laparoscopic group [32]. The authors cited the higher proportions of TME and distal rectal tumours as possible explanations. Several other comparative series that evaluated the rates of autonomic dysfunction showed similar, if not lower, rates of bladder and sexual dysfunction in the laparoscopic group [33-35]. Like the findings of the CLASSIC trial, bulkier and/or distal rectal tumours requiring TME were associated with higher rates of autonomic dysfunction [33-35].

The role of laparoscopic proctectomy for rectal cancer remains controversial and will likely be determined by the outcomes of upcoming large multi-centre randomised trials such as the American College of Surgeons Oncology Group (ACOSOG) Z6051, COLOR II, Japanese Clinical Oncology Group (JCOG) Study 0404 and the Australasian Laparoscopic Cancer of the Rectum Trial (ALaCaRT). These results will be able to validate the various short and long-term patient-oriented and oncologic outcomes of the laparoscopic approach.

Technique and Approaches

Several well standardized approaches to the conduct of laparoscopic colorectal resections have been described in the literature [36-39]. The lateral-to-medial approach is similar to the steps performed in the open approach, typically beginning with the release of the lateral peritoneum attachments along the white line of Toldt. The dissection is continued medially, freeing the colon and its enveloping mesentery off the retroperitoneal attachments. Vital structures such as the ureters, duodenum, gonadal vessels and pancreatic tail are identified so as to avoid iatrogenic injury. The division of the vascular pedicles can be performed either with laparoscopic staples, energy sources or in between clips. Restoration of bowel continuity is then complete with the anastomosis performed either intracorporeally or extracorporeally.

Other surgeons prefer a medial-to-lateral approach where the vascular pedicles are approached from the midline, isolated and ligated before continuing the dissection laterally, again freeing the mesocolon off the retroperitoneum.

Some recent studies have supported the medial-to-lateral approach because of various reported benefits such as shorter operative time, and quicker convalescence while attaining similar oncologic outcome as the lateral-to-medial approach [36-39]. There have not been any demonstratable differences in the peri-operative complications and oncologic outcomes between the two groups.

The theoretical oncologic advantage of early ligation of the vascular pedicle to avoid haematogenous tumour dissemination is another purported benefit, although this has never been proven. It is widely accepted that the approach should be individualised and dependent on the training and preference of the surgeon.

Hand Assisted Laparoscopic Surgery (HALS)

Following the results of the major trials supporting laparoscopic colectomy for colon cancer, widespread adoption remained limited [40-41]. The main reason behind this has been postulated to be the complexity of the technique [41]. Firstly, the two-dimensional images obtained by the laparoscope results in the loss of depth perception. The inability to physically manipulate the colon not only decreases proprioception significantly, it also requires a certain level of laparoscopic expertise in the surgical assistants in order to provide optimal retraction and counter-traction. In addition, the need to operate in multiple quadrants of the abdominal cavity, perform intra-corporeal colonic anastomosis and manipulate bulkier tumours only makes the procedure even more difficult.

In order to overcome these initial difficulties whilst at the same time retain the benefits of laparoscopic surgery, the idea of placing a hand into the abdomen to facilitate the surgery was conceived in the early to mid 1990s by several surgeons such as Boland, Dunn and Ou [42-45]. This was termed hand-assisted laparoscopic surgery (HALS). HALS essentially bridges the differences between open and laparoscopic surgery. The fundamental difference in HALS for colorectal surgery is that the incision which is intended for the extraction of the specimen is created at the beginning of the procedure to allow for the introduction of the hand device [45-47]. This allows the surgeon to regain tactile propioception [45-47]. In addition, the fingers also help to provide adequate countertraction and retraction of surrounding structures to optimize the laparoscopic view. Having the hand of a surgeon who may not be a master in standard laparoscopic techniques in the peritoneal cavity invariably restores a certain amount of confidence when performing the procedure [47-50].

Over the past twenty years, HALS has evolved significantly with increased awareness and technological advancement. Before commercially manufactured hand-access devices were available, various inventive ideas for HALS included tightening of the fascia around the wrist of the inserted hand before pneumoperitoneum was created, and using specially made abdominal wall retractors to replicate pneumoperitoneum [45-47]. Once the benefits of HALS were reported in its initial stages, the first generation hand-access devices were manufactured and made available. These include the Dexterity PneumoSleeve™ (Blue Bell, PA, USA), Handport™ (Smith-Nephew PLC, London, *England*) and the Omniport™ (*Advanced Surgical Concepts* Ltd., Dublin, Ireland). These devices all shared similar designs in having a phalange to protect the wound with an adhesive securing the device to the abdominal wall. The surgeon's hand can then be inserted through the device into the abdomen without any loss of pneumoperitoneum.

Following wider adoption of HALS using the first generation hand-access devices, several shortcomings became apparent. These were addressed by the second-generation, multifunction, hand-access devices such as the GelPort™ (Applied Medical, Rancho Santa Margarita, CA, USA) and LapDisc™ (Ethicon, Endosurgery, Cincinnati, OH, USA). One significant improvement has been the ability to hold the device in place without the use of adhesives and not compromising the quality of the airseal from the seepage of blood/fluid under the seal. Another significant improvement is the multifunction capability of the second generation hand-access devices. Not only do they maintain pneumoperitoneum after the surgeon's hand is removed, they also permit the insertion of a laparoscopic trocar to enable the surgeon to perform standard laparoscopy if required.

Two randomised controlled trials and several other comparative studies between HALS and conventional laparoscopic resections have been performed [50-59] (Table 4). It would appear that HALS is able to achieve similar operative and oncologic outcomes, and at the same time, reduce the rates of conversions, and possibly shorten the operative times. Although the incision lengths reported for HALS were longer than those reported for conventional laparoscopic techniques, the clinical impact of this has been shown to be minimal and long term results did not demonstrate a higher rate of incisional hernia or small bowel obstruction [52]. Another reported benefit of HALS include the ability to perform more difficult or complex cases such as proctectomy or total colectomy, which would have been challenging using conventional laparoscopic techniques [60].

Recent comparative series have confirmed the feasibility of using HALS in various colorectal resections, from right and left-sided colectomies, to high and low anterior resections with complete TME [56 - 59]. A novel approach in utilising the hand-port as the end-colostomy site in HALS APR has also been described [61]. The analyses of the costs between the two techniques did not demonstrate any sizeable difference as the shorter operative time, fewer conversions and reduced number of trocars used in HALS were found to balance the additional cost of the hand-device [51, 53, 60].

Robotic Assisted Laparoscopic Surgery

With the increasing adoption of laparoscopy in abdominal surgery, several inherent limitations became apparent. These include the diminished freedom of motion, two-dimensional optics, rigid instrumentation, reduced depth perception and the dependence on skilled assistants to provide retraction, counter-traction and control the laparoscope [62-64]. With the success of robotics seen in the field of urology, there has been a growing interest in replicating the same success in colorectal surgery [65].

The benefits of robotic assisted laparoscopic surgery include the ability to provide three-dimensional and high resolution images, filtering of hand tremors, allowance for fine dexterity with a superior range of motion, and motion scaling. It also enables better manoeuvrability and precision of dissection especially in confined spaces [62-68]. These advantages are perhaps best exemplified in the performance of TME in rectal cancer within the confines of a deep and narrow pelvis [65-67]. Reports of a reduced CRM positivity rate and a more complete TME have been reported [63-64, 68].

Furthermore, the robotic technology facilitates intra-corporeal suturing, especially in instances such as performing suture rectopexy or repairing of the bladder defect following enbloc resections. The superior optics rendered enables better visualisation of the autonomic nerves thereby reducing the risk of damage during dissection [63-64]. This well accepted advantage of performing laparoscopic intracorporeal suturing and knotting has even led robotic surgeons to perform novel techniques of intracorporeal bowel anastomosis and extraction of resected specimens through natural orifices [64-65]. Another purported benefit is the ergonomic advantages presented by the robot. This reduces the surgeons' fatigue and potential injuries contributed by the unnatural positions often adopted in standard laparoscopy [63-64, 68].

Table 4. Comparison between HALS (H) and conventional laparoscopic (L) colectomy and/or proctectomy

Study	Study period (year)	No. of patients (H vs. L)	Operative time (H vs. L) (minutes)	Conversion to open (H vs. L) (%)	Incision size (H vs. L) (cm)	Hospital stay (H vs. L) (Days)	Morbidity (H vs. L) (%)
RCT							
Marcello [50]	2005–2006 (Multicentre)	47: 48	175 vs. 208*	2 vs. 12.5	8.2 vs. 6.1*	5.7 vs. 5.2	21 vs. 19
Targarona [51]	2001 – 2002	27: 27	120 vs. 135	7 vs. 22	-	7.2 vs. 6.5	26 vs. 23
Non-RCT							
Sonoda [52]	2001 – 2006	266: 270	225 vs. 180*	3 vs. 1.5	7.5 vs. 4.5*	6 vs. 5*	6.8 vs. 4.8 (Wound infection)
Ozturk [53]	2005 – 2008	100: 100	168 vs. 163	3 vs. 4	-	4 vs. 4	16 vs. 32*
Cima [54]	2003 – 2006	373: 596	242 vs. 258*	3.4 vs. 15.3*	-	6 vs. 5*	15.4 vs. 13.6
Hassan [55]	2004 – 2005	109: 149	277 vs. 211*	15 vs. 11	-	6 vs. 5*	18 vs. 11
Vogel [56] (Right colectomy)	2006 – 2009	43: 84	122 vs. 126	5 vs. 6	-	5 vs. 5	30 vs. 30
Chang [57] (Sigmoid colectomy)	1997 – 2003	66: 85	189 vs. 205	0 vs. 13*	8.1 vs. 6.2*	5.2 vs. 5	21 vs. 23
Yun [58] (High anterior resection)	2000 -2006	118: 128	148 vs. 161*	2.5 vs. 3.1	-	7.5 vs. 7.3	5.9 vs. 3.9
Tjandra [59] (Ultralow anterior resection)	2005 – 2006	32: 31	170 vs. 188*	0 vs. 0	7.6 vs. 4.9*	5.9 vs. 5.8	31.3 vs. 25.8

*: Statistically Significant.

Table 5. Comparative studies between robotically assisted (R) and conventional laparoscopic (L) colectomy and/or proctectomy

Study	Study period (year)	No. of patients (R vs. L)	Operative time (R vs. L) (minutes)	Conversion to open (R vs. L) (%)	Hospital stay (R vs. L) (Days)	Morbidity (R vs. L) (%)
RCT Baik [67] (Low anterior resection)	2006 – 2007	18:16	203 vs.196	0 vs. 11.1	7 vs. 9*	22.2 vs. 5.5
Non-RCT Park [70] (Low anterior resection)	2007 – 2009	41: 82	232 vs. 169*	0 vs. 0	9.9 vs. 9.4	29.3 vs. 23.2
D'Annibale [71]	2001 – 2003	53: 53	240 vs. 222	11.3 vs. 5.7	10 vs. 10	16 vs. 32*
Rawlings [72] (Right colectomy)	2002 – 2005	17: 15	210 vs. 160*	0 vs. 13.3	4 vs. 4	5.9 vs. 13.3
Rawlings [72] (Sigmoid colectomy)	2002 – 2005	13: 12	226 vs. 198	15.4 vs. 0	4 vs. 4.5	38.5 vs. 16.7
Spinoglio [73] (Right colectomy)	2005 – 2007	50: 161	384 vs. 266*	4 vs. 4	7.7 vs. 8.3	14 vs. 17

*: Statistically Significant.

Ever since the first robotic assisted colectomy was performed in 2002, several comparative studies have been performed evaluating robotic assisted and conventional laparoscopic colorectal resections (Table 5) [67, 70-73]. All these demonstrated comparable patient-oriented and operative outcomes between the two groups. However, the long-term outcomes of robotic assisted resections for colorectal cancer remain to be seen.

Despite the reported benefits, several limitations need to be addressed before the increased adoption of the robotic technology can be seen. First and foremost, the significant start-up cost of acquiring the robot and the consumables remains a major impediment. Secondly, the significantly lengthier operative times with robotic approaches have also added to the total costs and proven to be a major deterrent to many interested surgeons. Suffice to say, while robotic assisted colorectal resections have been proven to be feasible and safe when performed by experienced surgeons, until well conducted randomised trials conclusively demonstrate significant benefits of robotically assisted laparoscopic colorectal resections, its adoption will remain low and confined to centers with the financial and technical abilities to afford it. Trials are ongoing to compare the quality of TME, bladder and sexual dysfunction, short and long-term differences between laparoscopic and robotic approaches.

Single Port Access Surgery

The benefits and successes noted with laparoscopic colorectal surgery spurred surgeons to look for approaches that require fewer or smaller trocars. This led to the introduction of single port access surgery in the field of colorectal surgery [74-75].

The basic principle of single port access surgery is to have all the laparoscopic working ports and the laparoscope entering the abdominal cavity through a single incision, often placed around the umbilicus [76]. With laparoscopic instruments converging towards a central point at the level of the abdominal wall, new technical challenges were encountered. These included the loss of triangulation and the 'criss-crossing' of the instruments either intra- or extra-corporeally creating what is often described as the 'chopstick' effect [74-78]. This has resulted in the development of articulating instruments which help to overcome these limitations [74-78]. And to overcome the loss of triangulation, the insertion of intra-abdominal sutures as a sling or more recently, the use of magnets placed on the abdominal wall to facilitate intracorporeal retraction with bowel clips have been described [76, 79-80].

The development of the flexible tip laparoscopes such as the EndoEYE (Olympus Surgical and Industrial America Inc, Center Valley, PA, USA) and the use of bariatric length laparoscopes to keep the instrument handles at varying levels have enabled the surgeon to experience less collisions extracorporeally as well [76, 79].

Single incision surgery began with surgeons inserting several trocars adjacent to each other through a small single incision around the umbilicus [81-82]. Since then, numerous single port access devices have been designed and manufactured, and made commercially available. These include the Triport or QuadPort (Advanced Surgical Concepts, Wicklow, Ireland), AirSeal (SurgiQuest, Orange, CT, USA), SILS port (Covidien, Inc, Norwalk, CT, USA), Uni-X Single-Port Access Laparoscopic System (Covidien, Inc, Norwalk, CT, USA), GelPoint (Applied Medical, Rancho Santa Margarita, CA, USA) and the SSL Access System (Ethicon Endo-Surgery, Inc, Cincinnati, OH, USA). Each device brings with it its own uniqueness and limitations [76, 79].

Beginning with initial case reports and small case series demonstrating the safety and feasibility of performing colectomy through the single port device in benign conditions, recent studies comparing single port access surgery to standard laparoscopic techniques in the management of colon cancer have begun to emerge [83-88].

The operative time for single port access surgery have been reported to be slightly longer. Conversions from this technique can often be to conventional laparoscopy by inserting additional trocars or even to HALS, instead of the traditional lengthy abdominal incisions [83-88]. These reports also did not demonstrate any significant differences in the resection margin positivity rate and number of lymph nodes harvested in oncologic resections. There was also no increased morbidity associated with this new technique. Some advantages reported include significantly smaller incision lengths, less narcotic usage and shorter lengths of stay [86-88].

Until maturing data emerge, the question that remains unanswered is whether technical feasibility should translate to widespread adoption.

Laparoscopy for Emergency Indications

Practising colorectal surgeons often encounter patients who present with acute complications arising from colorectal cancers. These include bowel obstruction and perforation on presentation, and adhesive intestinal obstruction and anastomotic leaks after prior surgery. Whilst open surgery in these situations remains the norm, several studies have demonstrated the safety and feasibility of adopting the laparoscopic approach in selected patients [89-93]. The only comparative study between emergency laparoscopic and open surgery for obstructed right sided colon cancers demonstrated a longer operative time but reduced blood loss in the laparoscopic group. Although the laparoscopic group did not demonstrate a shorter hospital stay, fewer post-operative complications were seen in this group [94].

Apart from the technically simpler laparoscopic proximal diverting loop enterostomy/colostomy for obstructing colorectal cancers, emergency laparoscopic colectomies for complications of colon cancers such as obstruction, haemorrhage and perforation have also been performed [93, 95-96]. Laparoscopic adhesiolysis for post-colectomy adhesive small bowel obstruction has also been shown to be safe and feasible [97-99]. Laparoscopic reversal of Hartmann's procedures has been associated with a shorter hospital stay and lower morbidity rate [100].

In recent years, the role of laparoscopy has been extended to the management of anastomotic leaks. Apart from being able to accurately diagnose the leak and enable copious irrigation, the creation of a proximal stoma can be performed laparoscopically in instances where the size of the anastomotic dehiscence is small [101-102]. In the hands of experienced laparoscopic colorectal surgeons, laparoscopic revision or re-anastomosis for anastomotic dehiscence can be performed with good outcome, preventing the need of a lengthy abdominal incision.

Sound clinical judgement, appropriate patient selection and advanced laparoscopic skills are all essential before adopting laparoscopy for the management of colorectal cancers in the emergency setting.

Conclusions

The role of laparoscopy in the surgical management of colorectal cancer is expanding. It continues to evolve in so many aspects and is likely to become an integral part of the colorectal surgeon's armamentarium in the management of these cancers.

References

[1] Monson JR, Hill AD, Darzi A. Laparoscopic colonic surgery. *Br. J. Surg.* 1995 Feb; 82(2): 150-7.

[2] Monson JR. Advanced techniques in abdominal surgery. *BMJ.* 1993 Nov; 307(6915): 1346-50.

[3] Hoffman GC, Baker JW, Doxey JB, Hubbard GW, Ruffin WK, Wishner JA. Minimally invasive surgery for colorectal cancer. Initial follow-up. *Ann. Surg.* 1996 Jun; 223(6): 790-6.

[4] Bleday R, Babineau T, Forse RA. Laparoscopic surgery for colon and rectal cancer. *Semin Surg Oncol.* 1993 Jan-Feb; 9(1): 59-64.

[5] Koopmann MC, Heise CP. Laparoscopic and minimally invasive resection of malignant colorectal disease. *Surg. Clin. North Am.* 2008 Oct; 88(5): 1047-72.

[6]   Lacy AM, García-Valdecasas JC, Delgado S, Castells A, Taurá P, Piqué JM, Visa J.
        Laparoscopy-assisted colectomy versus open colectomy for treatment of non-metastatic
        colon cancer: a randomised trial. *Lancet.* 2002 Jun 29; 359(9325): 2224-9.

[7]   Lacy AM, Delgado S, Castells A, Prins HA, Arroyo V, Ibarzabal A, Pique JM. The
        long-term results of a randomized clinical trial of laparoscopy-assisted versus open
        surgery for colon cancer. *Ann. Surg.* 2008 Jul; 248(1): 1-7.

[8]   Clinical Outcomes of Surgical Therapy Study Group. A comparison of laparoscopically
        assisted and open colectomy for colon cancer. *N. Engl. J. Med.* 2004 May; 350(20):
        2050-9.

[9]   Fleshman J, Sargent DJ, Green E, Anvari M, Stryker SJ, Beart RW Jr, Hellinger M,
        Flanagan R Jr, Peters W, Nelson H; for The Clinical Outcomes of Surgical Therapy
        Study Group. Laparoscopic colectomy for cancer is not inferior to open surgery based
        on 5-year data from the COST Study Group trial. *Ann. Surg.* 2007 Oct; 246(4): 655-62.

[10]   Guillou PJ, Quirke P, Thorpe H, Walker J, Jayne DG, Smith AM, Heath RM, Brown
        JM; MRC CLASICC trial group. Short-term endpoints of conventional versus
        laparoscopic-assisted surgery in patients with colorectal cancer (MRC CLASICC trial):
        multicentre, randomised controlled trial. *Lancet.* 2005 May; 365(9472): 1718-26.

[11]   Jayne DG, Thorpe HC, Copeland J, Quirke P, Brown JM, Guillou PJ. Five-year follow-
        up of the Medical Research Council CLASICC trial of laparoscopically assisted versus
        open surgery for colorectal cancer. *Br. J. Surg.* 2010 Nov; 97(11): 1638-45.

[12]   Veldkamp R, Kuhry E, Hop WC, Jeekel J, Kazemier G, Bonjer HJ, Haglind E, Påhlman
        L, Cuesta MA, Msika S, Morino M, Lacy AM; COlon cancer Laparoscopic or Open
        Resection Study Group (COLOR). Laparoscopic surgery versus open surgery for colon
        cancer: short-term outcomes of a randomised trial. *Lancet Oncol.* 2005 Jul; 6(7): 477-
        84.

[13]   Colon Cancer Laparoscopic or Open Resection Study Group, Buunen M, Veldkamp R,
        Hop WC, Kuhry E, Jeekel J, Haglind E, Påhlman L, Cuesta MA, Msika S, Morino M,
        Lacy A, Bonjer HJ. Survival after laparoscopic surgery versus open surgery for colon
        cancer: long-term outcome of a randomised clinical trial. *Lancet Oncol.* 2009 Jan;
        10(1): 44-52.

[14]   Bilimoria KY, Bentrem DJ, Merkow RP, Nelson H, Wang E, Ko CY, Soper NJ.
        Laparoscopic-assisted vs. open colectomy for cancer: comparison of short-term
        outcomes from 121 hospitals. *J. Gastrointest. Surg.* 2008 Nov; 12(11): 2001-9.

[15]   Tjandra JJ, Chan MK. Systematic review on the short-term outcome of laparoscopic
        resection for colon and rectosigmoid cancer. *Colorectal. Dis.* 2006 Jun; 8(5): 375-88.

[16]   Bilimoria KY, Bentrem DJ, Nelson H, Stryker SJ, Stewart AK, Soper NJ, Russell TR,
        Ko CY. Use and outcomes of laparoscopic-assisted colectomy for cancer in the United
        States. *Arch. Surg.* 2008 Sep; 143(9): 832-9.

[17]   Kennedy GD, Heise C, Rajamanickam V, Harms B, Foley EF. Laparoscopy decreases
        postoperative complication rates after abdominal colectomy: results from the national
        surgical quality improvement program. *Ann. Surg.* 2009 Apr; 249(4): 596-601.

[18]   Wexner SD, Cohen SM, Ulrich A, Reissman P. Laparoscopic colorectal surgery - are
        we being honest with our patients? *Dis. Colon. Rectum.* 1995 Jul; 38(7): 723-7.

[19]   Cirocco WC, Schwartzman A, Golub RW. Abdominal wall recurrence after
        laparoscopic colectomy for colon cancer. *Surgery.* 1994 Nov; 116(5): 842-6.

[20] Bonjer HJ, Hop WC, Nelson H, Sargent DJ, Lacy AM, Castells A, Guillou PJ, Thorpe H, Brown J, Delgado S, Kuhrij E, Haglind E, Påhlman L; Transatlantic Laparoscopically Assisted vs Open Colectomy Trials Study Group. Laparoscopically assisted vs. open colectomy for colon cancer: a meta-analysis. *Arch. Surg.* 2007 Mar; 142(3): 298-303.

[21] Zhou ZG, Hu M, Li Y, Lei WZ, Yu YY, Cheng Z, Li L, Shu Y, Wang TC. Laparoscopic versus open total mesorectal excision with anal sphincter preservation for low rectal cancer. *Surg. Endosc.* 2004 Aug; 18(8): 1211-5.

[22] Braga M, Frasson M, Vignali A, Zuliani W, Capretti G, Di Carlo V. Laparoscopic resection in rectal cancer patients: outcome and cost-benefit analysis. *Dis. Colon. Rectum.* 2007 Apr; 50(4): 464-71.

[23] Ng SS, Leung KL, Lee JF, Yiu RY, Li JC, Teoh AY, Leung WW. Laparoscopic-assisted versus open abdominoperineal resection for low rectal cancer: a prospective randomized trial. *Ann. Surg. Oncol.* 2008 Sep; 15(9): 2418-25.

[24] Lujan J, Valero G, Hernandez Q, Sanchez A, Frutos MD, Parrilla P. Randomized clinical trial comparing laparoscopic and open surgery in patients with rectal cancer. *Br. J. Surg.* 2009 Sep; 96(9): 982-9.

[25] Kang SB, Park JW, Jeong SY, Nam BH, Choi HS, Kim DW, Lim SB, Lee TG, Kim DY, Kim JS, Chang HJ, Lee HS, Kim SY, Jung KH, Hong YS, Kim JH, Sohn DK, Kim DH, Oh JH. Open versus laparoscopic surgery for mid or low rectal cancer after neoadjuvant chemoradiotherapy (COREAN trial): short-term outcomes of an open-label randomised controlled trial. *Lancet Oncol.* 2010 Jul; 11(7): 637-45.

[26] Nandakumar G, Fleshman JW. Laparoscopy for rectal cancer. *Surg. Oncol. Clin. N. Am.* 2010 Oct; 19(4): 793-802.

[27] Aziz O, Constantinides V, Tekkis PP, Athanasiou T, Purkayastha S, Paraskeva P, Darzi AW, Heriot AG. Laparoscopic versus open surgery for rectal cancer: a meta-analysis. *Ann. Surg. Oncol.* 2006 Mar; 13(3): 413-24.

[28] Breukink S, Pierie J, Wiggers T. Laparoscopic versus open total mesorectal excision for rectal cancer. *Cochrane Database Syst. Rev.* 2006 Oct; 4:CD005200.

[29] Gouvas N, Tsiaoussis J, Pechlivanides G, Tzortzinis A, Dervenis C, Avgerinos C, Xynos E. Quality of surgery for rectal carcinoma: comparison between open and laparoscopic approaches. *Am. J. Surg.* 2009 Nov; 198(5): 702-8.

[30] Safar B, Fleshman JW. Laparoscopic total mesorectal excision for rectal cancer. *Semin Colon Rectal Surg* 2010 June; 21(2): 75-80.

[31] Fleshman JW, Wexner SD, Anvari M, LaTulippe JF, Birnbaum EH, Kodner IJ, Read TE, Nogueras JJ, Weiss EG. Laparoscopic vs. open abdominoperineal resection for cancer. *Dis. Colon. Rectum.* 1999 Jul; 42(7): 930-9.

[32] Jayne DG, Brown JM, Thorpe H, Walker J, Quirke P, Guillou PJ. Bladder and sexual function following resection for rectal cancer in a randomized clinical trial of laparoscopic versus open technique. *Br. J. Surg.* 2005 Sep; 92(9): 1124-32.

[33] Morino M, Parini U, Allaix ME, Monasterolo G, Brachet Contul R, Garrone C. Male sexual and urinary function after laparoscopic total mesorectal excision. *Surg. Endosc.* 2009 Jun; 23(6): 1233-40

[34] Nitori N, Hasegawa H, Ishii Y, Endo T, Kitajima M, Kitagawa Y. Sexual function in men with rectal and rectosigmoid cancer after laparoscopic and open surgery. *Hepatogastroenterology.* 2008 Jul-Aug; 55(85): 1304-7.

[35] Asoglu O, Matlim T, Karanlik H, Atar M, Muslumanoglu M, Kapran Y, Igci A, Ozmen V, Kecer M, Parlak M. Impact of laparoscopic surgery on bladder and sexual function after total mesorectal excision for rectal cancer. *Surg. Endosc.* 2009 Feb; 23(2): 296-303.

[36] Poon JT, Law WL, Fan JK, Lo OS. Impact of the standardized medial-to-lateral approach on outcome of laparoscopic colorectal resection. *World J. Surg.* 2009 Oct; 33(10): 2177-82.

[37] Liang JT, Lai HS, Huang KC, Chang KJ, Shieh MJ, Jeng YM, Wang SM. Comparison of medial-to-lateral versus traditional lateral-to-medial laparoscopic dissection sequences for resection of rectosigmoid cancers: randomized controlled clinical trial. *World J. Surg.* 2003 Feb; 27(2): 190-6.

[38] Pigazzi A, Hellan M, Ewing DR, Paz BI, Ballantyne GH. Laparoscopic medial-to-lateral colon dissection: how and why. *J. Gastrointest. Surg.* 2007 Jun; 11(6): 778-82.

[39] Rotholtz NA, Bun ME, Tessio M, Lencinas SM, Laporte M, Aued ML, Peczan CE, Mezzadri NA. Laparoscopic colectomy: medial versus lateral approach. *Surg. Laparosc Endosc. Percutan. Tech.* 2009 Feb; 19(1): 43-7.

[40] Kemp JA, Finlayson SR. Nationwide trends in laparoscopic colectomy from 2000 to 2004. *Surg. Endosc.* 2008 May; 22(5): 1181-7.

[41] Marcello PW. Hand-assisted laparoscopic colectomy: a helping hand? *Clin Colon Rectal Surg.* 2004 May; 17(2): 125-9.

[42] Boland JP, Kusminsky RE, Tiley EH. Laparoscopic minilaparotomy with manipulation: the middle path. *Minim. Invasive Ther.* 1993; 2: 63–7.

[43] Dunn DC. Digitally assisted laparoscopic surgery. *Br. J. Surg.* 1994; 81: 474.

[44] Ou H. Laparoscopic-assisted mini laparotomy with colectomy. *Dis. Colon. Rectum* 1995; 38: 324–6.

[45] Ballantyne GH, Leahy PF. Hand-assisted laparoscopic colectomy: evolution to a clinically useful technique. *Dis. Colon. Rectum.* 2004 May; 47(5): 753-65.

[46] Iqbal M, Bhalerao S. Current status of hand-assisted laparoscopic colorectal surgery: a review. *J. Laparoendosc Adv. Surg. Tech. A.* 2007 Apr; 17(2): 172-9.

[47] Loungnarath R, Fleshman JW. Hand-assisted laparoscopic colectomy techniques. *Semin Laparosc Surg.* 2003 Dec; 10(4): 219-30.

[48] Schlachta CM, Mamazza J, Seshadri PA, Cadeddu M, Gregoire R, Poulin EC. Defining a learning curve for laparoscopic colorectal resections. *Dis. Colon. Rectum.* 2001 Feb; 44(2): 217-22.

[49] Kavic MS. Hand-assisted laparoscopic surgery (HALS): a bridge to complex laparoscopic procedures. *JSLS.* 2005 Apr-Jun; 9(2): 123-4.

[50] Marcello PW, Fleshman JW, Milsom JW, Read TE, Arnell TD, Birnbaum EH, Feingold DL, Lee SW, Mutch MG, Sonoda T, Yan Y, Whelan RL. Hand-assisted laparoscopic vs. laparoscopic colorectal surgery: a multicenter, prospective, randomized trial. *Dis. Colon. Rectum.* 2008 Jun; 51(6): 818-26.

[51] Targarona EM, Gracia E, Garriga J, Martínez-Bru C, Cortés M, Boluda R, Lerma L, Trías M. Prospective randomized trial comparing conventional laparoscopic colectomy with hand-assisted laparoscopic colectomy: applicability, immediate clinical outcome, inflammatory response, and cost. *Surg. Endosc.* 2002 Feb; 16(2): 234-9.

[52] Sonoda T, Pandey S, Trencheva K, Lee S, Milsom J. Longterm complications of hand-assisted versus laparoscopic colectomy. *J. Am. Coll Surg.* 2009 Jan; 208(1): 62-6.

[53] Ozturk E, Kiran RP, Geisler DP, Hull TL, Vogel JD. Hand-assisted laparoscopic colectomy: benefits of laparoscopic colectomy at no extra cost. *J. Am. Coll Surg.* 2009 Aug; 209(2): 242-7.

[54] Cima RR, Pattana-arun J, Larson DW, Dozois EJ, Wolff BG, Pemberton JH. Experience with 969 minimal access colectomies: the role of hand-assisted laparoscopy in expanding minimally invasive surgery for complex colectomies. *J. Am. Coll Surg.* 2008 May; 206(5): 946-50.

[55] Hassan I, You YN, Cima RR, Larson DW, Dozois EJ, Barnes SA, Pemberton JH. Hand-assisted versus laparoscopic-assisted colorectal surgery: Practice patterns and clinical outcomes in a minimally-invasive colorectal practice. *Surg. Endosc.* 2008 Mar; 22(3): 739-43.

[56] Vogel JD, Lian L, Kalady MF, de Campos-Lobato LF, Alves-Ferreira PC, Remzi FH. Hand-assisted laparoscopic right colectomy: how does it compare to conventional laparoscopy? *J. Am. Coll Surg.* 2011 Mar; 212(3): 367-72.

[57] Chang YJ, Marcello PW, Rusin LC, Roberts PL, Schoetz DJ. Hand-assisted laparoscopic sigmoid colectomy: helping hand or hindrance? *Surg. Endosc.* 2005 May; 19(5): 656-61.

[58] Yun HR, Cho YK, Cho YB, Kim HC, Yun SH, Lee WY, Chun HK. Comparison and short-term outcomes between hand-assisted laparoscopic surgery and conventional laparoscopic surgery for anterior resections of left-sided colon cancer. *Int J Colorectal Dis.* 2010 Aug; 25(8): 975-81.

[59] Tjandra JJ, Chan MK, Yeh CH. Laparoscopic- vs. hand-assisted ultralow anterior resection: a prospective study. *Dis. Colon. Rectum.* 2008 Jan; 51(1): 26-31.

[60] Aalbers AG, Biere SS, van Berge Henegouwen MI, Bemelman WA. Hand-assisted or laparoscopic-assisted approach in colorectal surgery: a systematic review and meta-analysis. *Surg. Endosc.* 2008 Aug; 22(8): 1769-80.

[61] Koh DC, Law CW, Kristian I, Cheong WK, Tsang CB. Hand-assisted laparoscopic abdomino-perineal resection utilizing the planned end colostomy site. *Tech. Coloproctol.* 2010 Jun; 14(2): 201-6.

[62] Zimmern A, Prasad L, Desouza A, Marecik S, Park J, Abcarian H. Robotic colon and rectal surgery: a series of 131 cases. *World J. Surg.* 2010; 34(8): 1954-8.

[63] Pigazzi A, Garcia-Aguilar J. Robotic colorectal surgery: for whom and for what? *Dis. Colon. Rectum.* 2010; 53(7): 969-70.

[64] Mirnezami AH, Mirnezami R, Venkatasubramaniam AK, Chandrakumaran K, Cecil TD, Moran BJ. Robotic colorectal surgery: hype or new hope? A systematic review of robotics in colorectal surgery. *Colorectal Dis.* 2010 Nov; 12(11): 1084-93.

[65] Baik SH. Robotic colorectal surgery. *Yonsei Med. J.* 2008 Dec 31; 49(6): 891-6.

[66] Delaney CP, Lynch AC, Senagore AJ, Fazio VW. Comparison of robotically performed and traditional laparoscopic colorectal surgery. *Dis. Colon. Rectum.* 2003; 46(12): 1633-9.

[67] Baik SH, Kwon HY, Kim JS, Hur H, Sohn SK, Cho CH, Kim H. Robotic versus laparoscopic low anterior resection of rectal cancer: short-term outcome of a prospective comparative study. *Ann. Surg. Oncol.* 2009; 16(6): 1480-7.

[68] Pigazzi A, Luca F, Patriti A, Valvo M, Ceccarelli G, Casciola L, Biffi R, Garcia-Aguilar J, Baek JH. Multicentric study on robotic tumor-specific mesorectal excision for the treatment of rectal cancer. *Ann. Surg. Oncol.* 2010; 17(6): 1614-20.

[69] Weber PA, Merola S, Wasielewski A, Ballantyne GH. Telerobotic-assisted laparoscopic right and sigmoid colectomies for benign disease. *Dis. Colon. Rectum.* 2002 Dec; 45(12): 1689-94.

[70] Park JS, Choi GS, Lim KH, Jang YS, Jun SH. Robotic-assisted versus laparoscopic surgery for low rectal cancer: case-matched analysis of short-term outcomes. *Ann. Surg. Oncol.* 2010 Dec; 17(12): 3195-202.

[71] D'Annibale A, Morpurgo E, Fiscon V, Trevisan P, Sovernigo G, Orsini C, Guidolin D. Robotic and laparoscopic surgery for treatment of colorectal diseases. *Dis. Colon. Rectum.* 2004 Dec; 47(12): 2162-8.

[72] Rawlings AL, Woodland JH, Vegunta RK, Crawford DL. Robotic versus laparoscopic colectomy. *Surg. Endosc.* 2007; 21(10): 1701-8.

[73] Spinoglio G, Summa M, Priora F, Quarati R, Testa S. Robotic colorectal surgery: first 50 cases experience. *Dis. Colon. Rectum.* 2008; 51(11): 1627-32.

[74] Remzi FH, Kirat HT, Kaouk JH, Geisler DP. Single-port laparoscopy in colorectal surgery. *Colorectal Dis.* 2008 Oct; 10(8): 823-6.

[75] Romanelli JR, Earle DB. Single-port laparoscopic surgery: an overview. *Surg. Endosc.* 2009 Jul; 23(7): 1419-27.

[76] Tsai AY, Selzer DJ. Single-port laparoscopic surgery. *Adv. Surg.* 2010; 44: 1-27.

[77] Remzi FH, Kirat HT, Geisler DP. Laparoscopic single-port colectomy for sigmoid cancer. *Tech. Coloproctol.* 2010 Sep; 14(3): 253-5.

[78] Ross H, Steele S, Whiteford M, Lee S, Albert M, Mutch M, Rivadeneira D, Marcello P. Early multi-institution experience with single-incision laparoscopic colectomy. *Dis. Colon. Rectum.* 2011 Feb; 54(2): 187-92.

[79] Canes D, Desai MM, Aron M, Haber GP, Goel RK, Stein RJ, Kaouk JH, Gill IS. Transumbilical single-port surgery: evolution and current status. *Eur. Urol.* 2008 Nov; 54(5): 1020-9.

[80] Uematsu D, Akiyama G, Narita M, Magishi A. Single-access laparoscopic low anterior resection with vertical suspension of the rectum. *Dis. Colon. Rectum.* 2011 May; 54(5): 632-7.

[81] Navarra G, Pozza E, Occhionorelli S, Carcoforo P, Donini I. One-wound laparoscopic cholecystectomy. *Br. J. Surg.* 1997 May; 84(5): 695.

[82] Piskun G, Rajpal S. Transumbilical laparoscopic cholecystectomy utilizes no incisions outside the umbilicus. *J. Laparoendosc Adv. Surg. Tech. A.* 1999 Aug; 9(4): 361-4.

[83] Waters JA, Guzman MJ, Fajardo AD, Selzer DJ, Wiebke EA, Robb BW, George VV. Single-port laparoscopic right hemicolectomy: a safe alternative to conventional laparoscopy. *Dis. Colon. Rectum.* 2010 Nov; 53(11): 1467-72.

[84] Champagne BJ, Lee EC, Leblanc F, Stein SL, Delaney CP. Single-incision vs straight laparoscopic segmental colectomy: a case-controlled study. *Dis. Colon. Rectum.* 2011 Feb; 54(2): 183-6.

[85] Adair J, Gromski MA, Lim RB, Nagle D. Single-incision laparoscopic right colectomy: experience with 17 consecutive cases and comparison with multiport laparoscopic right colectomy. *Dis. Colon. Rectum.* 2010 Nov; 53(11): 1549-54.

[86] Papaconstantinou HT, Sharp N, Thomas JS. Single-Incision Laparoscopic Right Colectomy: A Case-Matched Comparison with Standard Laparoscopic and Hand-Assisted Laparoscopic Techniques. *J. Am. Coll Surg.* 2011 Mar (Electronic Publication).

[87]   Gandhi DP, Ragupathi M, Patel CB, Ramos-Valadez DI, Pickron TB, Haas EM. Single-incision versus hand-assisted laparoscopic colectomy: a case-matched series. *J. Gastrointest Surg.* 2010 Dec; 14(12): 1875-80.

[88]   Chen WT, Chang SC, Chiang HC, Lo WY, Jeng LB, Wu C, Ke TW. Single-incision laparoscopic versus conventional laparoscopic right hemicolectomy: a comparison of short-term surgical results. *Surg. Endosc.* 2011 Feb. 2011 Jun;25(6):1887-92.

[89]   Marohn MR, Hanly EJ, McKenna KJ, Varin CR. Laparoscopic total abdominal colectomy in the acute setting. *J. Gastrointest Surg.* 2005; 9(7): 881-6.

[90]   White SI, Frenkiel B, Martin PJ. A ten-year audit of perforated sigmoid diverticulitis: highlighting the outcomes of laparoscopic lavage. *Dis. Colon. Rectum.* 2010 Nov; 53(11): 1537-41.

[91]   Champagne B, Stulberg JJ, Fan Z, Delaney CP. The feasibility of laparoscopic colectomy in urgent and emergent settings. *Surg. Endosc.* 2009 Aug; 23(8): 1791-6.

[92]   Stulberg JJ, Champagne BJ, Fan Z, Horan M, Obias V, Marderstein E, Reynolds H, Delaney CP. Emergency laparoscopic colectomy: does it measure up to open? *Am. J. Surg.* 2009 Mar; 197(3): 296-301.

[93]   Nash GM, Bleier J, Milsom JW, Trencheva K, Sonoda T, Lee SW. Minimally invasive surgery is safe and effective for urgent and emergent colectomy. *Colorectal Dis.* 2010 May; 12(5): 480-4.

[94]   Ng SS, Lee JF, Yiu RY, Li JC, Leung WW, Leung KL. Emergency laparoscopic-assisted versus open right hemicolectomy for obstructing right-sided colonic carcinoma: a comparative study of short-term clinical outcomes. *World J. Surg.* 2008 Mar; 32(3): 454-8.

[95]   Gash K, Chambers W, Ghosh A, Dixon AR. The role of laparoscopic surgery for the management of acute large bowel obstruction. *Colorectal Dis.* 2011 Mar; 13(3): 263-6.

[96]   Gonzalez R, Smith CD, Ritter EM, Mason E, Duncan T, Ramshaw BJ. Laparoscopic palliative surgery for complicated colorectal cancer. *Surg. Endosc.* 2005 Jan; 19(1): 43-6.

[97]   Szomstein S, Lo Menzo E, Simpfendorfer C, Zundel N, Rosenthal RJ. Laparoscopic lysis of adhesions. *World J. Surg.* 2006 Apr; 30(4): 535-40.

[98]   Wang Q, Hu ZQ, Wang WJ, Zhang J, Wang Y, Ruan CP. Laparoscopic management of recurrent adhesive small-bowel obstruction: Long-term follow-up. *Surg. Today.* 2009; 39(6): 493-9.

[99]   Kirshtein B, Roy-Shapira A, Lantsberg L, Avinoach E, Mizrahi S. Laparoscopic management of acute small bowel obstruction. *Surg. Endosc.* 2005 Apr; 19(4): 464-7.

[100] van de Wall BJ, Draaisma WA, Schouten ES, Broeders IA, Consten EC. Conventional and laparoscopic reversal of the Hartmann procedure: a review of literature. *J. Gastrointest Surg.* 2010 Apr; 14(4): 743-52.

[101] Pera M, Delgado S, García-Valdecasas JC, Pera M, Castells A, Piqué JM, Bombuy E, Lacy AM. The management of leaking rectal anastomoses by minimally invasive techniques. *Surg. Endosc.* 2002 Apr; 16(4): 603-6.

[102] Joh YG, Kim SH, Hahn KY, Stulberg J, Chung CS, Lee DK. Anastomotic leakage after laparoscopic protectomy can be managed by a minimally invasive approach. *Dis. Colon. Rectum.* 2009 Jan; 52(1): 91-6.

In: Laparoscopy: New Developments, Procedures and Risks   ISBN: 978-1-61470-747-9
Editor: Hana Terzic, pp. 185-203   © 2012 Nova SciencePublishers, Inc.

Chapter VIII

Laparoscopic Splenectomy

Ji Chung Tham, ConalQuah and Basil Ammori

Department of Surgery at North Manchester General Hospital,
Manchester, United Kingdom.

Abstract

Splenectomy is performed for various conditions such as benign and malignant haematological diseases, secondary hypersplenism and trauma. The first laparoscopic splenectomy (LS) was reported in 1991 [1], and the advances in minimally invasive surgery have given surgeons the option to perform the LS safely in both children and adults.

The current literature of comparative studies provide evidence that the laparoscopic approach to splenectomy offers advantages over open surgery in terms of reduced postoperative pain and complication rate, better cosmesis and shorter hospital stayas well as quicker recovery of gastrointestinal function [2-4] and reduced need for blood transfusion. Moreover, when quality of life was measured with the SF-36 survey, the laparoscopic approach to splenectomy was associated with better 'general health' and 'physical functioning' and lesser 'bodily pain' postoperatively compared to open surgery [5]. Although, the early experience with LS suggested that the laparoscopic approach was only safe for normal to mildly enlarged spleens, more recent evidence has shown the technique to be safe and beneficial in patients with massive and 'supramassive' (length >22cm and weight >1600g) spleen [6]. Additionally, the laparoscopic approach did not compromise the intraoperative assessment and detection of accessory spleen compared to open surgery [7]. In high volume centres, the laparoscopic approach to splenectomy was either of equal cost [2] or offered cost savings compared to open surgery [8].

As with any operative procedure, there are numerous considerations to be undertaken before performing this procedure and care should be taken when carrying it out on children and pregnant patients. Methods to search for the evasive splenunculi, pre-operatively, remain to be perfected and are yet to be vigorously tested and benefits of the radiological-guided splenic artery embolisation remains unclear.

LS should be classified as the gold standard procedure and the open splenectomy should only be done if absolutely necessary.

Introduction

Delaitre and Maignien [1] reported the first laparoscopic splenectomy(LS) in 1991 and since then the gold standard for splenectomies are done by laparoscopy. There has been debate regarding the benefits of laparoscopic surgery, not only for splenectomies but also for cholecystectomies and liver resections. Recent advances in minimally invasive surgery have enabled the procedure to be done with ease and must be considered in every case. The minimally invasive approach is as safe as the open approach but more importantly are the advantages it offers. This includes quicker recovery, better quality of life and comparable complication rate.

This chapter will initially discuss the indications, benefits, contraindications and limitations of the laparoscopic approach. Then, we will examine special considerations one would need to reflect upon when planning to operate on patients who are pregnant, obese and when planning to operate on children. This is then followed by a discussion of pre-operative considerations, the procedure including patient positioning, operative outcomes, post-operative recovery and haematological response. Finally, we will review the complications, splenunculectomy for recurrences and post-operative care.

Indications

The indications of having LS are essentially similar to that for an open splenectomy. The common indications can be divided into the following groups:

- Haematological:
  - o Increased platelet consumption: idiopathic thrombocytopaenia (ITP) refractory to medical therapy or medication producing unacceptable side-effects and refractory thrombotic thrombocytopaenicpurpura
  - o Increased red blood cell consumption: hereditary spherocytosis, thalassaemia, sickle cell disease and refractory autoimmune haemolyticanaemia
  - o Neoplastic: lymphoproliferative diseases, hairy cell leukaemia, Hodgkin and non-Hodgkin lymphoma
  - o Miscellaneous: myeloproliferative diseases

- Intrinsic splenic conditions:
  - o Benign parenchymal disorders: splenic cyst, splenic abscesses, Gaucher disease
  - o Splenic vascular disorders: splenic artery aneurysm, splenic vascular tumours
  - o Primary malignancy of the spleen: lymphangiosarcomas, haemangiosarcoma, splenic lymphoma
  - o Secondary malignancy of the spleen: metastatic ovarian cancer or melanoma
  - o Miscellaneous: splenic volvulus or the wandering spleen, portal hypertension secondary to splenic vein thrombosis.

- Splenic trauma [9]:
  - o Due to the current lack of quality evidence, one should be cautious about venturing into performing the splenectomylaparoscopically in the haemodynamically unstable trauma patients. The American Association for the Study of Trauma (AAST) splenic injury scale based on CT criteria can be used to grade the level and severity of injury to the spleen (Table 1) [10]. The more useful grading system is the guidelines set out by the Society for Surgery for the Alimentary Tract (SSAT) Patient Care Guidelines (Table 2) which states that patients should only be operated on if they are haemodynamically unstable despite resuscitation [11]. Selective arterial embolisation for trauma remains controversial and further studies are required.

Table 1. Spleen Injury Scale (1994 Revision) as described by the American Association for the Surgery Trauma (AAST) [10]

Grade		Injury Description
I	Haematoma	Subcapsular, < 10% surface area
	Laceration	Capsular tear, < 1cm parenchymal depth
II	Haematoma	Subcapsular, 10-50% surface area; intraparenchymal, <5cm in diameter
	Laceration	1-3cm parenchymal depth which does not involve a trabecular vessel
III	Haematoma	Subcapsular, >50% surface area or expanding ; ruptured subcapsular or parenchymal haematoma, or, Intraparenchymal haematoma >5cm or expanding
	Laceration	>3cm parenchymal depth or involving trabecular vessels
IV	Laceration	Involving segmental or hilar vessels producing major devascularisation (>25% of spleen)
V	Laceration	Completely shattered spleen Hilar vascular injury which devascularises spleen
	Vascular	

Table 2. Indications for surgery as depicted by the Society for Surgery for the Alimentary Tract (SSAT) Patient Care Guidelines[11]

Haemodynamic instability, Bleeding > 1000ml Transfusion of > 2 units of blood Or other evidence of on-going blood loss

- Staging or diagnostic purposes [12]: Recent advances in radiological imaging technology has made staging laparoscopy relatively redundant. However, computed tomography and ultrasound assessment of the spleen and related anatomy is necessary prior to embarking on performing the procedure. Further discussion is detailed below.

Benefits over the Open Approach

The smaller incisions of the minimal invasive approach to splenectomy and the reduced tissue manipulation while allowing for clearer dissection through magnification of the operating field are factors associated with the observed reductions in postoperative analgesia requirements, postoperative complications (particularly respiratory and wound) and hospital stay, as well as better cosmesis and quicker return to preoperative function compared with open surgery (please refer to the postoperative recovery section) [2-4, 13]. When quality of life was measured using the Short form SF-36 survey, LS was also associated with better 'general health' and 'physical functioning' and lesser 'bodily pain' postoperatively compared to open surgery group [5].

Additionally, the laparoscopic approach could be completed with operative time, intra-operative blood loss or need for transfusion that are comparable or advantageous over open surgery [4, 13-16], as indicated in Table 3.

Table 3. Studies of open versus laparoscopic splenectomy with regards to operative time, intra-operative blood loss and need for transfusion

Author, year	Groups (size)	Spleen weight (g)	Operative time, minutes	Intra-operative blood loss (ml)	Post-operative need for transfusion (No. of patients)
Watanabe et al, 2007[14]	OS (28)	$460 \pm 200g^\dagger$	$205 \pm 60^\ddagger$	$750 \pm 600^\ddagger$	2
	LS (25)	$525 \pm 300 \, g^\dagger$	$173 \pm 53^\ddagger$	$359 \pm 280^\ddagger$	0
		$p = NS$	$p = NS$	$p < 0,05$	$p < 0.01$
Konstadoula kiset al, 2006[13]	OS (14)	$631 \pm 353 \, g^\dagger$	$135 \pm 23^\dagger$	N/A	2
	LS (14)	$685 \pm 274 \, g^\dagger$	$188 \pm 42^\dagger$		7
		$p = 0.27$	$p < 0.001$		$p = NS$
Boddyet al, 2006[15]	OS (18)	$2448 \, g^\dagger$	$45^\dagger \, (25\text{-}85)^*$	$200^\dagger \, (0\text{-}5120)^*$	N/A
	LS (11)	$2000 \, g^\dagger$	$90^\dagger \, (45\text{-}225)^*$	$800^\dagger \, (20\text{-}5120)^*$	
		$p = NS$	$p < 0.001$	$p < 0.05$	
Kucuket al, 2005 [16]	OS (38)	$212.1 \pm 156 \, g^\ddagger$	$81.4 \pm 30.8^\ddagger$	$188.2 \pm 93.7^\ddagger$	0
	LS (30)	$187.3 \pm 132 \, g^\ddagger$	$148.2 \pm 63.8^\ddagger$	$216.4 \pm 128.9^\ddagger$	0
		$p = NS$	$p < 0.01$	$p = NS$	
Doniniet al, 1999 [4]	OS (56)	$732 \pm 1184 \, g^\ddagger$	$133 \pm 42^\ddagger$	$347 \pm 511^\ddagger$	15
	LS (44)	$773 \pm 1113 \, g^\ddagger$	$130 \pm 62^\ddagger$	$295 \pm 279^\ddagger$	2
		$p = 0.86$	$p = 0.76$	$p = 0.67$	$p = 0.004$

OS: open splenectomy, LS: laparoscopic splenectomy, N/A: not available, NS: not significant.
‡mean, †median, $\pm$ standard deviation, *range.

Since the laparoscopic approach was shown to be, at least, comparable to the open approach with regards to intra-operative parameters but yet provided better postoperative results, it would be reasonable to conclude that the laparoscopic option is the superior choice.

Limitations and Contraindications

However, there are contraindications to the laparoscopic approach, which can be grouped into:

- General:
  - o   The need for laparotomy for concurrent procedures.

- Supermassive splenomegaly:
  - o   The supermassive splenomegaly has been defined as a spleen with a diameter of more than 22cm [6, 17]. Laparoscopy in patients with such a sizable spleen is technically challenging due to the limited working space that restricts manipulation and the difficulty in retrieving the spleen. The hand-assisted approach to LS (HALS) can be considered, and there is some evidence to show that it reduced operating times, conversion rates and complications compared to the pure laparoscopic and open approaches [18-20].

- Portal hypertension:
  - o   Portal hypertension might be considered a relative contraindication as there is a considerable risk of bleeding from varices with the need to convert to an open operation [21]. However, there are reports on the safety of LS in patients with cirrhosis and portal hypertension [22, 23]. Careful preoperative patient counselling is necessary, and the use of pre-operative splenic artery embolization may make patients with portal hypertension amenable to surgery [24].

Special Considerations

- Pregnancy:

It is extremely rare to have a pressing need for splenectomy to arise during pregnancy and any surgery should be postponed during pregnancy. Rarely, immune thrombocytopaenicpurpura and haemolysis secondary to a red corpuscular disorder may worsen during pregnancy necessitating a splenectomy [25, 26]. Additionally, a splenectomy may be necessary if there is splenic injury from blunt trauma that does not settle with conservative treatment. The laparoscopic technique has been described to be safe during the second trimester [12]. The laparoscopic technique still retains its benefits; one case study reported the feasibility of LS in a 24-week primigravida patient and two systematic reviews described the safety of laparoscopic surgery, including LS, in pregnancy[26-28].

- Morbid obesity:

Morbid obesity used to be a relative contraindicated in laparoscopic surgery. However, in recent years, there has been an exponential increase in bariatric operations with proven safety record [29]. Hence, it is no longer considered contraindicative. In fact, one might argue that it could be easier to perform LS in the morbidly obese than to perform open surgery due to the improved exposure and access.

- Children:

The benefits of the laparoscopic approach in children is similar to those in adults [12, 30]. However, it is quite important to preserve the spleen in children whenever possible due to the risk of overwhelming sepsis, which is quoted at 77% with a 50% mortality at an age younger than 2 years [12]. A literature review noted that the infection rate in children age 16 and younger were 4.4% with a mortality rate of 2.2% [31]. A report on post-splenectomy patients with sickle cell disease showed a 5.7% sepsis rate within a strict protocol of vaccination and antibiotic prophylaxis [32].

Preoperative Considerations

- Imaging:
  - o Ultrasound: Evaluation of the splenic size ultrasonically is beneficial. In benign disease, ultrasound assessment is adequate to assess the spleen size, vasculature and synchronous conditions [12]. The information obtained will help in weighing the risk and benefits of performing the operation laparoscopically.
  - o Computed tomography (CT): In malignant disease however, CT should be performed to evaluate anatomical conditions (spleen size, presence of splenic infarct and inflammation in surround tissues) as well as to stage the disease [33]. Additionally, for accessory spleens, numerous studies have showed that preoperative detection by CTs are inconsistent with a sensitivity and specificity of 60% and 95.6% and it should instead only be used to complement intraoperative accessory spleen detection, though intraoperative laparoscopic detection alone might suffice as it has a sensitivity and specificity of 93.3% and 100% [34, 35]. A more detailed discussion about accessory spleen detection will be discussed later in the chapter.
  - o Other recent methods for locating accessory spleens might include 99m-technetium-labelled heat-damaged red blood cells [36] or the use of intravenous contrast-enhanced ultrasound [37]. However, these methods are new and have not had the necessary amount of vigorous reviews to validate them.
- Haematological assessment:
  - o All patients should have a full blood count test done. Patients should ideally have a platelet count above $50 \times 10^9/l$ prior to surgery to minimise the risk of massive intraoperative bleeding. Although there is a report of patients being operated on with platelet counts below $20 \times 10^9/l$ (as low as $1 \times 10^9/l$) for immune thrombocytopaenicpurpura [38], one should explore all modalities to improve the patient's platelet count before embarking on what might turn out to be a high risk procedure. Pre-operative and/or intra-operative (after division of the vascular pedicle) platelet transfusion may be needed.

o   Consideration should be given to pre-operative transfusion of packed red blood cells in patients with a haemoglobin level of less than 8-10g/dl.

- Vaccination:
  o   Since the spleen is responsible for assisting the white blood cells to clear encapsulated bacteria, post-splenectomy patients are at a relatively high risk of overwhelming sepsis from organisms such as *Streptococcus pneumoniae*, *Neisseria meningitides* (group C meningococcus)and *Haemophilusinfluenzae*type B, with anoverall incidence of about 3.2% and a mortality rate of 40-50% [12].
  o   The standard pneumococcal vaccine that should be used is the 23-valent pneumococcal vaccine as stated by the British Committee for Standards in Haematology [39]. The risk of post-splenectomy sepsis is highest amongst patients older than 50 years of age, those with malignancy of the spleen, patients requiring splenectomy secondary to iatrogenic injury, and patients with thalassaemia major and sickle-cell anaemia [40, 41]. Hence, vaccination against *Streptococcus pneumoniae*, *Haemophilus influenza* and *Neisseria meningitides* at 15 days prior to surgery or within 30 days of surgery is a necessity [39]. An exception to preoperative vaccination is patients on high dose steroids or immunosuppressive therapy who might not mount an adequate antibody response to vaccination; immunisation could be deferred until the dose of such drug therapy has been reasonably reduced following a response to splenectomy [42].

- Operative antibiotic prophylaxis:
  o   The European Association for Endoscopic Surgery (EAES) recommends antibiotic prophylaxis of cefazolin or clindamycin at induction of anaesthesia [39].

- Embolization of splenic artery:
  o   Currently, there are no randomized controlled trials that suggest pre-operative splenic artery embolisation is effective in reducing the difficulty of the splenectomy or operative complications. However, there are studies which document its use in children and adults with splenomegaly [43, 44], in portal hypertension [24] and in trauma [45].
  o   The use of pre-operative splenic artery embolization has been shown to be safe but perhaps should be reserved to patients with massive splenomegaly [spleens larger than 20 cm) [43, 46], though it might be of limited benefit in those with spleens larger than 30 cm.
  o   Reso*et al* demonstrated that the use of pre-operative splenic artery embolization with HALS resulted in a shorter operative time, less blood loss and lower conversion rate [46].
  o   Romano *et al* reports that after embolization, an average of 71% devascularisation and 68% reduction in spleen weight can be achieved in patients with portal hypertension [24]. Currently, the EAES [12] suggest that portal hypertension is a contraindication to splenectomy. However, if pre-operative embolization can

reduce splenic size and risk of bleeding, this may allow LS to be performed safely.

Patient Positioning

- Anterior or supine:
    - o This is a less commonly used position in which the patient is placed in a modified lithotomy position which is in a semi-frog-leg position whilst lying supine. This would allow the surgeon to stand between the patient's leg with the laparoscopic stack placed on the left just by the patient's head while the assistant and scrub nurse standing on either side of the patient [1].
    - o This position allows excellent access for a diagnostic laparoscopy and access to the spleen, stomach, body and tail of pancreas, and the colonic splenic flexure. Hence, it is excellent for patients requiring simultaneous operations like a concurrent cholecystectomy or laparoscopic biopsy. Also, a midline laparotomy can be performed if a conversion is necessary.
    - o However, this position is limited in patients with massive splenomegaly where exposure of the splenic hilum, ligaments and vasculature becomes restricted. Nevertheless, the table can be tilted to achieve the semi-lateral position to facilitate the splenectomy by allowing it to 'hang down' with gravity; an approach described as the 'hanging spleen technique'[47].
    - o 4 to 5 ports with at least one 10mm port and one 12 mm port are needed for this position.
    - o The 10mm port is placed for the camera, whilst the 12mm port is placed for usage of the linear stapler.

- Right lateral:
    - o The patient is placed on the right lateral position with the waist at the 'break' of the table allowing the space between the costal margin and the iliac crest to be opened when the table is placed in the slight 'jack-knife' configuration. The operating surgeon is positioned on the patient's right with the laparoscopic stack placed by the patient's head on the left.
    - o This position allows safe vascular control as dissection of the ligaments and hilar structures is made easier with the abdominal viscera and spleen lying more medially and with the spleen hanging from its ligamental attachments. It also allows good visualisation of the tail of pancreas.
    - o If a conversion to the open approach is needed, the patient can be tilted to the 45° angle to allow a left subcostal incision to be made.
    - o Three ports may be sufficient for this position with at least one 10mm port and one 12mm port.

- Semi-lateral:
    - o This position is a hybrid between the supine and the right lateral position and the patient lies on the right side at 45°. Operating staff and laparoscopic

stack positioning is similar to the right lateral position. The port placement is also similar to the port positions used in the right lateral position.

   o   In this position, both the benefits of the supine and right lateral position can be achieved simply by tilting the table.

   o   Similar to the right lateral position, usually only 3 ports are required with at least one 10mm port and one 12mm port.

The Procedure

The use of a 30° or 45° angled laparoscope allows better visualisation as compared to a 0° laparoscope. It is vital to have a suction device at hand in case of bleeding, and the use of ultrasonic dissection device facilitates dissection. Vascular structures can be ligated using an ultrasonic device, endoscopic linear staplers, electrothermal bipolar vessel sealer, locking clips or ligatures.

The principals to a splenectomy are to circumferentially mobilise the splenic hilum cautiously and avoid damaging the splenic capsule. The circumferential mobilisation helps 'thin' out the hilum and allows stapling devices to be used to ligate the vessels present within it. The usual approach is to dissect the peritoneal covering of the splenocolic ligament (Figure 1), followed by mobilising the splenocolic ligament.

Then, the gastrosplenic ligament is mobilised; this ligament can be visualised by lifting the spleen up (Figure 2) and pulling the stomach medially or by opening up the lesser sac. Next, the splenophrenic and splenorenal ligament can be dissected.

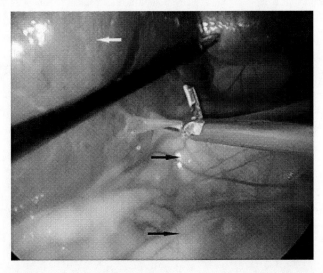

Figure 1. Laparoscopic image showing the ultrasonic dissector being used to dissected the peritoneal covering of the splenocolic ligament. White arrow indicates the spleen and the black arrow indicates colon.

Once the spleen is fully mobilised, an endoscopic stapling device can be used to ligate the hilum but care should be taken to avoid including the tail of pancreas and not to superimpose the vein and artery. Haemostatic clips can be placed on small splenic artery branches to help thin down the hilum (Figure 3). Superimposition of the artery and vein can result in arteriovenous fistula formation. The tail of pancreas can be excluded by stapling as close to the hilum as possible (Figure 4). Sometimes, there may be some posterior attachment of the upper pole of the spleen to the abdominal wall; the stapling device, ultrasonic device or electrothermal bipolar vessel sealer can be used to divide these structures. Alternatively, the splenic vessels or their branches may be tackled head-on after minimal splenic mobilisation and ligated or clipped individually.

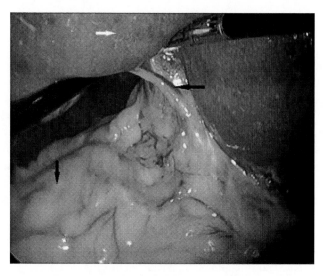

Figure 2. Laparoscopic image depicting the visualisation of the gastrosplenic ligament. The white arrow indicates the spleen, the horizontal black arrow indicates a branch of the splenic artery in the gastrosplenic ligament and the downward black arrow indicates the stomach.

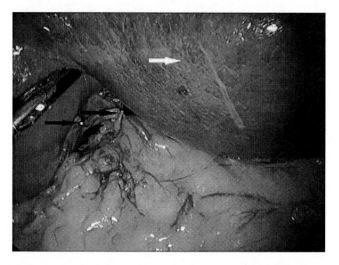

Figure 3. Laparoscopic image showing haemostatic clip ligation to help 'thin down' the hilum. The white arrow indicates the spleen and the black arrows indicate the haemostatic clips on a branch of the splenic artery.

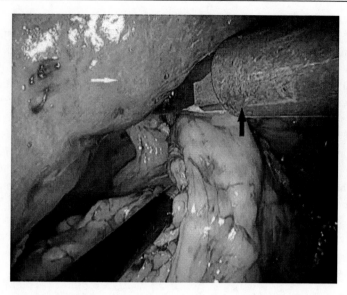

Figure 4. Laparoscopic image showing the usage of a linear stapler to ligate the splenic hilum. The white arrow indicates the spleen and the black arrow indicates the linear stapling device which clamping onto the splenic hilum. Care should be taken not to include any clips within the staple line as these could result in stapler failure and bleeding.

Some surgeons use specialised laparoscopic retractors [48] to enhance exposure and facilitate a difficult dissection and hence reduce bleeding, particularly for enlarged spleens. Others have found that the hand-assisted technique useful in enhancing retraction, easing the learning curve, and allowing the enlarged spleen to be removed with a smaller incision as compared to a formal laparotomy [19, 49]. In patients with massive splenomegaly or previous abdominal surgery, the hand-assisted approach has been shown to shorten operating times, lower conversion rates and reduce perioperative complications compared to the completely laparoscopic technique [15, 50]. However, the surgeon's hand or forearm could hamper certain manoeuvres due to the limited intra-abdominal space and hand fatigue can be problematic to the surgeon.

Placement of drains is not advised, and there is no good evidence to show that it makes any therapeutic difference.

Accessory spleens:

As discussed earlier, CT detection of the accessory spleen is unreliable and hence a combination of pre-operative localisation and intra-operative localisation should be performed to detect them. Preoperative detection by CT has a sensitivity and specificity of 60% and 95.6% respectively and intra-operative laparoscopic detection has a sensitivity and specificity of 93.3% and 100% respectively [34, 35]. The commonest sites for accessory spleens are at the lower pole or hilum of the spleen [34]. However, accessory spleens might be present anywhere in the abdominal cavity even within the parenchyma of the pancreas [2, 36]; possibly due to the close proximity of the two organs during embryological development.

Intraoperative localisation of accessory spleens should be done prior to splenic mobilisation. Up to 16% of patients with ITP will have accessory spleens and unless removed during splenectomy, could result in inadequate haematological response or disease relapse [7].

Spleen retrieval techniques:

Once the spleen has been amputated, difficulty may be faced when the specimen is too large to be removed through the incision site. The following strategies described may help to ease the removal of the spleen.

The specimen should be removed using a strong bag, such as those made of ripcord nylon. To prevent recurrences in benign or more importantly in malignant disease, care must be taken to avoid spillage of splenic material in order to avoid implantation.

If the specimen must be removed whole to avoid spillage of malignant cells or is required for histopathological examination such as with an intrasplenictumour, a mini-laparotomy can be used or the specimen can be removed via the hand port if the hand-assisted technique was employed. Otherwise, the spleen can be removed piecemeal or could be morcellated. To morcellate the specimen, one can use a morcellator or any blunt instrument but it must be done within a strong bag to avoid bag rupture [3]. Additionally, vacuum suction devices have been employed for the removal of massive spleens in patients with benign disease such as a liposuction device or suction curette [51, 52].

Operative outcomes:

- It is well establish that the laparoscopic approach is superior to the open splenectomy in terms of reductions in operative blood loss, perioperative complications and operative times [12].
- The operative difficulty and time of LS increase with corresponding increase in the size of the spleen from standard size, to moderate and further massive splenomegaly (Table 4) [13].

Table 4. Effect of spleen size on operative outcomes of laparoscopic splenectomy [13]

Size*	Operative time (minutes): mean (± SD)	Conversion rate (%)	Complication rate (%)
Standard	143 (± 50)	4	11
Moderate	179 (± 77)	0	27
Massive	176 (± 56)	23	27

*Standard size spleen is arbitrarily defined as weighing less than 400g, moderate as between 400 to 1000 g and massive as more than 1000 g (up to 3500g).

- Conversion to the open procedure is most commonly due to uncontrolled bleeding from blood vessels or from the parenchyma, and a rate of around 10% is not uncommon[4]. Also, conversions are commonly due to a large spleen obstructing the operative field, with some studies quoting a high conversion rate for spleens with a diameter larger than 22 cm, spleens that reach the anterior superior iliac spine or crosses the midline, or spleens weighing more than 2000 g [53-55].
- Complications of LS might include [12]:

  o Bleeding as a result of capsular tear or vessel injury
  o Visceral injury such as gastric, diaphragmatic and pancreatic damage
  o Cell spillage, e.g. due to perforation of the retrieval bag, resulting in recurrence of benign or malignant disease

Postoperative recovery:

When compared to open splenectomy, patients return to oral diet quicker and have shorter hospital stays [3, 4, 7, 13, 56] (Table 5):

Table 5. Postoperative recovery following laparoscopic versus open splenectomy

Author, year	Groups (size)	Spleen size/weight	Return to oral diet (day)	Duration of intravenous analgesia use, days	Length of hospital stay (day)
Sampath *et al*, 2007[7]	OS (54) LS (51)	12 cm[‡] 11 cm[‡] $p = 0.27$	N/A	N/A	10[‡] 3[‡] $p = 0.0003$
Konstadoula kis *et al*, 2006[13]	OS (14) LS (14)	631 ± 353 g[†] 685 ± 274 g[†] $p = 0.27$	N/A	N/A	6.5 ± 1.2[†] 5.0 ± 2.4[†] $p = 0.035$
Owera *et al*, 2006[56]	OS (13) LS (15)	1100[†] (1000-3800)* g 1300[†] (1000-3600)* g $p = 0.618$	3[†] (2-5)* 1[†] (1-3)* $p = 0.017$	4[†] (3-5.5)* [β] 1[†] (0-2)* [β] $p < 0.001$	10[†] (6-20)* 3[†] (2-40)* $p = 0.0001$
Cordera *et al*, 2003[3]	OS (44) LS (42)	273[†] (55-1320)* g 157[†] (40-530)* g $p = $ N/A	4.02 ± 0.99[†] 2.33 ± 0.28[†] $p = 0.000$	2.42 ± 0.99[†] 1.24 ± 0.15[†] $p = 0.000$	5.34 ± 2.52[†] 3.31 ± 0.72[†] $p = 0.000$
Donini *et al*, 1999[4]	OS (56) LS (44)	732 ± 1184 g[‡] 773 ± 1113 g[‡] $p = 0.86$	3.6 ± 0.8[‡] 1.7 ± 0.8[‡] $p < 0.0001$	4 ± 2.8[‡□] 2.4 ± 1.7[‡□] $p < 0.0001$	7.2 ± 2.1[‡] 5.1 ± 2.7[‡] $p = 0.0002$

OS: open splenectomy, LS: laparoscopic splenectomy, N/A: not available, [‡]mean, [†]median, ± standard deviation, *range, [α]number of vials of analgesia.

- Cordera *et al* reported significantly shorter duration of need for parenteral analgesia with LS compared with open surgery (mean days, 1.24 vs. 2.42 days, $p < 0.01$)[3], while Velanovich *et al* showed that LS was associated with significantly less 'bodily pain' compared to open surgery (mean pain scores on the SF-36 survery, 55.5 vs. 88 , $p < 0.01$) [5].

Haematological response:

- Failure in normalisation of the platelet count or a relapse in ITP patients, may be due to missing an accessory spleen. Sampath *et al* [7], found no difference in the recurrence rate of ITP after LS versus those who had the open procedure.They described complete recurrences (refractory to medical therapy) in 28% of 54 open splenectomy patients compared to 15% of 51 laparoscopic cases ($p = 0.222$); four (7%) recurrencesin the open group were due to missing an accessory spleen as compared to one (2%) in the laparoscopic group.
- A systematic review of short and long-term failure of LS in adult ITP [57] revealed that short-term failure, defined as no platelet response or initial response with a relapse, at approximately 8% and long-term failure, defined as a relapse after 5 years, at approximately 44 per 1,000 patient years of follow-up, with a cumulative failure rate of 28% at 5 years.

- For other indications for splenectomy, Balaguéet al[58] reported 83% complete remission when thrombocytopenic purpura was secondary to human immunodeficiency virus infection, 100% remission in patients with Evans syndrome and hereditary spherocytosis, and a 70% remissionin patients with autoimmune haemolyticanaemia.

Complications

Postoperative complications may include:

- General: haemorrhage, postoperative ileus, pneumonia, deep vein thrombosis.
- Specific: gastric dilatation, intra-abdominal collection, portal vein thrombosis, damage to the tail of pancreas and pancreatic fistula, leucocytosis and thrombocytosis, gastric fistula, post-splenectomysepticaemia.

Laparoscopic Splenunculectomy for Disease Recurrence

Currently, the pathophysiology of recurrence of haematological conditions after an initial response to splenectomy, such as in ITP, is poorly understood. Although a missed accessory spleen might be a contributor, this has been found to be untrue in the majority of cases, and the aetiology of recurrence is more likely to be multi-factorial [12]. Nonetheless, a search for accessory spleens, especially in patients with recurrent ITP who fail to respond to re-introduction of medical therapy, is necessary [7]. Computed tomography with or without radio-labelled red blood cells, followed by percutaneous injection of methylene blue dye at the target site, or the administration of 99m-technetium-labelled heat-damaged red blood cells pre-operatively and their detection intra-operatively within splenunculi using an gamma probe have been described [36].

Repeat laparoscopy in an attempt to remove accessory spleens should be reserved to patients who fail medical therapy or suffer significant side-effects of therapy [36]. Laparoscopic access to the accessory spleen might be facilitated by the paucity of adhesions following a previous laparoscopic procedure (LS) compared with open splenectomy.

Postoperative Care

- Postoperative haematological assays are essential to assess platelet counts, especially in patients with thrombocytopaenia, and to detect post-splenectomy thrombocytosis. If the platelet count rises to above 1000×10^9/l, aspirin should be prescribed. However, if the patients are at high risk of thrombosis such as patients who have a supramassive splenomegaly, myeloproliferative disorder with hypercoagulopathy, haemolyticanaemia and haematological malignancy, then 4 weeks of anticoagulation prophylaxis is recommended [12]. If venous thrombosis ensues despite these prophylactic measures, warfarin therapy for 6 months with an international normalised ratio between 2 and 3 is advised [59, 60].

- Antibiotic prophylaxis: The EAES recommends oral penicillin V or erythromycin for at least 2 years in the adult or 5 years in children, and that asplenic patients should take intravenous amoxicillin or equivalent alternatives when they suffer from any flu-like symptoms (Table 6) [12, 39]. Lifelong prophylaxis should be offered to all patients, especially to children up to the age of 16 and in any patients with other underlying impaired immune function[39].

Table 6. Recommended antibiotic prophylaxis in post-splenectomy patients [39]

Oral Penicillin V	
Adults	250-500 mg twice a day
Children aged 5-14	250 mg twice a day
Children aged < 5	125 mg twice a day
Oral Erythromycin	
Adults and children aged > 8	250-500 mg twice a day
Children aged 2-8	250 mg twice a day
Children aged < 2	125 mg twice a day

Conclusion

We believe that the gold standard for splenectomies is to remove the spleen laparoscopically. It is evident that LS confers benefits and have comparable complications to the open splenectomy. However, one should still be weary when approaching the 'supramassive' spleen with more evidence required in the literature including techniques to assist in reducing the size of the spleen pre-operatively. Additionally, more evidence is required regarding splenunculi detection pre-operatively and when searching for a source of recurrence; so does pre-operative splenic artery embolisation.

References

[1] Delaitre B, Maignien B. [Splenectomy by the laparoscopic approach. Report of a case. *Presse Med*. 1991;20:2263.

[2] Park A, Marcaccio M, Sternbach M, Witzke D, Fitzgerald P. Laparoscopic vs open splenectomy. *Arch. Surg*. 1999;134:1263-9.

[3] Cordera F, Long KH, Nagorney DM, McMurtry EK, Schleck C, Ilstrup D, et al. Open versus laparoscopic splenectomy for idiopathic thrombocytopenic purpura: clinical and economic analysis. *Surgery*. 2003;134:45-52.

[4] Donini A, Baccarani U, Terrosu G, Corno V, Ermacora A, Pasqualucci A, et al. Laparoscopic vs open splenectomy in the management of hematologic diseases. *Surg. Endosc.* 1999;13:1220-5.

[5] Velanovich V. Laparoscopic vs open surgery: a preliminary comparison of quality-of-life outcomes. *Surg. Endosc.* 2000;14:16-21.

[6] Grahn SW, Alvarez J, Kirkwood K. Trends in laparoscopic splenectomy for massive splenomegaly. *Arch. Surg.* 2006;141:755-61; discussion 61-2.

[7] Sampath S, Meneghetti AT, MacFarlane JK, Nguyen NH, Benny WB, Panton ON. An 18-year review of open and laparoscopic splenectomy for idiopathic thrombocytopenic purpura. *Am. J. Surg.* 2007;193:580-3; discussion 3-4.

[8] Reddy VS, Phan HH, O'Neill JA, Neblett WW, Pietsch JB, Morgan WM, et al. Laparoscopic versus open splenectomy in the pediatric population: a contemporary single-center experience. *Am. Surg.* 2001;67:859-63; discussion 63-4.

[9] Carobbi A, Romagnani F, Antonelli G, Bianchini M. Laparoscopic splenectomy for severe blunt trauma: initial experience of ten consecutive cases with a fast hemostatic technique. *Surg. Endosc.* 2010;24:1325-30.

[10] Moore EE, Cogbill TH, Jurkovich GJ, Shackford SR, Malangoni MA, Champion HR. Organ injury scaling: spleen and liver (1994 revision). *J. Trauma.* 1995;38:323-4.

[11] (SSAT) PCCoTSfSotAT. Surgical treatment of injuries and diseases of the spleen. J *Gastrointest* Surg. 2005;9:453-4.

[12] Habermalz B, Sauerland S, Decker G, Delaitre B, Gigot JF, Leandros E, et al. Laparoscopic splenectomy: the clinical practice guidelines of the European Association for Endoscopic Surgery (EAES). *Surg. Endosc.* 2008;22:821-48.

[13] Konstadoulakis MM, Lagoudianakis E, Antonakis PT, Albanopoulos K, Gomatos I, Stamou KM, et al. Laparoscopic versus open splenectomy in patients with beta thalassemia major. *J. Laparoendosc Adv. Surg. Tech. A.* 2006;16:5-8.

[14] Watanabe Y, Horiuchi A, Yoshida M, Yamamoto Y, Sugishita H, Kumagi T, et al. Significance of laparoscopic splenectomy in patients with hypersplenism. *World J. Surg.* 2007;31:549-55.

[15] Boddy AP, Mahon D, Rhodes M. Does open surgery continue to have a role in elective splenectomy? *Surg. Endosc.* 2006;20:1094-8.

[16] Kucuk C, Sozuer E, Ok E, Altuntas F, Altunbas F, Yilmaz Z. Laparoscopic versus open splenectomy in the management of benign and malign hematologic diseases: a ten-year single-center experience. *J. Laparoendosc Adv. Surg. Tech. A.* 2005;15:135-9.

[17] Heniford BT, Park A, Walsh RM, Kercher KW, Matthews BD, Frenette G, et al. Laparoscopic splenectomy in patients with normal-sized spleens versus splenomegaly: does size matter? *Am. Surg.* 2001;67:854-7; discussion 7-8.

[18] Rosen M, Brody F, Walsh RM, Ponsky J. Hand-assisted laparoscopic splenectomy vs conventional laparoscopic splenectomy in cases of splenomegaly. *Arch. Surg.* 2002;137:1348-52.

[19] Targarona EM, Balague C, Cerdán G, Espert JJ, Lacy AM, Visa J, et al. Hand-assisted laparoscopic splenectomy (HALS) in cases of splenomegaly: a comparison analysis with conventional laparoscopic splenectomy. *Surg. Endosc.* 2002;16:426-30.

[20] Barbaros U, Dinççağ A, Sümer A, Vecchio R, Rusello D, Randazzo V, et al. Prospective randomized comparison of clinical results between hand-assisted laparoscopic and open splenectomies. *Surg. Endosc.* 2010;24:25-32.

[21] Ohta M, Nishizaki T, Matsumoto T, Shimabukuro R, Sasaki A, Shibata K, et al. Analysis of risk factors for massive intraoperative bleeding during laparoscopic splenectomy. *J. Hepatobiliary Pancreat. Surg.* 2005;12:433-7.

[22] Zhu JH, Wang YD, Ye ZY, Zhao T, Zhu YW, Xie ZJ, et al. Laparoscopic versus open splenectomy for hypersplenism secondary to liver cirrhosis. *Surg. Laparosc. Endosc. Percutan Tech.* 2009;19:258-62.

[23] Hashizume M, Tomikawa M, Akahoshi T, Tanoue K, Gotoh N, Konishi K, et al. Laparoscopic splenectomy for portal hypertension. *Hepatogastroenterology.* 2002 2002 May;49:847-52.

[24] Romano M, Giojelli A, Capuano G, Pomponi D, Salvatore M. Partial splenic embolization in patients with idiopathic portal hypertension. *Eur. J. Radiol.* 2004;49:268-73.

[25] Griffiths J, Sia W, Shapiro AM, Tataryn I, Turner AR. Laparoscopic splenectomy for the treatment of refractory immune thrombocytopenia in pregnancy. *J. Obstet. Gynaecol. Can.* 2005;27:771-4.

[26] Allran CF, Weiss CA, Park AE. Urgent laparoscopic splenectomy in a morbidly obese pregnant woman: case report and literature review. *J. Laparoendosc Adv. Surg. Tech. A.* 2002;12:445-7.

[27] Nezhat FR, Tazuke S, Nezhat CH, Seidman DS, Phillips DR, Nezhat CR. Laparoscopy during pregnancy: a literature review. *JSLS.* 1997;1:17-27.

[28] Jackson H, Granger S, Price R, Rollins M, Earle D, Richardson W, et al. Diagnosis and laparoscopic treatment of surgical diseases during pregnancy: an evidence-based review. *Surg. Endosc.* 2008;22:1917-27.

[29] Dominguez EP, Choi YU, Scott BG, Yahanda AM, Graviss EA, Sweeney JF. Impact of morbid obesity on outcome of laparoscopic splenectomy. *Surg. Endosc.* 2007;21:422-6.

[30] Rescorla FJ, Breitfeld PP, West KW, Williams D, Engum SA, Grosfeld JL. A case controlled comparison of open and laparoscopic splenectomy in children. *Surgery.* 1998;124:670-5; discussion 5-6.

[31] Reihneŕ E, Brismar B. Management of splenic trauma--changing concepts. *Eur. J. Emerg. Med.* 1995;2:47-51.

[32] Lesher AP, Kalpatthi R, Glenn JB, Jackson SM, Hebra A. Outcome of splenectomy in children younger than 4 years with sickle cell disease. *J. Pediatr Surg.* 2009;44:1134-8; discussion 8.

[33] Heniford BT, Matthews BD, Answini GA, Walsh RM. Laparoscopic splenectomy for malignant diseases. *Semin Laparosc. Surg.* 2000;7:93-100.

[34] Quah C, Ayiomamitis GD, Shah A, Ammori BJ. Computed tomography to detect accessory spleens before laparoscopic splenectomy: is it necessary? *Surg. Endosc.* 2011;25:261-5.

[35] Stanek A, Stefaniak T, Makarewicz W, Kaska L, Podgórczyk H, Hellman A, et al. Accessory spleens: preoperative diagnostics limitations and operational strategy in laparoscopic approach to splenectomy in idiopathic thrombocytopenic purpura patients. *Langenbecks Arch. Surg.* 2005;390:47-51.

[36] Altaf AM, Sawatzky M, Ellsmere J, Bonjer HJ, Burrell S, Abraham R, et al. Laparoscopic accessory splenectomy: the value of perioperative localization studies. *Surg. Endosc.* 2009 Jan. Epub ahead of publication

[37] von Herbay A, Vogt C, Häussinger D. [The ultrasound contrast agent levovist helps with the differentiation between accessory spleen and lymph nodes in the splenic hilum: a pilot study]. *Z. Gastroenterol.* 2004;42:1109-15.

[38] Keidar A, Sagi B, Szold A. Laparoscopic splenectomy for immune thrombocytopenic purpura in patients with severe refractory thrombocytopenia. *Pathophysiol. Haemost. Thromb.* 2003 2003;33:116-9.

[39] Guidelines for the prevention and treatment of infection in patients with an absent or dysfunctional spleen. Working Party of the British Committee for Standards in Haematology Clinical Haematology Task Force. *BMJ.* 1996;312:430-4.

[40] Bisharat N, Omari H, Lavi I, Raz R. Risk of infection and death among post-splenectomy patients. *J. Infect.* 2001;43:182-6.

[41] Kyaw MH, Holmes EM, Toolis F, Wayne B, Chalmers J, Jones IG, et al. Evaluation of severe infection and survival after splenectomy. *Am. J. Med.* 2006;119:276.e1-7.

[42] Shatz DV, Schinsky MF, Pais LB, Romero-Steiner S, Kirton OC, Carlone GM. Immune responses of splenectomized trauma patients to the 23-valent pneumococcal polysaccharide vaccine at 1 versus 7 versus 14 days after splenectomy. *J. Trauma.* 1998;44:760-5; discussion 5-6.

[43] Poulin EC, Mamazza J, Schlachta CM. Splenic artery embolization before laparoscopic splenectomy. An update. *Surg. Endosc.* 1998;12:870-5.

[44] Hickman MP, Lucas D, Novak Z, Rao B, Gold RE, Parvey L, et al. Preoperative embolization of the spleen in children with hypersplenism. *J Vasc Interv Radiol.* 1992;3:647-52.

[45] Schnüriger B, Inaba K, Konstantinidis A, Lustenberger T, Chan LS, Demetriades D. Outcomes of proximal versus distal splenic artery embolization after trauma: a systematic review and meta-analysis. *J. Trauma.* 2011;70:252-60.

[46] Reso A, Brar MS, Church N, Mitchell P, Dixon E, Debru E. Outcome of laparoscopic splenectomy with preoperative splenic artery embolization for massive splenomegaly. *Surg. Endosc.* 2010;24:2008-12.

[47] Delaitre B, Bonnichon P, Barthes T, Dousset B. [Laparoscopic splenectomy. The "hanging spleen technique" in a series of nineteen cases]. *Ann. Chir.* 1995;49:471-6.

[48] Machado MA, Makdissi FF, Herman P, Montagnini AL, Sallum RA, Machado MC. Exposure of splenic hilum increases safety of laparoscopic splenectomy. *Surg. Laparosc.Endosc. Percutan Tech.* 2004;14:23-5.

[49] Handoscopic surgery: a prospective multicenter trial of a minimally invasive technique for complex abdominal surgery. Southern Surgeons' Club Study Group. *Arch. Surg.* 1999;134:477-85; discussion 85-6.

[50] Kercher KW, Matthews BD, Walsh RM, Sing RF, Backus CL, Heniford BT. Laparoscopic splenectomy for massive splenomegaly. *Am. J. Surg.* 2002;183:192-6.

[51] Leonello D, Aspinall S, Kollias J. Laparoscopic spleen extraction--a simple technique. *Ann. R. Coll Surg. Engl.* 2009;91:435.

[52] Lai PB, Leung KL, Ho WS, Yiu RY, Leung BC, Lau WY. The use of liposucker for spleen retrieval after laparoscopic splenectomy. *Surg. Laparosc. Endosc. Percutan Tech.* 2000;10:39-40.

[53] Terrosu G, Baccarani U, Bresadola V, Sistu MA, Uzzau A, Bresadola F. The impact of splenic weight on laparoscopic splenectomy for splenomegaly. *Surg. Endosc.* 2002;16:103-7.

[54] Park AE, Birgisson G, Mastrangelo MJ, Marcaccio MJ, Witzke DB. Laparoscopic splenectomy: outcomes and lessons learned from over 200 cases. *Surgery.* 2000;128:660-7.

[55] 55.Targarona EM, Espert JJ, Cerdán G, Balagué C, Piulachs J, Sugrañes G, et al. Effect of spleen size on splenectomy outcome. A comparison of open and laparoscopic surgery. *Surg. Endosc.* 1999;13:559-62.

[56] Owera A, Hamade AM, Bani Hani OI, Ammori BJ. Laparoscopic versus open splenectomy for massive splenomegaly: a comparative study. *J. Laparoendosc. Adv. Surg. Tech. A.* 2006;16:241-6.

[57] Mikhael J, Northridge K, Lindquist K, Kessler C, Deuson R, Danese M. Short-term and long-term failure of laparoscopic splenectomy in adult immune thrombocytopenic purpura patients: a systematic review. *Am. J. Hematol.* 2009;84:743-8.

[58] Balagué C, Targarona EM, Cerdán G, Novell J, Montero O, Bendahan G, et al. Long-term outcome after laparoscopic splenectomy related to hematologic diagnosis. *Surg. Endosc.* 2004;18:1283-7.

[59] Ikeda M, Sekimoto M, Takiguchi S, Kubota M, Ikenaga M, Yamamoto H, et al. High incidence of thrombosis of the portal venous system after laparoscopic splenectomy: a prospective study with contrast-enhanced CT scan. *Ann. Surg.* 2005;241:208-16.

[60] Pietrabissa A, Moretto C, Antonelli G, Morelli L, Marciano E, Mosca F. Thrombosis in the portal venous system after elective laparoscopic splenectomy. *Surg. Endosc.* 2004;18:1140-3.

In: Laparoscopy: New Developments, Procedures and Risks   ISBN: 978-1-61470-747-9
Editor: Hana Terzic, pp. 205-218   © 2012 Nova Science Publishers, Inc.

Chapter IX

Robotic-Assisted Procedures in General Surgery

Richdeep S. Gill[1], Kevin Whitlock[2], David P. Al-Adra[1],
Chad Ball[3] and Shazheer Karmali[4]

[1] Department of Surgery, University of Alberta, Edmonton, Alberta, Canada.
[2] Faculty of Medicine and Dentistry, University of Alberta, Edmonton, Alberta, Canada.
[3] Department of Surgery, University of Calgary, Calgary, Alberta, Canada.
[4] Center for Advancement of Minimally Invasive Surgery (CAMIS),
Royal Alexandria Hospital, Edmonton, Alberta, Canada.

Abstract

General surgery has advanced into a multitude of subspecialties over the last two decades including, but not limited to, colorectal and upper gastrointestinal (UGI). Advancements in surgical procedures in each field, specifically laparoscopic or minimally invasive surgery (MIS), have been partially responsible for this specialization. Minimally invasive surgery within each subspecialty has evolved and in many cases is advantageous or comparable to open surgery. The advantages of MIS can be demonstrated by improved recovery and subsequently shorter hospital stay following fundoplication or decreased blood loss following total mesorectal excision. As surgical procedures continue to progress in complexity, further advancements in surgical techniques are necessary to maintain safety and efficiency. Robotic-assisted surgical procedures may be the next evolution in minimally invasive surgery. With improved three-dimensional visualization and surgical instruments with seven degrees-of-freedom, robotic-assisted colorectal, UGI and biliary surgery has been shown to be safe and feasible in both comparative studies and case series. However, further studies are needed to define a clear patient benefit that justifies the increased operational impact and costs associated with robotic-assisted surgery in General Surgery.

Introduction

The definition of a general surgeon has evolved over the last two decades [1]. Initially defined a surgeon capable of performing a multitude of surgical procedures on many different organ systems in the body, including upper gastrointestinal (UGI), colorectal, biliary surgery, among others [2]. However, the role of a general surgeon has slowly been changing with further subspecialization within the field, seemingly focused on specific patient populations or organ systems [3]. Surgical fellowship training has provided general surgery trainees to further enhance their surgical skills by a focused approach to increase competency in particular surgical procedures [4]. In colorectal surgery, fellowship training is thought to enhance surgical skills to allow precise mesorectal dissection to improve rectal cancer surgery. The second factor to contribute to further specialization has been the progression of minimally invasive surgery (MIS) [3]. MIS procedures such as laparoscopic surgery have rapidly grown, since the first laparoscopic cholecystectomy in France in 1987 [5]. Despite improved postoperative pain and shorter duration of hospital stay, limitations of laparoscopic surgery exist [6]. Robotic-assisted surgery is hailed as the next evolution of MIS surgery. In this review, we will explore this progression in MIS surgery, by assessing the use of robotic surgery in general surgery.

Laparoscopic Cholecystectomy

Despite the first laparoscopic cholecystectomy (LC) being performed in France in 1987 [5], widespread use of laparoscopic surgery did not occur immediately. Initially concern was raised about the safety of such procedures. Also, unfamiliarity with new surgical equipment and surgeon inexperience served as barriers. LC was considered a demanding procedure with a long learning curve [7]. In fact it took an average of 200 operations to reach a plateau for the operation time [7]. However, as the literature and experience emerged, acceptance of LC became widespread. Schulze et al reported improved pulmonary peak flow and pain scores following LC in 53 patients [8]. They speculated that these factors might explain the shorter hospital stay of these patients. Bisgaard et al reported that following uncomplicated LC, there is no pathophysiologic basis for more than two to three days of convalescence [9]. Furthermore, resumption of daily physical activities postoperatively may occur in a week in 50% of patients with appropriate encouragement [10]. A recent meta-analysis of five randomized controlled trials, including 215 patients, reported LC as day surgery to be safe in elective cases [11]. Consequently, there are over half a million cholecystectomy procedures performed in North America every year and the number continues to increase [12]. Therefore, LC has become a standard of care for gallbladder disease in symptomatic patients. The steady progression has occurred over a decade in early 21st century. Currently there is debate as to whether robotic cholecystectomy surgery is effective and safe. Surgeons are trying to determine the feasibility of this young technology in replacing the established laparoscopic procedure.

Robotic Surgery

Robotic surgery is deemed the next evolution of MIS surgery. It is believed by supporters that it too will progress, similar to laparoscopic surgery in the past. The limitations to conventional laparoscopic surgery may be driver of this phenomenon. Limitations to laparoscopic surgery include restricted movement and impaired dexterity, especially in overweight or obese patients [13]. Furthermore, the range of movements may be restricted by the location of operation, such as the pelvis. The surgeon is restricted from performing or placing highly accurate sutures [14]. The visualization is reduced by the two-dimensional image on the flat monitor. Lastly, the surgeon is placed in irregular positions and undergoes undesired fatigue and stress. Robotic surgery, which most commonly utilizes the Da Vinci robot or Zeus robot systems, allows the surgeon to go beyond these restrictions. These robot systems function as master-slave devices. The surgeon operates the robotic system from a console away from the patients. Visualization of the intra-abdominal anatomy is improved with the 3-dimensional image and magnification [15]. Also, the robotic arms are free of any physiologic tremor of the operating surgeon, and have increased flexibility compared to standard laparoscopic instruments [16,17]. Additionally, the operating console in robotic surgery relieves the ergonomic strain on the surgeon's trunk, neck and upper extremities from laparoscopic surgery [18]. Despite these potential benefits of robotic-assisted surgery, safety and efficacy are key determinants in the advancement of robotics in general surgery.

Robotic Cholecystectomy

Satava and Green first described robotic-telesurgical laparoscopic surgery in 1992 [19]. The same year SRI International developed an early system to test their concept [20]. Then in 1996, Bowersox and colleagues validated the robotic surgical concept by performing vascular anastomoses on animals [21]. The robotic technique allowed for stereoscopic vision and improved dexterity [22]. Robotic-assisted surgery was first introduced by the first tele-surgical laparoscopic cholecystectomy performed in 1997 [13]. Since it introduction, robotic-assisted cholecystectomies have been performed by a multitude of surgeons at various centers. Giulianotti et al performed 52 robotic-assisted cholecystectomies over a 2-year period [14]. They utilized four ports and reported a mean operative time of 85 min. They also reported a relatively reduced operative time during the second period of performing robotic-assisted cholecystectomy of 66 min. They attributed the reduction in time to gains in operative experience. Vidovszky et al performed 51 robotic cholecystectomies over a 1-year period [23]. They reported high rates of successful completion of the robotic procedure, with only 3 conversions to either conventional laparoscopic or open surgery. Conversion from robotic to open cholecystectomy is an important consideration, as it is seen as undesirable from an efficiency standpoint. A recent systematic review found there to be no significant difference in the conversion rates between conventional laparoscopy and robotic cholecystectomy [24-27]. As well, there are numerous supportive studies that report 0% conversion rates for robotic cholecystectomy [14,28,29], including those following completion of 50 robotic cholecystectomies [14,30]. Hence, the literature supports that robotic-assisted cholecystectomy may be performed with low conversion rates.

Mortality and morbidity are important considerations for any surgical procedure. A recent systematic review found that none of the included trials reported any mortality following robotic cholecystectomy [24]. Two of the trials in the aforementioned systematic review reported morbidity [25,26]. However, the complications were only associated with the surgery itself in one of those studies. The complication in that study was arterial bleeding; however there was no significant difference between the robotic and laparoscopic groups [26]. Furthermore, after reviewing other robotic studies, morbidity rates are generally very low [31]. A postoperative bile duct leak and laceration of the left superior epigastric artery have been reported [30,32]. But, in those studies the complications occurred in a single case. It is generally considered that the complication rate with robotic cholecystectomy is comparable to laparoscopic cholecystectomy [24].

The goal of any surgical procedure is to use time efficiently in the operating room. This involves balancing speed with safety, to minimize complications. So, does using a robot alter operative time? It has been speculated that, although fatigue of the surgeon would be reduced, the operating time would increase when performing robotic cholecystectomy. Furthermore, operator experience relates closely with performance and speed; so does using more complicated technology prolong the learning curve? A recent meta-analysis of four studies, reported that operating time was not significantly different when comparing robotic to conventional laparoscopy [24-27,33]. Concurrently, a recent study comparing 50 robotic to 50 laparoscopic cholecystectomies reported similar findings [30]. However, operating times may be quite variable among different surgical centers [34]. Possible explanations to this occurrence may be related to how operating time is reported. For instance, operating time may sometimes include robot set-up time, while in other cases; only actual procedural time is reported. Furthermore, the associated learning curve for robotic cholecystectomies seems to be important [23,32]. Published results that include early robotic operative experience usually report increased operative times. On the other hand, studies that report later experience typically have decreased operative times. However, based on available literature, it appears that following the initial learning curve, robotic cholecystectomy is comparable to laparoscopic cholecystectomy in regard to operative time.

The cost associated with robotic cholecystectomy remains a major hindrance. With the cost of the Da Vinci robotic system estimated to be $1 to $2 million, the introduction of the technique to a surgical center is a significant investment. Furthermore, the need for a specialized surgical team to efficiently use the robotic system needs to be considered. Unfortunately, only a limited number of studies have reported operating and total costs of robotic cholecystectomy. However, these studies consistently describe robotic cholecystectomy to be more expensive than the conventional laparoscopic approach [28,30,31]. With the objective of cost-effective medicine, the overall cost of robotic cholecystectomy that at this point is a considerable barrier. However the increased cost of robotic surgery may reflect the early stage of its evolution. Similar hesitations were present when the introduction of laparoscopic cholecystectomy, thus it remains to seen if this barrier will be overcome. Currently, use of robotic cholecystectomy for routine use is difficult to justify. Nevertheless, it has been suggested that it may serve as a bridge to performing advanced robotic procedures [34]. Jayaraman et al have suggested that robotic cholecystectomy allows a surgeon in practice to develop and gain experience with the robotic system, which may facilitate them performing more advanced robotic procedures [34].

Robotic Fundoplication

Nissan fundoplication has emerged as the treatment option of choice for gastro-esophageal reflux disease (GERD) that is resistant to medical treatment. Gastroesophageal reflux disease (GERD) is defined as a 'condition which develops when the reflux of stomach contents causes troublesome symptoms and/or complications' by the Montreal Consensus [35]. Also, in North American, GERD is a common condition; with 36% of healthy persons suffering from heartburn at least once a month and 7% experience symptoms of heartburn once a day [36]. Additionally, 2% of adults suffer from complicated GERD, which includes histological or macroscopic injury to the esophagus [36].

Often the only solution for a mechanical disorder is surgical treatment. Fundoplication is indicated in patients with complications of GERD, such as Barrett's esophagus or peptic stricture [37]. Furthermore, extra-esophageal manifestations such as asthma, hoarseness, cough, chest pain, and aspiration are also indications for surgery [38,39]. However, surgical management may also be chosen by patients wishing to avoid long-term medications or if medical management has failed [40].

Interestingly, this surgical technique has been around for more than 50 years. In 1956, Rudolph Nissen wrapped the gastric fundus around the distal esophagus as an anti-reflux treatment; this was called the "open Nissen fundoplication" [41]. This procedure was the optimal surgical option until the early 1990s, when Dallenmagne first described the laparoscopic Nissen fundoplication [42]. The laparoscopic approach was proposed to decrease complications, improve recovery time, and improve cosmesis [43]. However, surgeons were initially skeptical of the minimally invasive approach.

The original shortcomings of laparoscopic fundoplication were bowel perforations, vascular injury, a lengthy learning curve, greater cost, and longer operation times [43]. Initial studies reported complications and questioned the benefits of laparoscopic fundoplication [44-47]. However, the results were often conflicting and many centers continued to use laparoscopy. Recently a meta-analysis looked at 17 years of research, comparing open and laparoscopic fundoplication. The laparoscopic approach was found to have lower complication rates, reduced length of stay, and allowed for earlier return to normal activity [43]. Furthermore, both techniques have similar long-term outcomes [43]. Thus, laparoscopic fundoplication is considered a safe and effective treatment of GERD.

The benefits of robotic fundoplication compared to the laparoscopic approach include improved ergonomic positioning and enhanced three-dimensional view [48,49]. This addresses two limitations of conventional laparoscopy, including the two dimensional view screens and often-cumbersome ergonomics. However, before robotic fundoplication gains acceptance, it must be shown to improve patient's symptoms, allow discontinuation of reflux medications with minimal morbidity.

In terms of mortality, a recent systematic review found there was no reported mortality with robotic fundoplication [48,50-55]. Furthermore, this review reported no significant difference in the number of intraoperative complications between robotic to laparoscopic fundoplication [48,50,51,55]. Within this review, three of the included trials reported no intraoperative complications associated with robotic fundoplication [52-54]. As well, other studies have found that robotic and laparoscopic fundoplication have comparably low morbidity rates [14,56]. These findings support the safety and feasibility of robotic fundoplication.

The systematic review by Markar et al, did not analyze conversion rates following robotic fundoplication [50]. However upon reviewing individual studies, the conversion rate to open fundoplication was similar between the robotic and laparoscopic techniques [14,49]. However the conversion rate from robotic to laparoscopic fundoplication is a new consideration. According to several studies, this occurs 0 - 11% of the time [14,49,51,53,54,56]. An important consideration is the experience of the surgeons performing the fundoplication. Two studies found the conversion rate from robotic fundoplication to conventional laparoscopy to be 2.4 – 5.1% [14,49]. Furthermore, Hartmann et al, found that their conversion rate went from 20% in the first 30 procedures to 0% in the last 88 cases [49]. Thus it appears that conversion rates may be inversely related to experience. Overall, the conversion rates from robotic to laparoscopic or open fundoplication are low and comparable to traditional laparoscopy.

The systematic review by Marker et al, also reported significantly longer operative times for robotic fundoplication compared to laparoscopic fundoplication [48,50-55]. However, the review recognized significant statistical heterogeneity and statistical bias when analyzing operating times [50]. So, it is questionable as to whether their conclusion about robotic fundoplication is valid. However, other primary studies have reported that operative times to be significantly longer with robotic surgery [49,52]. Some of the larger studies have reported times ranging from 92 – 207 min [14,32,49,53]. Therefore, there is evidence to suggest that robotic surgery may extend operative time. This once again may be related to operative experience. Giulianotti et al postulated that there was a sharp learning curve associated with robotic fundoplication [14]. They observed that their operating times decreased progressively with each case [14].

Resolution of pre-operative symptomatology is one of the key measures of a successful fundoplication procedure. Postoperative dysphagia is one of the most common complications following fundoplication. Markar et al, reported no significant difference between the robotic and laparoscopic fundoplication in terms of postoperative dysphagia [50,52,53,55]. Furthermore, the review reported no statistical evidence of heterogeneity, but insufficient data for calculation of statistical bias [50]. However, only 3 primary studies were included in the calculation. Nonetheless, other studies report similar finding [51,56,57]. The actual rate of post-operative dysphagia is quite variable among studies, ranging from 0 - 18% prevalence [53,56,57]. The study by Draaisma et al revealed that mucosal healing, lower esophageal sphincter tone, and reduction in esophageal acid exposure were similar between robotic and laparoscopic fundoplication [51]. Specifically, the rate of esophagitis dropped from 76% to 13% and 24 hour esophageal pH monitoring demonstrated that percentage of time with pH < 4.0 went from 13.5% to 0.7% after robotic fundoplication [51]. So although the data is limited at this time, there is qualitative and quantitative evidence supporting equivocal rates of postoperative dysphagia following robotic fundoplication.

Another measure of successful fundoplication is discontinuation of anti-reflux medication including proton-pump inhibitor (PPI) therapy. According to Muller-Stich et al, 15% of the patients following robotic fundoplication resumed PPI therapy within 30 days of the surgery [55] compared to 10% in the laparoscopic group; however the difference was not statistically significant [55]. Hartmann et al, reported that the majority of patients discontinued PPI intake postoperatively with both surgical techniques [49]. It appears, that either MIS approach, generally allows patients to cease their PPI therapy following fundoplication. Overall, both approaches to fundoplication have good and comparable postoperative outcomes for the majority of patients.

Cost remains a major obstacle to the routine use of robotics in performing minimally invasive fundoplication. Currently, a paucity of data exists with regards to cost analysis. In a recent review, two trials reported appropriate cost analysis, however meta-analysis was not possible [50]. Robotic fundoplication was reported to be €501 to €1806 more expensive than laparoscopic fundoplication [53,55]. As well, numerous other studies have cited high costs as barriers to adopting this new technology [31,58,59].

The estimated cost per robotic fundoplication ranges from €3157 to €6973 [53-55,57]. Unfortunately, the calculation of cost is highly variable between studies. Some include operating room personnel, length of stay, investment, and material costs, while others only consider operative billing costs. This makes cost comparison between studies difficult. However, regardless of cost reporting, the literature suggests that cost is increased for robotic fundoplication. Currently, it is controversial whether the robotic technique provides enough additional benefits to outweigh the financial barriers. Perhaps in time as the technology becomes more affordable, it may lead to greater utilization.

Robotic Colorectal Surgery

Laparoscopic colorectal resection involves a range of surgical procedures depending on the anatomical region to be resected. Colon resections involve right, transverse, left and sigmoid colon resections. Rectal resections can range from a low anterior resection (removal of the rectum with preservation of the sphincter complex) to abdominoperineal resection (en bloc removal of rectum and sphincter complex). Overall, laparoscopic colorectal surgery has been slower to gain acceptance compared to both cholecystectomy and fundoplication. There have been concerns regarding oncologic outcomes. Early trials suggested that laparoscopic colon resection might lead to tumor dissemination [60,61]. This has lead to a number of clinical trials to assess these concerns. Lacy et al randomized 219 patients over a five-year period to receive either laparoscopic-assisted colectomy or traditional open colectomy [62]. Patients treated with the laparoscopic approach had significantly less blood loss, length of hospital stay, postoperative wound infections and ileus compared to the open approach. However, the laparoscopic procedure was longer by approximately twenty minutes. The primary outcome of this study, which was cancer-related survival, was significantly increased in the laparoscopic group. Interestingly, the improvement in cancer-related survival was most prominent for stage III colon cancer. The Clinical Outcomes of Surgical Therapy Study Group conducted a multicentre non-inferiority study and randomized 872 patients with median follow-up of 4.4 years to assess time to tumor recurrence [63]. They reported similar rates of recurrence between the two groups (16% vs. 18%). Also, recurrence rates within surgical wounds were less than 1% in both groups. Similar to other studies comparing laparoscopic and open colectomy, they're results revealed shorter hospital stays and less use of post-operative narcotics in the laparoscopic treated patients. Laparoscopic rectal resection (LAR or APR) was compared to open rectal resection in the United Kingdom Medical Research Council CLASICC trial [64]. They recruited 794 patients and randomized them in a

2:1 ratio favoring laparoscopic resection. This translated into 128 patients in the open rectal resection group and 253 in the laparoscopic rectal resection group. They reported a similar overall survival at 3-year follow-up between both groups. Local recurrence rates were also similar between groups at approximately 10%. Since laparoscopic colorectal resection now has strong evidence to suggest that it is an equivocal oncologic procedure as the open approach, future progression is capable. The next stage of development seems to be robotic colectomy and rectal resection.

Weber et al described the first robotic-assisted laparoscopic colectomies in 2002 [65]. They performed a right and sigmoid colectomy for recurrent episode of diverticulitis. Since then interest and experience in robotic colectomy has been steadily increasing. Spinoglio et al described their initial experience with robotic colorectal surgery and compared it to laparoscopic colorectal resections during the same time period [66]. Of the 50 patients enrolled, the majority was for cancer. The reported a mean operative time of 339 min compared to 266 min for robotic vs. laparoscopic resection, respectively. Though robotic resection was associated with a longer operative time, the mean operative time was significantly decreased during the last 25 cases compared to the initial 25 cases. Rawlings et al compared 30 robotic colectomies (right and sigmoid) to 27 laparoscopic colectomies [67]. They also reported significantly increased operative time for right hemicolectomy in the robotic group (219 vs. 169 min). However, there was no significant difference in operative time between robotic and laparoscopic sigmoid resection. Luca et al reported a mean operative time of 290 ± 69 min for 55 robotic left colon and rectal cancer resections [68]. Unfortunately, they did not separately assess operative time for robotic rectal cancer resection. However, Park et al performed total robotic rectal resection for cancer including splenic flexure mobilization on 45 patients and reported an operative time of 294 ± 80 min [69]. This group utilized a six-port robotic system, which allows assess from the splenic flexure to the pelvic diaphragm without need to reposition the patient. Thus, it is possible to avoid time delays related to repositioning the patient and moving the robot.

Conversion from robotic colectomy to either laparoscopic or open colectomy has been reported by a number of studies. Huettner et al reported 8 conversions out of 70 robotic colectomies (right and sigmoid) performed by a single surgeon [70]. Reasons for conversion ranged from robotic malfunction to difficult dissection secondary to adhesions or bleeding. In performing robotic right hemicolectomy, D'Annibale et al reported no conversions following 50 consecutive resections [71]. Luca et al, reported no conversions following 55 left colon or rectal resections [68]. For totally robotic rectal resection, Park et al reported one conversion to laparscopic resection for iliac artery injury [69]. Interestingly, a recent systematic review comparing robotic to laparoscopic colorectal surgery, reported a combined conversion rate of 6% (16/288) [72].

According to the review by Mirnezami et al, no intra-operative or 30-day mortality has been reported [72]. They determined that the overall complication rate was 11% from a total of 288 robotic procedures. Major complications, such as anastomotic leak or intra-operative bowel injury, were estimated to occur in 2.1% and 1.1% of cases, respectively. Cardiovascular complications occurred in five patients (1.8%). Minor complications such as wound infections (1.8%) and atelectasis (1.1%) were also reported. Huettner et al reported a total of 8 complications in their series of 70 robotic colectomies (11%) [70]. Of these, three were major complications including anastomotic leak, transverse colonic and cecal injury presumed secondary to unrecognized thermal injury. Luca et al reported a relatively higher anastomotic leak rate of 12.7% (7/55) following robotic left colon and rectal resection for cancer [68]. Five of the seven cases of leak were for rectal operations. However, they also stated that all of these cases were treated successively with pelvic drainage and antibiotic therapy. In contrast, Park et al reported one anastomotic leak following 45 robotic rectal resections for cancer, which was managed with re-operation and diverting ileostomy [69].

The hospital length of stay (LOS) following robotic colon or rectal resection is variable in the literature, which makes comparison challenging. Following robotic right hemicolectomy, D'Annibale et al reported a mean hospital LOS of 7 ± 1.2 days [71]. While Huettner et al reported a median LOS of 3 and 4 days following robotic right hemicolectomy and sigmoid colectomy, respectively. Following robotic left colon or rectal resection; mean LOS was estimated to be 7.5 ± 2.8 days [68]. Park et al reported an increased LOS of 9.8 ± 5.2 days following robotic rectal resection for cancer [69]. The indications for colorectal surgery and the differences in involvement of the robotic system make it difficult to determine the contribution of the robotic system to LOS in these patients. This is an important consideration when we are considering the overall cost of robotics. It is unclear if the additional costs of the robotic system translate into saving in other areas of healthcare, such as hospital costs related to LOS.

The additional costs of robotic surgery remain an obstacle in colorectal surgery. Rawlings et al compared costs of laparoscopic and robotic right hemicolectomies, assessing total hospital and operating room costs [67]. They reported mean total hospital costs (US$) of robotic surgery to be $9,255 \pm 5,075$ compared to $8,073 \pm 2,805$ for laparoscopic surgery. The difference between the two groups was not significant, however the sample size was small with a total of 32 patients. On the other hand, total operating room costs, operating room personnel, supply and time costs were significantly greater in the robotic right colectomy group. Interestingly, when comparing robotic and laparoscopic sigmoid colectomy, total OR costs were similar. However, sample size was again very small with a total of 25 sigmoid colectomies. Clearly, further studies are needed to clarify the financial burden of robotic colorectal surgery, with focus on operating room and other hospital related costs.

Conclusion

Advanced robotic procedures have entered the domain of general surgery. The drive behind robotics may be limitation of laparoscopic surgery, patient demand, or ongoing specialization. The increased technical fluidity, visualization and range of motion of the robotic system are difficult to deny. However, the cost to benefit ratio of robotic surgery within general surgery remains controversial. The increased cost of robotic cholecystectomy may not be routinely justifiable, however, it may serve as an excellent bridge to more advanced robotic procedures. The same has been suggested of robotic right hemicolectomies. Though is natural in the evolution of surgery to be skeptical of change, especially due to technology. The progression of robotic surgery may indeed be similar to the advancement to laparoscopic surgery that occurred a decade before. There are numerous benefits to minimally invasive surgery, however the specific advantages of robotic surgery in general surgery warrant further investigation.

References

[1]   Fischer JE. The Impending Disappearance of the General Surgeon. *JAMA* 2007;298(18):2191-2193.

[2]   Santry HP, Chokshi N, Datrice N, Guitron J, Moller MG. General surgery training and the demise of the general surgeon. *Bull Am. Coll Surg.* 2008 Jul;93(7):32-38.

[3]   Jurkovich GJ, Rozycki GS. Acute care surgery: real or imagined threat to the general surgeon. *Am. J. Surg.* 2010 Jun;199(6):862-863.

[4]   Borman KR, Vick LR, Biester TW, Mitchell ME. Changing demographics of residents choosing fellowships: longterm data from the American Board of Surgery. *J. Am. Coll. Surg.* 2008 May;206(5):782-8; discussion 788-9.

[5]   Perissat J. Invited Commentary. *Surgical Endoscopy* 1990;4:149.

[6]   Reddick EJ, Olsen DO. Outpatient laparoscopic laser cholecystectomy. *Am. J. Surg.* 1990 Nov;160(5):485-7; discussion 488-9.

[7]   Voitk AJ, Tsao SG, Ignatius S. The tail of the learning curve for laparoscopic cholecystectomy. *Am. J. Surg.* 2001 Sep;182(3):250-253.

[8]   Schulze S, Thorup J. Pulmonary function, pain, and fatigue after laparoscopic cholecystectomy. *Eur. J. Surg.* 1993 Jun-Jul;159(6-7):361-364.

[9]   Bisgaard T, Klarskov B, Kehlet H, Rosenberg J. Recovery after uncomplicated laparoscopic cholecystectomy. *Surgery* 2002 Nov;132(5):817-825.

[10]   Wasowicz-Kemps DK, Slootmaker SM, Kemps HM, Borel-Rinkes IH, Biesma DH, van Ramshorst B. Resumption of daily physical activity after day-case laparoscopic cholecystectomy. *Surg. Endosc.* 2009 Sep;23(9):2034-2040.

[11]   Gurusamy K, Junnarkar S, Farouk M, Davidson BR. Meta-analysis of randomized controlled trials on the safety and effectiveness of day-case laparoscopic cholecystectomy. *Br. J. Surg.* 2008 Feb;95(2):161-168.

[12]   Livingston EH, Rege RV. A nationwide study of conversion from laparoscopic to open cholecystectomy. *Am. J. Surg.* 2004 Sep;188(3):205-211.

[13]   Himpens J, Leman G, Cadiere GB. Telesurgical laparoscopic cholecystectomy. *Surg. Endosc.* 1998 Aug;12(8):1091.

[14]   Giulianotti PC, Coratti A, Angelini M, Sbrana F, Cecconi S, Balestracci T, et al. Robotics in general surgery: personal experience in a large community hospital. *Arch. Surg.* 2003 Jul;138(7):777-784.

[15]   Jourdan IC, Dutson E, Garcia A, Vleugels T, Leroy J, Mutter D, et al. Stereoscopic vision provides a significant advantage for precision robotic laparoscopy. *Br. J. Surg.* 2004 Jul;91(7):879-885.

[16]   Dakin GF, Gagner M. Comparison of laparoscopic skills performance between standard instruments and two surgical robotic systems. *Surg. Endosc.* 2003 Apr;17(4):574-579.

[17]   Bodner J, Schmid T, Wykypiel H, Bodner E. First experiences with robotic-assisted laparoscopic cholecystectomies. *European Surgery* 2002;34(3):166-169.

[18]   Berguer R, Forkey DL, Smith WD. Ergonomic problems associated with laparoscopic surgery. *Surg. Endosc.* 1999 May;13(5):466-468.

[19]   Satava RM, Green PS. The next generation: telepresence surgery: current status and implications for endoscopy. *Gastrointestinal Endoscopy* 1992;38:277.

[20] Green PS, Satava RM, Hill JR, Simon IB. Telepresence: advanced teleoperator technology for minimally invasive surgery. *Surgical Endoscopy* 1992;6:90.

[21] Bowersox JC, Shah A, Jensen J, Hill J, Cordts PR, Green PS. Vascular applications of telepresence surgery: initial feasibility studies in swine. *J. Vasc. Surg.* 1996 Feb;23(2):281-287.

[22] Yohannes P, Rotariu P, Pinto P, Smith AD, Lee BR. Comparison of robotic versus laparoscopic skills: is there a difference in the learning curve? *Urology* 2002 Jul;60(1):39-45; discussion 45.

[23] Vidovszky TJ, Smith W, Ghosh J, Ali MR. Robotic cholecystectomy: learning curve, advantages, and limitations. *J. Surg. Res.* 2006 Dec;136(2):172-178.

[24] Gurusamy KS, Samraj K, Fusai G, Davidson BR. Robot assistant for laparoscopic cholecystectomy. *Cochrane Database Syst. Rev.* 2009 Jan 21;(1)(1):CD006578.

[25] Aiono S, Gilbert JM, Soin B, Finlay PA, Gordan A. Controlled trial of the introduction of a robotic camera assistant (EndoAssist) for laparoscopic cholecystectomy. *Surg. Endosc.* 2002 Sep;16(9):1267-1270.

[26] den Boer KT, Bruijn M, Jaspers JE, Stassen LP, Erp WF, Jansen A, et al. Time-action analysis of instrument positioners in laparoscopic cholecystectomy. *Surg. Endosc.* 2002 Jan;16(1):142-147.

[27] Zhou HX, Guo YH, Yu XF, Bao SY, Liu JL, Zhang Y, et al. Zeus robot-assisted laparoscopic cholecystectomy in comparison with conventional laparoscopic cholecystectomy. *Hepatobiliary Pancreat Dis. Int.* 2006 Feb;5(1):115-118.

[28] Heemskerk J, van Dam R, van Gemert WG, Beets GL, Greve JW, Jacobs MJ, et al. First results after introduction of the four-armed da Vinci Surgical System in fully robotic laparoscopic cholecystectomy. *Dig. Surg.* 2005;22(6):426-431.

[29] Kim VB, Chapman WH, Albrecht RJ, Bailey BM, Young JA, Nifong LW, et al. Early experience with telemanipulative robot-assisted laparoscopic cholecystectomy using da Vinci. *Surg. Laparosc. Endosc. Percutan Tech* 2002 Feb;12(1):33-40.

[30] Breitenstein S, Nocito A, Puhan M, Held U, Weber M, Clavien PA. Robotic-assisted versus laparoscopic cholecystectomy: outcome and cost analyses of a case-matched control study. *Ann. Surg.* 2008 Jun;247(6):987-993.

[31] Bodner J, Augustin F, Wykypiel H, Fish J, Muehlmann G, Wetscher G, et al. The da Vinci robotic system for general surgical applications: a critical interim appraisal. *Swiss. Med. Wkly.* 2005 Nov 19;135(45-46):674-678.

[32] Ruurda JP, Draaisma WA, van Hillegersberg R, Borel Rinkes IH, Gooszen HG, Janssen LW, et al. Robot-assisted endoscopic surgery: a four-year single-center experience. *Dig. Surg.* 2005;22(5):313-320.

[33] Kraft BM, Jager C, Kraft K, Leibl BJ, Bittner R. The AESOP robot system in laparoscopic surgery: increased risk or advantage for surgeon and patient? *Surg. Endosc.* 2004 Aug;18(8):1216-1223.

[34] Jayaraman S, Davies W, Schlachta CM. Getting started with robotics in general surgery with cholecystectomy: the Canadian experience. *Can. J. Surg.* 2009 Oct;52(5):374-378.

[35] Vakil N, van Zanten SV, Kahrilas P, Dent J, Jones R, Global Consensus Group. The Montreal definition and classification of gastroesophageal reflux disease: a global evidence-based consensus. *Am. J. Gastroenterol.* 2006 Aug;101(8):1900-20; quiz 1943.

[36] Toward Optimized Practice. Treatment of Gastroesophageal Reflux Disease (GERD) in Adults. 2009; Available at: http://www.topalbertadoctors.org/informed_practice/ clinical_practice_guidelines/complete%20set/GERD/gerd_guideline.pdf.

[37] Lagergren J, Bergstrom R, Lindgren A, Nyren O. Symptomatic gastroesophageal reflux as a risk factor for esophageal adenocarcinoma. *N. Engl. J. Med.* 1999 Mar 18;340(11):825-831.

[38] Lindstrom DR, Wallace J, Loehrl TA, Merati AL, Toohill RJ. Nissen fundoplication surgery for extraesophageal manifestations of gastroesophageal reflux (EER). *Laryngoscope* 2002 Oct;112(10):1762-1765.

[39] Rakita S, Villadolid D, Thomas A, Bloomston M, Albrink M, Goldin S, et al. Laparoscopic Nissen fundoplication offers high patient satisfaction with relief of extraesophageal symptoms of gastroesophageal reflux disease. *Am. Surg.* 2006 Mar;72(3):207-212.

[40] Stefanidis D, Hope WW, Kohn GP, Reardon PR, Richardson WS, Fanelli RD, et al. Guidelines for surgical treatment of gastroesophageal reflux disease. *Surg. Endosc.* 2010 Nov;24(11):2647-2669.

[41] Nissen R. [A simple operation for control of reflux esophagitis]. *Schweiz. Med. Wochenschr.* 1956 May 18;86(Suppl 20):590-592.

[42] Dallemagne B, Weerts JM, Jehaes C, Markiewicz S, Lombard R. Laparoscopic Nissen fundoplication: preliminary report. *Surg. Laparosc. Endosc.* 1991 Sep;1(3):138-143.

[43] Peters MJ, Mukhtar A, Yunus RM, Khan S, Pappalardo J, Memon B, et al. Meta-analysis of randomized clinical trials comparing open and laparoscopic anti-reflux surgery. *Am. J. Gastroenterol.* 2009 Jun;104(6):1548-61; quiz 1547, 1562.

[44] Cadiere GB, Houben JJ, Bruyns J, Himpens J, Panzer JM, Gelin M. Laparoscopic Nissen fundoplication: technique and preliminary results. *Br. J. Surg.* 1994 Mar;81(3):400-403.

[45] Watson DI, Jamieson GG, Mitchell PC, Devitt PG, Britten-Jones R. Stenosis of the esophageal hiatus following laparoscopic fundoplication. *Arch. Surg.* 1995 Sep;130(9):1014-1016.

[46] Dallemagne B, Weerts JM, Jehaes C, Markiewicz S. Causes of failures of laparoscopic antireflux operations. *Surg. Endosc.* 1996 Mar;10(3):305-310.

[47] Hinder RA, Filipi CJ, Wetscher G, Neary P, DeMeester TR, Perdikis G. Laparoscopic Nissen fundoplication is an effective treatment for gastroesophageal reflux disease. *Ann. Surg.* 1994 Oct;220(4):472-81; discussion 481-3.

[48] Cadiere GB, Himpens J, Vertruyen M, Bruyns J, Germay O, Leman G, et al. Evaluation of telesurgical (robotic) NISSEN fundoplication. *Surg. Endosc.* 2001 Sep;15(9):918-923.

[49] Hartmann J, Menenakos C, Ordemann J, Nocon M, Raue W, Braumann C. Long-term results of quality of life after standard laparoscopic vs. robot-assisted laparoscopic fundoplications for gastro-oesophageal reflux disease. A comparative clinical trial. *Int. J. Med. Robot.* 2009 Mar;5(1):32-37.

[50] Markar SR, Karthikesalingam AP, Hagen ME, Talamini M, Horgan S, Wagner OJ. Robotic vs. laparoscopic Nissen fundoplication for gastro-oesophageal reflux disease: systematic review and meta-analysis. *Int. J. Med. Robot.* 2010 Jun;6(2):125-131.

[51] Draaisma WA, Ruurda JP, Scheffer RC, Simmermacher RK, Gooszen HG, Rijnhart-de Jong HG, et al. Randomized clinical trial of standard laparoscopic versus robot-assisted

laparoscopic Nissen fundoplication for gastro-oesophageal reflux disease. *Br. J. Surg.* 2006 Nov;93(11):1351-1359.

[52] Melvin WS, Needleman BJ, Krause KR, Schneider C, Ellison EC. Computer-enhanced vs. standard laparoscopic antireflux surgery. *J. Gastrointest. Surg.* 2002 Jan-Feb;6(1):11-5; discussion 15-6.

[53] Nakadi IE, Melot C, Closset J, DeMoor V, Betroune K, Feron P, et al. Evaluation of da Vinci Nissen fundoplication clinical results and cost minimization. *World J. Surg.* 2006 Jun;30(6):1050-1054.

[54] Morino M, Pellegrino L, Giaccone C, Garrone C, Rebecchi F. Randomized clinical trial of robot-assisted versus laparoscopic Nissen fundoplication. *Br. J. Surg.* 2006 May;93(5):553-558.

[55] Muller-Stich BP, Reiter MA, Wente MN, Bintintan VV, Koninger J, Buchler MW, et al. Robot-assisted versus conventional laparoscopic fundoplication: short-term outcome of a pilot randomized controlled trial. *Surg. Endosc.* 2007 Oct;21(10):1800-1805.

[56] Ayav A, Bresler L, Brunaud L, Boissel P. Early results of one-year robotic surgery using the Da Vinci system to perform advanced laparoscopic procedures. *J. Gastrointest Surg.* 2004 Sep-Oct;8(6):720-726.

[57] Heemskerk J, van Gemert WG, Greve JW, Bouvy ND. Robot-assisted versus conventional laparoscopic Nissen fundoplication: a comparative retrospective study on costs and time consumption. *Surg. Laparosc. Endosc. Percutan. Tech.* 2007 Feb;17(1):1-4.

[58] Hartmann J, Jacobi CA, Menenakos C, Ismail M, Braumann C. Surgical treatment of gastroesophageal reflux disease and upside-down stomach using the Da Vinci robotic system. A prospective study. *J. Gastrointest. Surg.* 2008 Mar;12(3):504-509.

[59] Costi R, Himpens J, Iusco D, Sarli L, Violi V, Roncoroni L, et al. [Robotic fundoplication for gastro-oesophageal reflux disease]. *Chir. Ital.* 2004 May-Jun;56(3):321-331.

[60] Berends FJ, Kazemier G, Bonjer HJ, Lange JF. Subcutaneous metastases after laparoscopic colectomy. *Lancet* 1994 Jul 2;344(8914):58.

[61] Vukasin P, Ortega AE, Greene FL, Steele GD, Simons AJ, Anthone GJ, et al. Wound recurrence following laparoscopic colon cancer resection. Results of the American Society of Colon and Rectal Surgeons Laparoscopic Registry. *Dis. Colon Rectum.* 1996 Oct;39(10 Suppl):S20-3.

[62] Lacy AM, Garcia-Valdecasas JC, Delgado S, Castells A, Taura P, Pique JM, et al. Laparoscopy-assisted colectomy versus open colectomy for treatment of non-metastatic colon cancer: a randomised trial. *Lancet* 2002 Jun 29;359(9325):2224-2229.

[63] Clinical Outcomes of Surgical Therapy Study Group. A comparison of laparoscopically assisted and open colectomy for colon cancer. *N. Engl. J. Med.* 2004 May 13;350(20):2050-2059.

[64] Jayne DG, Guillou PJ, Thorpe H, Quirke P, Copeland J, Smith AM, et al. Randomized trial of laparoscopic-assisted resection of colorectal carcinoma: 3-year results of the UK MRC CLASICC Trial Group. *J. Clin. Oncol.* 2007 Jul 20;25(21):3061-3068.

[65] Weber PA, Merola S, Wasielewski A, Ballantyne GH. Telerobotic-assisted laparoscopic right and sigmoid colectomies for benign disease. *Dis. Colon. Rectum.* 2002 Dec;45(12):1689-94; discussion 1695-6.

[66] Spinoglio G, Summa M, Priora F, Quarati R, Testa S. Robotic colorectal surgery: first 50 cases experience. *Dis. Colon. Rectum.* 2008 Nov;51(11):1627-1632.

[67] Rawlings AL, Woodland JH, Vegunta RK, Crawford DL. Robotic versus laparoscopic colectomy. *Surg. Endosc.* 2007 Oct;21(10):1701-1708.

[68] Luca F, Cenciarelli S, Valvo M, Pozzi S, Faso FL, Ravizza D, et al. Full robotic left colon and rectal cancer resection: technique and early outcome. *Ann. Surg. Oncol.* 2009 May;16(5):1274-1278.

[69] Park YA, Kim JM, Kim SA, Min BS, Kim NK, Sohn SK, et al. Totally robotic surgery for rectal cancer: from splenic flexure to pelvic floor in one setup. *Surg. Endosc.* 2010 Mar;24(3):715-720.

[70] Huettner F, Rawlings AL, McVay WB, Crawford DL. Robot-assisted laparoscopic colectomy: 70 cases - one surgeon. *Journal of Robotic Surgery* 2008;2(4):227-234.

[71] D'Annibale A, Pernazza G, Morpurgo E, Monsellato I, Pende V, Lucandri G, et al. Robotic right colon resection: evaluation of first 50 consecutive cases for malignant disease. *Ann. Surg. Oncol.* 2010 Nov;17(11):2856-2862.

[72] Mirnezami AH, Mirnezami R, Venkatasubramaniam AK, Chandrakumaran K, Cecil TD, Moran BJ. Robotic colorectal surgery: hype or new hope? A systematic review of robotics in colorectal surgery. *Colorectal Dis.* 2010 Nov;12(11):1084-1093.

In: Laparoscopy: New Developments, Procedures and Risks   ISBN: 978-1-61470-747-9
Editor: Hana Terzic, pp. 219-229   © 2012 Nova Science Publishers, Inc.

Chapter X

The Challenges of Laparoscopic Rectal Cancer Surgery

M. Chand[*1] *and A. Parvaiz*[2]
[1] Royal Marsden Hospital
Downs Road, Surrey
[2] Queen Alexandra Hospital
National Laparoscopic Colorectal Surgery Training Centre
Southwick Hill Road, Cosham, Portsmouth.

Introduction

Laparoscopic surgical resection has been universally accepted in the management of colon cancer since its inception in 1991 [1]. Laparoscopic surgery for colon cancer has been well proven by randomized studies to benefit patients; the procedure results in earlier recovery of bowel function, reduced blood loss, less postoperative pain, and decreased hospital stay compared with conventional open colectomy [2, 3]. Most of these studies have also shown adequate lymph node yields and tumor clearance in addition to the improved short-term outcomes in terms of reduced post operative pain, shorter hospital stay, reduced ileus and comparable long-term clinical outcomes. While the minimally invasive approach for colonic resections has become well established and accepted, its role in management of rectal cancer is evolving and remains contentious [4].

The concept of total mesorectal excision (TME) during rectal resection was introduced by Heald in 1979 [5]. The goal of TME is the excision of the rectum along with its blood vessels and surrounding lymph nodes within an intact visceral fascial envelope. Preserving the integrity of this mesorectal fascial envelope and obtaining a negative circumferential margin are the key elements in minimizing pelvic recurrence. Later refinements included preservation of the pelvic automomic nerves and nerve plexuses. Heald reported rates of local recurrence

---

[*] Corresponding author MC: Email mans001@aol.com

as low as 2.7% after potentially curative resection for rectal cancer. He simultaneously showed that it was possible to perform a restorative resection in as many as 90% of rectal cancers with a permanent stoma rate of less than 10%. Nonetheless, such major pelvic dissection with low colorectal or coloanal anastomoses has been associated with considerable morbidity. Anastomotic leak rates of > 15% have been commonly reported and most TME surgeons advocate temporary defunctioning of these anastomoses in order to reduce the consequences if not the frequency of anastomotic leakage [6] Low anterior resection with TME has become the gold standard in the surgical management of rectal cancer [7].

However, applying laparoscopic surgery to rectal cancer is a different proposition. The high rates of morbidity and mortality of patients with local recurrence of rectal cancer are the understandable concerns of the skeptics. Currently there is no evidence to suggest that laparoscopic surgery for rectal cancer in appropriately selected patients leads to this. We review the challenges associated with laparoscopic surgery of the rectum.

Anatomical Considerations and the Importance of MRI

The rectum is intimately surrounded by neurovascular, lymphatic and visceral structures within a confined space. Even the minimal disturbance of these structures can lead to profound physiological and functional consequences. The complexity of the rectum's anatomical relations is compounded by the pathological spread of rectal cancer. Tumor spread is not only longitudinal but circumferential. Quirke identified that circumferential margin involvement following surgery correlated with the development of local recurrence [8]. The pursuit of a precise and bloodless operation which allowed for a clean muscle tube in preparation of circular stapling devices of the late 1970's led to the now universally accepted total mesorectal excision. Preserving the integrity of this mesorectal fascial envelope and obtaining a negative circumferential margin are the key elements in minimizing pelvic recurrence.

The advent of high spatial resolution magnetic resonance imaging (MRI) has provided important information when deciding the merits of curative surgery. MRI has become an integral part of the staging process in rectal cancer in the UK. In comparison with endoluminal techniques, it offers detailed assessment of all tumors including bulky and stricturing tumours. Furthermore, it allows assessment of the entire mesorectum and accuracy in depth of invasion, tumor sub-type (eg mucinous) and extra-mural venous invasion. This is particularly important when deciding the appropriateness of laparoscopic resection.

Patient Selection

Appropriate choice of patient is necessary to perform successful laparoscopic surgery. Patients with significant co-morbidity, high BMI, locally advanced cancers or who have undergone pre-operative long course chemo-radiotherapy, all present distinct challenges with regard to rectal cancer surgery. These factors may preclude laparoscopic surgery for some surgeons [9, 10].

Clearly, there is some degree of subjectivity in patient selection and this may be related to the experience of the surgeon. Appropriate selection will mean less likelihood of conversion or other sub-optimal outcomes. For example, patients with cardio-respiratory co-morbidity benefit from shorter operating time and may be adversely affected by table positioning, eg reverse Trendelenburg, and pneumoperitoneum. Yet conversely, they are also likely to benefit from a faster recovery which laparoscopic surgery provides.

Patients with locally advanced rectal cancers who require multivisceral resection or where the bulk of the tumor is large, may not have much to gain from a laparoscopic pelvic dissection. However, in progressive colorectal units, this will be a relatively small proportion of all rectal cancers.

Potential of Laparoscopic Surgery

Improvements in image quality and the development of newer instruments have allowed the surgeons to expand the horizon in laparoscopic colorectal surgery. Rectal resection for cancer is no exception. Laparoscopy allows for a more precise anatomical TME dissection. High definition laparoscopes with increased viewing angles, means that the abdominal and pelvic cavity can be inspected with much greater visualization. The surgeon is able to view areas of the pelvis which are inaccessible to the naked eye in open surgery. For example, dissection in a narrow male pelvis is often difficult to complete under direct vision and can require several position changes to complete the operation safely. Furthermore, the laparoscopic view is also well illuminated and magnified making it easier to follow surgical planes and anticipate bleeding.

1) More precise anatomical TME dissection. No part of a laparoscopic TME need be completed blind, a 30 degree camera allows a clear view even low in the pelvis. In contrast, conventional TME dissection, especially low posteriorly in a male pelvis is often difficult to complete under direct vision. The laparoscopic view is also well illuminated and magnified making it easier to see and follow surgical planes.

2) Reduced trauma to the oncologic specimen with less inadvertent compromise of specimen quality. Laparoscopic operating tends to displace the rectum and mesorectum gently from side to side. The camera can operate in a very confined space and illuminates its view. In contrast, considerable traction is required to obtain lighting and a view low in the pelvis in conventional resection. Such handling and retraction of the oncologic specimen can cause tears into the mesorectum or even into the lumen. Once a tear begins it tends to progress because traction on the specimen is difficult to avoid during open operations. Rates of R0 resection might be higher following laparoscopic resection.

3) Faster postoperative recovery. Laparoscopic resection offers the potential for reduced blood transfusion requirements, reduced surgical trauma, a less marked inflammatory response, earlier return of gut function and shorter hospital stay compared with conventional operating.

Laparoscopic surgery reduces the trauma to the oncologic specimen with less inadvertent handling. Laparoscopic operating tends to displace the rectum and mesorectum gently from side to side. The camera can operate in a very confined space and illuminates its view. In contrast, considerable traction is required to obtain lighting and a view low in the pelvis in conventional open surgery. Such handling and retraction of the oncologic specimen can cause tears into the mesorectum or even into the lumen. Once a tear begins it tends to progress because traction on the specimen is difficult to avoid during open operations. Rates of "R0" – tumor free, resection might be higher following laparoscopic resection.

Laparoscopic resection offers the potential for reduced blood transfusion requirements, reduced surgical trauma, a less marked inflammatory response, earlier return of gut function and shorter hospital stay compared with conventional operating. All these factors contribute to faster recovery in the majority of patients.

Oncological Safety

The main opposition to laparoscopic rectal resection is a fear of oncological inadequancy. The increased, but wholly justifiable, scrutiny of pathological specimens allows the resection to be qualitatively assessed [11]. The literature suggests that local recurrence, lymph node harvest and oncological clearance are not being compromised [12]. However, many of the studies reporting laparoscopic TME include small numbers of patients and follow up of less than 3 years. In addition, some studies that claim to have performed TME have not consistently provided information regarding height of tumor from anal verge, oncological data such as distance from distal margin, clearance of circumferential margin and selection/exclusion criteria [13].

Bretagnol et al reported a prospective series of 144 laparoscopic TMEs with low colorectal or coloanal anastomosis for mid and low rectal cancers of stage T3 N1 or less [14]. Their conversion rate was 14%. Clear distal and circumferential margins were achieved in 98% and 94% respectively. Two patients developed local recurrence and the 3-year overall and disease-free survival rates were 89% and 77% respectively. Zhou et al reported excellent results of laparoscopic resection for rectal cancer with TME and sphincter preservation in their randomized trial [15]. Their overall morbidity rate was 6.1%, anastomotic leakage rate was 1.2%, mean operative blood loss was 20 mL, and mean operating time was 120 min. However, the report provided no details on method of randomization or definition and rate of conversion, nor whether the analysis was performed on an intention-to-treat basis. Lujan et al have reported a single centre randomized controlled trial in which 204 patients with mid and low rectal cancers were randomized between open and laparoscopic resection [16]. Patients in the laparoscopic group had earlier return of gut function and shorter hospital stay at mean of 2.8 days and 8.2 days respectively. There were fewer anastomotic leaks in the laparoscopic group, CRM positivity was 4%, five-year local recurrence was 4.8%, disease-free survival was 84.8% and overall survival 72.1%. Overall, the results demonstrated oncological equivalence but with significantly faster return of gut function, decreased transfusion requirements and shorter hospital stay following laparoscopic resection.

The CLASICC trial offers substantial evidence on laparoscopic resection for rectal cancer [2]. It included patients with colorectal cancers from 27 centers in United Kingdom and provided detailed subgroup analysis of short- and long-term outcomes of patients with rectal cancer. 242 laparoscopic rectal resections were performed, of which 129 were TMEs. The benefits with laparoscopic surgery of lower intra-operative blood loss, less pain, early return of gut function and less narcotic use were confirmed. Hospital stay was 11 days and was shorter than the 13 days for open TME group. This trial has been criticized for high conversion rates of 34% and high rates of circumferential resection margin (CRM) positivity of 16%. A subsequent 3 year update of this trial revealed equivalent oncologic and quality of life outcomes for the laparoscopic and open groups (overall survival 74.6% laparoscopic and 66.7% open). In addition, the trend toward increased CRM positivity seen in the laparoscopic group did not result in an increased rate of local recurrence (7.8% laparoscopic and 7.0% open) and the administration of neoadjuvant chemoradiation and adjuvant chemotherapy was equivalent in both groups.

A recent systematic review and meta-analysis comparing short and medium term outcomes of over 1400 laparoscopic versus 1755 open TMEs concluded that there were no oncological differences between laparoscopic and open resections for treatment of primary rectal cancer [12]. Laurent et al emphasized the importance of specialization in TME in their series of 238 laparoscopic TMEs with 5-year follow up (median follow up = 52 months) [17]. More than 80% of their rectal resections were for mid and low tumors. All patients were treated with curative intent. Their conversion rate was 15%. The local recurrence rate was 3.8% in laparoscopic completed and no worse (3.5%) in laparoscopic converted cases, both these figures being lower than the 5.5% observed for their open TMEs. These results are in line with the observations of other groups showing that adequately trained laparoscopic surgeons can obtain equivalent long term oncologic results to open TME surgeons. Additionally, a notable observation made by Laurent et al was that the overall survival at 5 years was better in the laparoscopic group than in the open group, especially in Stage III cancers. This impact of laparoscopic surgery on survival requires further investigation.

These reports from surgeons and centres at the leading edge of developments in laparoscopic colorectal cancer surgery show that laparoscopic resection for rectal cancer with TME can be achieved without oncologic compromise and with potential benefits in terms of transfusion requirements, return of gut function, R0 resection rates, and length of stay when compared to conventional resection.

Splenic Flexure Mobilization

Mobilization of the splenic flexure for anterior resection has been disputed in open surgery. Selective mobilization of the splenic flexure only where there are concerns in the integrity of the anastomsosis, does not lead to a higher rate of anastomotic leak or recurrence [18]. Furthermore, the use of the sigmoid colon as the proximal anastomotic end has been shown to be safe. The evolution of laparoscopic rectal surgery provides an opportunity to challenge traditional surgical dogma. The same principles of safe surgery apply in laparoscopy, and if there is no suggestion of tension or compromise on the anastomosis, the splenic flexure may be left alone. Clearly, the closer the tumor is to the anal verge, the more relevant this issue becomes. But it is not a given that the splenic flexure must be mobilized during an ultra-low dissection.

Defunctioning Stomas

Defunctioning stomas are used to prevent the clinical consequences of an anastomotic leak. The use of defunctioning stomas are specific to the operating surgeon although are somewhat dictated by the operative conditions and tumour location. Height of tumor from the anal verge is a known risk factor for anastomotic dehiscence [19]. It is therefore more likely to perform a defunctioning stoma during an ultra-low anterior resection. It is difficult to theorize which patients will need a stoma prior to surgery however it is important to note that overall anastomotic leak rates are lower with laparoscopic rectal cancer surgery than open resection.

Challenges and Morbidity

Conventional cross stapled anastomosis is more difficult to achieve laparoscopically than in open surgery because the available staplers for laparoscopic use are not able to flex sufficiently to allow easy placement of a staple line across the rectum at right angles. Frequently it is necessary to use a number of firings of the stapler to transect the rectum along a more oblique line than intended.

Indeed, Leroy et al in an attempt to explain their 17% clinical leak rate, hypothesized that such a long staple line increases the risk of leakage [20]. They postulated that refinement of the staplers and the technique of stapling in order to enable the stapling device to be applied perpendicular to the bowel would result in a short staple line and a potential reduction in the leak rate. Brannigan et al examined the technique of laparoscopic rectal stapling following TME using a virtual model and simulation of laparoscopic stapling. They concluded that the minimal angulation of the stapler head required for successful transverse stapling of the rectum was 62-68° [21].

For adequate clearance below a low rectal cancer a transverse rather than an oblique transaction of the rectum is optimal. In order to compensate for the limited angulation of current laparoscopic staplers it is necessary to employ special techniques to ensure adequate clearance and safe anastomosis for very low rectal cancers. These include perineal pressure to render the lowest part of the rectum more accessible for staple-transection, dissection into the pelvic funnel in the intersphincteric plane to allow the somewhat oblique staple line to adequately clear the low neoplasm and transanal division of the rectum and hand- sutured coloanal anastomosis.

Rectal cancer resections are generally associated with a significant rate of morbidity and mortality. Several large published series of laparoscopic TME suggest rates in the order of 1-2 % which compares favourably with the 3-8% range reported in open surgery (Dutch trial).

Some of the large series have reported leak rates ranging from 10 – 17% after laparoscopic TME. However, with increasing experience, anastomotic leak rates appear to be declining. In a case-control study comparing laparoscopic and open TME, Breukink et al reported 9% anastomotic leakage in the laparoscopic group vs 14% in the open group [22]. Lujan et al in their recently published single centre randomized trial of laparoscopic versus open TMEs for mid and low rectal cancers, reported anastomotic leak rates of 6% in the laparoscopic group as against 12 % in the open TME group [16]. Similarly, Tsang al from

Hong Kong had only 1 anastomotic leak in their series of 105 laparoscopic rectal cancer resections [23]. Results in our own unit are in agreement with these figures with a leak rate of 0.9% following laparoscopic TME ($n = 106$) as against 3.3 % ($n = 60$) after conventional TME.

Laparoscopic TME has the potential to achieve better preservation of the pelvic autonomic nervous system because the magnified operative view allows easier identification of pelvic nerves. Liang et al studied 98 patients with T3 mid or low rectal cancers undergoing laparoscopic TME following neo-adjuvant chemo-radiotherapy [24]. Patients underwent pre and postoperative assessment of urinary and sexual function with the help of a standardized questionnaire. Any patients with abnormal urinary or sexual function preoperatively were excluded. They reported that it was possible for the majority of their patients to retain satisfactory genitourinary function following a laparoscopic TME with autonomic nerve preservation technique. Similarly, Asoglu et al, in their series of 34 laparoscopic and 29 open TMEs, found that the open technique was associated with a significantly higher incidence of sexual dysfunction, but not bladder dysfunction compared with laparoscopic TME [25].

However, Jayne et al in the only randomized trial investigating genitourinary function post laparoscopic TME, found worse overall sexual and erectile function in men undergoing laparoscopic TME than after open TME [26]. There was no difference in urinary function between the two groups and in both sexes. These results may be due to the learning curve associated with the technique. Further randomized studies are expected to help address this matter conclusively.

Conversion to Open Surgery

Conversion rate ranges widely. The most common reasons cited for conversion include technical difficulties secondary to tumour fixity, dense adhesions or inadequate visualization due to obesity, uncertainties regarding the oncological completeness or hemorrhage. It has also been suggested that male sex and stapled anastomosis are independent risk factors for conversion [27]. However, the definition of conversion in laparoscopic rectal surgery has varied between authors with some describing hybrid operations in which the rectum is mobilized by an open technique where others would consider these as conversions. We believe that requirement of open technique to mobilize the rectum during any part of the laparoscopic TME should be regarded as a conversion.

The experience of the operating surgeon is a major determinant of the conversion rate. Conversion rates have generally decreased over recent years, attributable to a combination of improved instrumentation, imaging technology, increasing experience and perhaps better patient selection. Tsang et al had 2 conversions in 105 Laparoscopic TMEs and Leroy et al in their series of 102 laparoscopic TMEs involving patients across all T stages reported a conversion rate of 3% [20, 23]. The conversion rate in our unit for laparoscopic TME surgery is 3.7 % with satisfactory oncological outcomes.

A German prospective study found an association between high conversion rates and poor oncological outcome in terms of local recurrence [28]. In their study of 389 patients, 114 laparoscopic rectal resections were attempted. There were 25 conversions (21.9%). Of the 89 laparoscopic completed resections, 47.2% were TMEs. The local recurrence rate was 16% in the converted group as against 6.9% and 9.5% in the laparoscopic completed and the open group respectively. Main reasons for conversion were tumor fixity and rectal perforation. It is interesting to note that 76% of the conversions ($n = 19$) occurred within the first half of the inclusion period between 1998 and 2001, reflecting the learning curve of the operating surgeons. The other possible explanation for this could be that these very locally advanced tumors necessitating conversions had bad biology and hence increased local recurrence rates.

It is likely that conversion will not increase local recurrence rates provided the decision to convert is made before there is any compromise of resection planes or resection margins (as may have happened in the study quoted). A misguided laparoscopic "trial dissection" that compromises an oncological resection that would have been straightforward conventionally may condemn the patient to an R1 resection and local recurrence and should be avoided. It is more important to complete the operation in an oncologically sound and radical manner than to complete it laparoscopically.

Learning Curves

Laparoscopic rectal resection with TME requires advanced laparoscopic skills, a secure grounding in conventional TME techniques and a sound understanding of surgical oncological principles. Technically, this is challenging surgery and requires intense concentration over a prolonged period, sequential operating in several surgical fields and meticulous technique to achieve a perfect TME.

The single most reason for the reduction in local recurrence rates in the last 30 years has been safe oncological surgery along the principles of TME. Laparoscopic resection of rectal cancer must adhere to these principles and match the local recurrence rates of open surgery. The learning curve for this type of laparoscopic surgery is high. The number of cases required to reach a plateau in terms of speed, morbidity rate, conversion rate and, of course, oncological adequacy is debatable. Competence in laparoscopic colonic surgery is mandatory. Supervision and preceptorship by an experienced laparoscopic surgeon is required to gain the necessary confidence in the more challenging pelvic surgery.

One of the main advantages of laparoscopic surgery which is not always as well publicized as the more popular benefits of shorter hospital stay, faster recovery and smaller incisions, is the use of laparoscopy as a teaching tool. Traditionally, experience in open pelvic surgery has been a consequence of hours at the operating table assisting more senior surgeons. However, laparoscopy allows more than just the immediate operators to gain a view and furthermore allows recording and use as teaching videos. This allows faster recognition of anatomical patterns and identification of the important neurovascular structures of the pelvis.

Similar to laparoscopic cholecystectomy, several early reports ignored the effect of the steep learning curve on the results. The principles of good open surgery are relevant to laparoscopy. Traction and counter-traction allow for precise dissection as in open surgery but understanding how to achieve this requires practise and time. Learning curves do not only affect technique but the outcome of the operation eg, lymph node harvest, intra-operative complications and conversion rates [29]. Standardization of technique resulting in an operation that is reproducible and predictable and therefore easier to teach is becoming accepted. The evolution of the "masterclass" is a consequence of this and by teaching a reproducible technique, oncological outcome is less likely to be compromised [30].

Robotic Surgery and the Future

The first robotic laparoscopic colectomy was reported by Weber et al in 2001 [31]. Since then, a wide range of colorectal operations have been performed for both benign and malignant disease. Short-term results seem encouraging and the development of more powerful technology will no doubt improve things further.

Full robotic and robotic-assisted surgery overcomes the technical difficulties in complex and difficult laparoscopic surgery by providing tridimensional imaging, instruments with seven degrees of freedom that mimic hand movements and dexterity. It also eliminates hand tremors, which further enhances precision. However, many authors still prefer to use a hybrid technique and take advantage of the robotic precise dissection only during the total mesorectal excision, as multi-quadrant operation in left colonic resection will increase operative time as the robotic cart has to be moved twice. Despite its potential advantages, robotic TME surgery is not established as standard practice and issues such as hybrid operations, (laparoscopy with robotic surgery), second intervention, conversion, cost, standardization of technique and training will have to be addressed before its use can become widespread.

Conclusion

Laparoscopic colonic resection has become accepted as a safe and viable alternative to open surgery. Whether or not laparoscopy is appropriate for rectal resection remains contentious. The main opposition to laparoscopic rectal surgery stems from the potential compromise of oncological safety and high rates of local recurrence. Currently, there is no evidence which supports this skepticism but long-term data is still not available. There is no doubt that laparoscopic rectal surgery is difficult and may not be suitable for all surgeons and patients, but in appropriately selected cases there are clear benefits. Furthermore, laparoscopy provides improved access, anatomical view and supercedes the limitations of manual dexterity when in experienced hands.

References

[1]   Jacobs, M., J.C. Verdeja, and H.S. Goldstein, Minimally invasive colon resection (laparoscopic colectomy). *Surgical laparoscopy and endoscopy*, 1991. 1(3): p. 144-50.

[2]   Guillou, P.J., et al., Short-term endpoints of conventional versus laparoscopic-assisted surgery in patients with colorectal cancer (MRC CLASICC trial): multicentre, randomised controlled trial. *Lancet,* 2005. 365(9472): p. 1718-26.

[3] Veldkamp, R., et al., Laparoscopic surgery versus open surgery for colon cancer: short-term outcomes of a randomised trial. *The lancet oncology*, 2005. 6(7): p. 477-84.

[4] Chand, M. and R.J. Heald, Laparoscopic rectal cancer surgery. *The British journal of surgery*, 2011. 98(2): p. 166-7.

[5] Heald, R.J., A new approach to rectal cancer. *British journal of hospital medicine*, 1979. 22(3): p. 277-81.

[6] Matthiessen, P., et al., Defunctioning stoma reduces symptomatic anastomotic leakage after low anterior resection of the rectum for cancer: a randomized multicenter trial. *Annals of surgery*, 2007. 246(2): p. 207-14.

[7] MacFarlane, J.K., R.D. Ryall, and R.J. Heald, Mesorectal excision for rectal cancer. *Lancet*, 1993. 341(8843): p. 457-60.

[8] Quirke, P., et al., Local recurrence of rectal adenocarcinoma due to inadequate surgical resection. Histopathological study of lateral tumour spread and surgical excision. *Lancet*, 1986. 2(8514): p. 996-9.

[9] Senagore, A.J., et al., A national comparison of laparoscopic vs. open colectomy using the National Surgical Quality Improvement Project data. *Diseases of the colon and rectum*, 2009. 52(2): p. 183-6.

[10] Tan, P.Y., et al., Laparoscopically assisted colectomy: a study of risk factors and predictors of open conversion. *Surgical endoscopy*, 2008. 22(7): p. 1708-14.

[11] Quirke, P., Training and quality assurance for rectal cancer: 20 years of data is enough. *The lancet oncology*, 2003. 4(11): p. 695-702.

[12] Anderson, C., G. Uman, and A. Pigazzi, Oncologic outcomes of laparoscopic surgery for rectal cancer: a systematic review and meta-analysis of the literature. European journal of surgical oncology : *the journal of the European Society of Surgical Oncology and the British Association of Surgical Oncology*, 2008. 34(10): p. 1135-42.

[13] Anthuber, M., et al., Outcome of laparoscopic surgery for rectal cancer in 101 patients. *Diseases of the colon and rectum*, 2003. 46(8): p. 1047-53.

[14] Bretagnol, F., et al., The oncological safety of laparoscopic total mesorectal excision with sphincter preservation for rectal carcinoma. *Surgical endoscopy*, 2005. 19(7): p. 892-6.

[15] Zhou, Z.G., et al., Laparoscopic versus open total mesorectal excision with anal sphincter preservation for low rectal cancer. *Surgical endoscopy*, 2004. 18(8): p. 1211-5.

[16] Lujan, J., et al., Randomized clinical trial comparing laparoscopic and open surgery in patients with rectal cancer. *The British journal of surgery*, 2009. 96(9): p. 982-9.

[17] Laurent, C., et al., Laparoscopic versus open surgery for rectal cancer: long-term oncologic results. *Annals of surgery*, 2009. 250(1): p. 54-61.

[18] Brennan, D.J., et al., Routine mobilization of the splenic flexure is not necessary during anterior resection for rectal cancer. *Diseases of the colon and rectum*, 2007. 50(3): p. 302-7; discussion 307.

[19] Moran, B.J., Predicting the risk and diminishing the consequences of anastomotic leakage after anterior resection for rectal cancer. *Acta chirurgica Iugoslavica*, 2010. 57(3): p. 47-50.

[20] Leroy, J., et al., Laparoscopic total mesorectal excision (TME) for rectal cancer surgery: long-term outcomes. *Surgical endoscopy*, 2004. 18(2): p. 281-9.

[21] Brannigan, A.E., et al., Intracorporeal rectal stapling following laparoscopic total mesorectal excision: overcoming a challenge. *Surgical endoscopy*, 2006. 20(6): p. 952-5.

[22] Breukink, S.O., et al., Laparoscopic vs open total mesorectal excision for rectal cancer: an evaluation of the mesorectum's macroscopic quality. *Surgical endoscopy*, 2005. 19(3): p. 307-10.

[23] Tsang, W.W., et al., Laparoscopic sphincter-preserving total mesorectal excision with colonic J-pouch reconstruction: five-year results. *Annals of surgery*, 2006. 243(3): p. 353-8.

[24] Liang, J.T., H.S. Lai, and P.H. Lee, Laparoscopic pelvic autonomic nerve-preserving surgery for patients with lower rectal cancer after chemoradiation therapy. *Annals of surgical oncology*, 2007. 14(4): p. 1285-7.

[25] Asoglu, O., et al., Impact of laparoscopic surgery on bladder and sexual function after total mesorectal excision for rectal cancer. *Surgical endoscopy*, 2009. 23(2): p. 296-303.

[26] Jayne, D.G., et al., Bladder and sexual function following resection for rectal cancer in a randomized clinical trial of laparoscopic versus open technique. *The British journal of surgery*, 2005. 92(9): p. 1124-32.

[27] Laurent, C., et al., Laparoscopic approach in surgical treatment of rectal cancer. *The British journal of surgery*, 2007. 94(12): p. 1555-61.

[28] Strohlein, M.A., et al., Comparison of laparoscopic vs. open access surgery in patients with rectal cancer: a prospective analysis. *Diseases of the colon and rectum*, 2008. 51(4): p. 385-91.

[29] Park, I.J., et al., Multidimensional analysis of the learning curve for laparoscopic colorectal surgery: lessons from 1,000 cases of laparoscopic colorectal surgery. *Surgical endoscopy*, 2009. 23(4): p. 839-46.

[30] Lindsetmo, R.O. and C.P. Delaney, A standardized technique for laparoscopic rectal resection. *Journal of gastrointestinal surgery : official journal of the Society for Surgery of the Alimentary Tract*, 2009. 13(11): p. 2059-63.

[31] Weber, P.A., et al., Telerobotic-assisted laparoscopic right and sigmoid colectomies for benign disease. *Diseases of the colon and rectum*, 2002. 45(12): p. 1689-94; discussion 1695-6.

In: Laparoscopy: New Developments, Procedures and Risks   ISBN: 978-1-61470-747-9
Editor: Hana Terzic, pp. 231-242   © 2012 Nova SciencePublishers, Inc.

Chapter XI

The Potential Role of 'NOTES' in Gynaecological Oncology Surgery and Sentinel Lymph Nodes Detection

Mohamed K. Mehasseb and Robin A. F. Crawford

Addenbrooke's hospital, Department of Gynaecological Oncology,
Hills road, Cambridge, CB2 0QQ, UK.

Abstract

Although still considered an experimental alternative to traditional and laparoscopic surgery, Natural Orifice Transluminal Endoscopic Surgery (NOTES) is quickly emerging as a new concept of minimally invasive surgery. The concept of NOTES advocates the lack of abdominal incisions and their related complications by combining endoscopic and laparoscopic techniques to diagnose and treat abdominal pathologies. Although still in its early days, NOTES is developing rapidly and is attracting a considerable interest from the surgical communities in all specialties. In much the same way as laparoscopy was originally developed, NOTES defies conventional surgical practices and has been the subject of understandable scepticism. The registered base of research in humans is still scarce; however, the porcine model experimental studies hold great promise.

In this work, we explore the concept of NOTES from a gynaecological oncologist's perspective, highlighting its potential use in the field of gynaecological oncology and sentinel lymph nodes detection.

Introduction

Natural Orifice Transluminal Endoscopic Surgery (NOTES) has emerged as a new concept of minimally invasive surgery, and is still considered an experimental alternative to traditional surgical techniques. NOTES advocates the lack of abdominal incisions and their related complications by combining endoscopic and laparoscopic techniques to diagnose and treat abdominal pathology [1]. At present, there is rapid development in NOTES and the technique is attracting a considerable interest from the surgical communities in all specialties. In much the same way as minimal access surgery many years ago, NOTES defies conventional surgical practices and has been the subject of understandable scepticism. The registered base of research in humans is yet scarce; however, the porcine and cadaveric experimental studies hold a great promise. In this article we explore the concept of NOTES from a gynaecologist's perspective, highlighting its potential application to the field of gynaecological oncology surgery.

Historical Perspective

Since the introduction of the very first endoscope by Philipp Bozzini in 1805 [2] endoscopy evolved over more than two centuries. In 1901, the first experimental laparoscopy that introduced a cystoscope into a dog's abdominal cavity, was reported by the German surgeon George Kelling[3].Developments have progressed from flexible endoscopy in the 1950s, to endoscopic retrograde cholangiopancreatography in the 1970s, to endoscopic ultrasound, and percutaneous endoscopic fine-needle techniques in the 1980s. The first laparoscopic cholecystectomy was performed on 12 September 1985 [4] moving the endoscopic technology from the purely diagnostic purposes to the therapeutic world. The most widely accepted opinion is that the first true NOTES was performed in 2004 by Kallooet al. from Johns Hopkins Hospital. They described a NOTES procedure for a transgastric peritoneal exploration with liver biopsy in a porcine model [5]. This was described as a revolutionary step in therapeutic endoscopy. Although several variations of natural orifice operations predate the work of Kallooet al., it was their first experiment that initiated the current interest in NOTES.

Although it remains *unpublished*, the first *human* NOTES procedure was performed in India in 2004, where Reddy and Rao performed a transgastric endoscopic appendicectomy for a patient with a severe burn injury to the abdominal wall (unpublished data presented at the 45th Annual Conference of the Society of Gastrointestinal Endoscopy of India, February 28–29, 2004; Jaipur, India. Paper titled *Per oral transgastric endoscopic appendectomy in human*).

The first *publishedhuman* NOTES was a transvaginal endoscopic cholecystectomy that was carried out by Zorron, University Hospital of Teresopolis, Brazil, on 13 March 2007 [6, 7]. Several days later, another two transvaginal endoscopic cholecystectomies were respectively performed by Bessler, Columbia University Medical Center, USA; and Marescaux, University Louis Pasteur, France[8, 9].

Many NOTES procedures have now been performed using the porcine model including nephrectomy [10], distal pancreatectomy[11], and cholecystectomy [12], with favourable results published in the literature. A recent review by Flora et al. [13] only identified four reports of NOTES performed in humans until 2007. In the past few years, many centres have published their experiences using NOTES and hybrid NOTES procedures with humans. Tubal ligation, cholecystectomy, gastrojejunostomy, splenectomy and oophorectomy were performed [8].

Fundamental Techniques
for Gynaecological NOTES

Peritoneal Access

For more than 100 years, transvaginal endoscopy, later known as *culdoscopy*, has been performed to visualize the abdominal and pelvic cavity. Transvaginal access has been used for years by gynaecologists for diagnostic and therapeutic purposes (e.g. hysterectomy, myomectomy, adnexectomy and fertiloscopy) [8]. Now recent interest in NOTES has resulted in a reconsideration of culdoscopy as an entry point to the surgical approach [14].In 2007, Tsin et al. published a collective review of 100 combined culdoscopy/laparoscopy operations, which the authors referred to as minilaparoscopy-assisted natural orifice surgery (MANOS) [15]. They reported on salpingo-oophorectomy, myomectomy, ovarian cystectomy, appendectomy, cholecystectomy, and "culdolaparoscopy" during vaginal hysterectomy. In these 100 patients, the only complication was postoperative fever [15]. Transvaginal extraction of the gall bladder, colon, spleen, and kidney have been previously described for laparoscopic operations [16].

Creation of Pneumoperitoneum and Maintaining Intra-Abdominal Pressure

Similar to laparoscopic surgery, NOTES requires a pneumoperitoneum to create a working space. However, the efficacy of maintaining and monitoring pneumoperitoneum using flexible endoscopy is largely untested in humans, and although several procedures have been performed successfully, porcine studies have suggested that this method is associated with marked variation of intra-abdominal pressure and major increases in peak inspiratory pressure with deleterious effects on haemodynamic and pulmonary function [17, 18].

Platform and Instruments for NOTES

The efficiency of intra-abdominal manipulation during NOTES depends on the endoscopes and accessory instrumentation. The current flexible endoscopes were designed to allow visual inspection of the visceral lumens. Thus, they pose several problems when used outside the confined environment of a luminal structure, as they are mainly used for diagnostic and limited therapeutic purposes within the gastrointestinal tract. Their drawbacks for NOTES include having only one or two narrow working channels with less than adequate light intensity in the peritoneal cavity. Retraction and dissection are virtually impossible because there is no triangulation of instruments at the tip of the endoscope. The simple push and torque techniques used in flexible endoscopy limit the reliable movement of the endoscope tip. These constraints have limited the further development of NOTES. Orientation remains a problem, as the operator at times has less visual cues and unfamiliar viewing angles compared to conventional laparoscopy. In addition, the camera view rotates with rotation of the instruments, disorientating the operator even more. Thus, natural orifice surgery requires more instruments adaptability, surgical training and capability than current endoscopic practice offers [19].

Potential Advantages of NOTES

NOTES offers distinct advantages described in table 1. The benefits of a vaginal approach will hopefully extend to NOTES potentially increasing patients' acceptance of such surgical approach. So far, there are no randomized trials comparing NOTES with laparoscopic surgery, either in an experimental or clinical setting. Without the support of sound data, the potential advantages of NOTES remain theoretical.

Every surgery involves the risk of complications (table 2). Management of these complications with difficult 'manoeuvring' in the small field may prove troublesome in the management of different "accidents" and mishaps.

Table 1. Advantages of Transvaginal Natural Orifice Transluminal Endoscopic Surgery (adapted from [20])

Minimises surgical site infections
Eliminates postoperative complications related to abdominal incisions
Reduces stimuli for adhesions and postoperative abdominal sequelae
Potentially more cost-effective by shortening postoperative recovery, reducing the need for inpatient admission, and subsequently decreasing inpatient complications such as nosocomial infection and venous thromboembolism
Less breach of peritoneal cavity with possibly improved oncologic and infectious outcomes
Use of high-level disinfection rather than sterilization
Potentially suitable for high surgical risk / unfit for surgery patients

Table 2. Disadvantages of Transvaginal Natural Orifice Transluminal Endoscopic Surgery (adapted from [20])

Potential introduction of vaginal commensals to peritoneal cavity
Troublesome bleeding that is difficult to control
Reduced operative field and lack of triangulation of instruments
Concerns about fertility with risks of infection and bleeding
Steep learning curve

Although the risk of peritoneal infection after puncturing the vagina is possible, sterilizing the vagina before surgery seems to reduce this risk to minimal level. Clearly, it is critical to evaluate and consider this potential unknown risk of a transvaginal NOTES procedure with further studies. It is worthwhile remembering that the transvaginal approach has been used for oocyte retrieval for more than 20 years [21-23]. The risk of infertility after transvaginal NOTES procedures is unknown, but avoidance of bleeding and inflammation to the pelvis should minimize this potential risk.

There are mainly challenges facing NOTES use and development (Table 3).The main challenge in NOTES development is training. There is no economic analysis of NOTES available in the literature, however, there is likely to be a considerable capital cost incurred with starting offering a NOTES service.

Table 3.Transvaginal Natural Orifice Transluminal Endoscopic Surgery:
Barriers to clinical practice (adapted from [24])

Safest entry and closure of the transluminal access site
Prevention of infection
Intracorporeal suturing devices
Spatial orientation
Instrument development
Management of complications
Removing resected organs
Training of providers

While transvaginal NOTES is argued to be a promising access, the gynaecologists'opinions remain divided on the potential advantages and risks of NOTES. In a survey involving the heads of the gynaecological departments of 181 university and major teaching hospitals across Germany, Austria, and Switzerland, gynaecologists raised concerns about postoperative infection, visceral lesions, infertility, and adhesions as conceivable complications [25].

Of the respondents, 69.2 % classified transvaginal access for extrapelvic abdominal surgery as ethical; the remaining 30.8 % described it as experimental. Only 28.8 % would recommend NOTES to their patients if NOTES presented the same surgical risks as the laparoscopic approach. When asked about NOTES-associated complications, 73.1 % mentioned the risk of infection, 61.5 % visceral lesions, 44.2 % infertility, and 34.6 % adhesions. In terms of long-term problems, gynaecologists are concerned about dyspareunia and infertility.

Adopting their patients' point of view, 17.3 % voted the lack of scarring compared to laparoscopy as important and 57.6 % as unimportant. Since long-term experience has not yet been achieved, potential problems such as dyspareunia, infertility, and the spread of pre-existing endometriosis remain theoretical complications [25].

However, the patients' perspectives are different. In a survey of 100 women who were given a written description of minimally invasive surgery and NOTES surgery exploring their concerns and opinions regarding transvaginal surgery, it seemed that women had a positive perception of transvaginal procedures and would want such procedures if they were found to be equivalent to laparoscopic surgeries [26].

The majority of women (68%) indicated that they would want a transvaginal procedure in the future because of decreased risk of abdominal wall incisional hernia and decreased operative pain (90 and 93%, respectively), while only 39% were concerned with the improved cosmesis of NOTES surgery.

Of the women polled, nulliparous women and those under 45 years were significantly more often concerned with how transvaginal surgery may affect healthy sexual life and fertility issues. Of the women who would not prefer transvaginal surgery, a significant number indicated concerns over infectious issues. Women who would want transvaginal surgery for themselves more often reported that they would recommend the procedure to their female family members [26].

Application of NOTES in Gynaecologic Oncology Surgery

Given the increased survivorship in gynaecological oncology patients, and with improved prognosis, surgeons should pay particular attention to the quality of life during surgical convalescence and chemotherapy/radiotherapy treatment. Shortening the recovery period and avoiding unnecessary delays between surgery and adjuvant therapy is also an important issue. With the introduction of the principles of Enhanced Recovery Programmes for gynaecological oncology surgery, the concept of NOTES becomes even more appealing.

Laparoscopy is now a reliable method for staging pelvic malignancies, directing the management, and avoiding unnecessary laparotomy and recent interest clearly demonstrates that laparoscopic techniques must now be part of the armamentarium of the gynaecologic oncologist [27, 28]. Retroperitoneal pelvic and para-aortic lymphadenectomy is widely accepted, as a staging and/or prognostic procedure in gynaecologic malignancies Laparoscopic retroperitoneal lymph node dissection has been shown to be a safe and efficacious procedure with better outcome, recovery and quality of life compared to open retroperitoneal lymphadenectomy [29]. The extraperitoneal approach is equally feasible and safe laparoscopically, although this approach is traditionally undertaken through a laparotomy. [30].

Associated morbidity ranges from 2 to 13% of cases [31], bearing in mind that some of those women will undergo intensivepostoperative treatment. In that respect, one should try to minimize the impact of surgery in all women, and NOTES may offer potential advantages [32]. The role of diagnostic transvaginal NOTES for staging gynaecological cancer, especially ovarian malignancies, remains to be explored and compared to the standard diagnostic techniques.

The first reported case of clinical diagnostic application of transvaginal NOTES for cancer staging is attributed to Zorrón et al. in 2007 [32]. In a 50-year-old female patient presenting with ascites, diffuse abdominal pain, and weight loss for 2 months, diagnosis of peritoneal carcinomatosis was suspected, which was also found when a CT scan was performed. Transvaginal NOTES was used for diagnostic staging of the patient, using a colonoscope introduced into the abdomen through a small incision in the vagina. Biopsies of liver, diaphragm, ovaries, and peritoneum were successfully performed. Operative time was 105 min, vaginal access and closure was obtained in 15 min. The patient was discharged 48 hours after the procedure without complications [32].Although this technique allowed direct visualization and biopsies of the lesions, it is yet to compete with radiological guided biopsies to establish the diagnosis in term of invasiveness, short duration of procedure, and quick recovery. However, the advantage of visual staging puts NOTES more en par with laparoscopic-guided biopsies, when indicated.

To the best of our knowledge, the use of NOTES for retroperitoneal pelvic and para-aortic lymph nodes dissection has never been considered in a clinical setting, while transperitoneal laparoscopic procedures were done in humans [8]. A recent feasibility study of extraperitoneal lymphadenectomy using transvaginal NOTES in a porcine survival model was conducted by Nassif et al [33]. Using a transvaginal access to the retroperitoneum, they successfully performed retroperitoneal lymphadenectomies in six female pigs (three pelvic lymph node excision and three others in the laterocaval, interaorticocaval and para-aortic regions). Colpotomy was closed with interrupted absorbable sutures. They experienced one accidental peritoneal perforation, one diffuse anterior abdominal wall emphysema, one abdominal wall bleeding secondary to electrical muscle stimulation and two pneumoperitoneums evacuated by Veress needle insertion. All animals thrived until three weeks after the initial intervention. On laparoscopic second look there were no abscess, no infection and no adhesions even with the accidental peritoneal perforation. On laparotomy, no retroperitoneal abscess was found, but there was a small amount of fibrosis at the lymphadenectomy sites. All colpotomies were inspected and had healed well. The authors suggested that cadaveric experiments would test its feasibility in humans. The sentinel lymph node technique could be a potential application of NOTES lymphadenectomy in humans [33].

As the lymph node dissection itself is associated with significant morbidity, sentinel lymph node (SLN) techniques using dye and/or radioactive tracers (e.g. Technetium) have been successfully assessed, validated and used in vulvar cancer [34] and are now being assessed in cervical and endometrial carcinomas [35] to try and diminish the surgical trauma. Performing sentinel lymph node dissection with NOTES could reduce the impact of oncologic surgery [36].

The management of *vulvar* carcinoma is increasingly being performed with less radical surgical intervention. Vulvar cancer itself would not seem likely to benefit from the advantages of NOTES since it is a superficial lesion that can be removed by classical surgical excision and SLN reduces the impact of the traditional inguino-femoral lymph nodes dissection. The use of transvaginal NOTES approach for pelvic lymph node dissection or sentinel lymph node in *vaginal* cancer could be an option since the upper two-thirds of the vagina is drained by lymphatics to the pelvic nodes, with the lymphatics paralleling the course of the uterine artery and the vaginal artery to the obturator, internal and external iliac nodes. The lower third of the vagina however drains to the inguinalefemoral nodes. SLN biopsy in *cervical* cancer is also emerging as an accurate staging tool [37, 38]. The SLN will be found mainly in the external iliac and obturator regions [39]. NOTES could potentially be used for sentinel lymph node biopsy for cervical cancer and be used to orientate chemo radiotherapy as adjuvant treatment. When it comes to SLN mapping of *endometrial* carcinoma [40, 41] many problems arise. First, the lymphatic drainage of the uterus is considerably more ambiguous than vulva and cervix. Second, there is no easily accessible or visible lesion in endometrial cancer as there is in vulvar or cervical cancers, making injection difficult. Third, the variation of reported locations of sentinel nodes ranges from the parametrium to the para-aortic region on either side of the body. These issues regarding the primary tumor and the patterns of lymphatic drainage make sentinel lymph node biopsy for endometrial carcinoma less practical. Although the value of lymphadenectomy in *ovarian* cancer remains controversial, an extraperitoneal lymph node exploration to remove sentinel lymph node or suspected positive node on imaging for advanced ovarian cancer, may be the most promising application for NOTES in gynaecological malignancies. However, it is often difficult to specify a single node as the sentinel in ovarian cancer [42].

A study by Bourdel et al. assessed the feasibility of sentinel lymph node (SLN) biopsy in gynecologic malignancies using natural orifices transluminal endoscopic surgery (NOTES) in a porcine model [43].In their study, ten female pigs were operated. Patent blue dye was injected in the paracervical region. The endoscope was introduced through a right lateral colpotomy. Internal iliac vessels were visualized followed by the identification of external iliac vessels. Bilateral dissection was performed to achieve visualization of the aorta and the vena cava. SLN colored in blue were bluntly dissected and then excised. The mean operative time was 56±16 minutes. The mean number of SLN retrieved was 1.75±1.28. All but one SLN were identified by NOTES procedure. No major complication was observed in this series. A total of 19 SLN were harvested, of which 11 from the left side and 8 from the right side. Fifteen lymph nodes were obtained from the iliac vessels or the promontory and 4 from the lateral aortic or preaortic region. This study confirmed the feasibility of the SLN technique by NOTES. However, prospective randomized series are necessary to establish the safety and the real benefits of this new technique [43].

The principles of oncologic surgery providence have to preserved at all times, as well as the need to ensure any potential for tumour seeding is absolutely minimized (e.g. by respecting 'no-touch' principles or careful bagging of specimens prior to retrieval) [44]. Although very promising, the precise usefulness and real indications of NOTES in gynaecologic oncology surgery will be established once the technique and instrument advances have taken place. Therefore, in the first instance, it seems pertinent to focus on feasibility and safety studies, with the ultimate aim of conducting randomized controlled trials using comparisons with the current gold standard for that particular procedure, which in many cases will be a laparoscopic technique. At present, access via multiple "unnatural" portals seems to have significant advantages over single-portal access, although single-port laparoscopic portals and instruments are emerging as a strong player in the field. A combined approach gives better visualization and orientation; and easier retraction, triangulation and manipulation of abdominal organs [11, 45, 46].

Conclusions

In conclusion, NOTES as an evolving approach to minimal access surgery is still in its infancy, but it is gathering momentum. Before achieving widespread use, it is paramount to provide evidence that NOTES procedures are at least equal to the currently available accepted techniques. The onus must be to first show that transluminal abdominal surgery is consistent with safe operative performance. Only then can subsequent experience be expected to discriminate comfort and acceptability (if not preference) of this new approach. In exchange for reduced abdominal access, the surgeon is clearly required to give up some degrees of comfort and perhaps safety due to the constraints imposed by limited space and reduced capacity for instrument triangulation. With collaboration among surgeons, engineers and computer scientists; accompanied by the development of instrumentation and miniature *in vivo* robots, NOTES, the new dimension of minimally invasive surgery, might herald a promising future. It is worth noting that the concept of single-incision laparoscopic surgery is evolving at a rapid rate [47] and may very well serve as a bridge in the introduction of techniques and new technology ultimately used for NOTES procedures. As NOTES procedures are introduced for humans, it seems sensible to use single-port laparoscopic access in early trials to ensure safety. The advent of robotic-assisted surgery may also facilitate the introduction and use of NOTES in the future.

References

[1]   McGee MF, Rosen MJ, Marks J, al. e. A primer on natural orifice transluminal endoscopic surgery: building a new paradigm. *Surg. Innov.*2006;13: 86-93.

[2]   Morgenstern L. The 200th anniversary of the first endoscope: Philipp Bozzini (1773-1809). *Surg. Innov.*2005;12: 105-106.

[3]   Litynski GS. Endoscopic surgery: the history, the pioneers. *World J. Surg*1999;23: 745-753.

[4]   Reynolds W. The first laparoscopic cholecystectomy. *JSLS*2001;5: 89-94.

[5]   Kalloo AN, Singh VK, Jagannath BS, al. e. Flexible transgastric peritonesocopy: a novel approach to diagnostic and therapeutic interventions in the peritoneal cavity. *Gastrointest. Endosc.*2004;60: 287-292.

[6]   Zorron R, Filgueiras M, Maggioni LC, Pombo L, Lopes Carvalho G, Lacerda Oliveira A. NOTES.Transvaginal cholecystectomy: report of the first case. *Surg. Innov.*2007;14: 279-83.

[7]   Zorron R, Maggioni LC, Pombo L, Oliveira AL, Carvalho GL, Filgueiras M. NOTES transvaginal cholecystectomy: preliminary clinical application. *Surg. Endosc.*2008;22: 542-7.

[8]   Marescaux J, Dallemagne B, Perretta S, Wattiez A, Mutter D, Coumaros D. Surgery without scars. Report of transluminal cholecystectomy in a human being. *Arch Surg*2007;142: 823-827.

[9]   Bessler M, Stevens PD, Milone L, Parikh M, Fowler D. Transvaginal laparoscopically assisted endoscopic cholecystectomy: a hybrid approach to natural orifice surgery. *Gastrointest. Endosc.*2007;66: 1243-5.

[10]   Isariyawongse JP, McGee MF, Rosen MJ, Cherullo EE, Ponsky LE. Pure natural orifice transluminal endoscopic surgery (NOTES) nephrectomy using standard laparoscopic instruments in the porcine model. *J Endourol*2008;22: 1087-91.

[11]   Ryou M, Fong DG, Pai RD, Tavakkolizadeh A, Rattner DW, Thompson CC. Dual-port distal pancreatectomy using a prototype endoscope and endoscopic stapler: a natural orifice transluminal endoscopic surgery (NOTES) survival study in a porcine model. *Endoscopy*2007;39: 881-7.

[12]   Scott DJ, Tang SJ, Fernandez R, Bergs R, Goova MT, Zeltser I, Kehdy FJ, Cadeddu JA. Completely transvaginal NOTES cholecystectomy using magnetically anchored instruments. *Surg. Endosc.*2007;21: 2308-2316.

[13]   Flora ED, Wilson TG, Martin IJ, O'Rourke NA, Maddern GJ. A review of natural orifice translumenal endoscopic surgery (NOTES) for intra-abdominal surgery: experimental models, techniques, and applicability to the clinical setting. *Ann. Surg.*2008;247: 583-602.

[14] Christian J, Barrier BF, Schust D, Miedema BW, Thaler K. Culdoscopy: a foundation for natural orifice surgery--past, present, and future. *J. Am. Coll. Surg.*2008;207: 417-22.

[15] Tsin DA, Colombero LT, Lambeck J, Manolas P. Minilaparoscopy-assisted natural orifice surgery. *JSLS*2007;11: 24-9.

[16] Ghezzi F, Raio L, Mueller MD, al. e. Vaginal extraction of pelvic masses following operative laparoscopy. *Surg. Endosc.*2002;16: 1691-1696.

[17] von Delius S, Huber W, Feussner H, Wilhelm D, Karagianni A, Henke J, Preissel A, Schneider A, Schmid RM, Meining A. Effect of pneumoperitoneum on hemodynamics and inspiratory pressures during natural orifice transluminal endoscopic surgery (NOTES): an experimental, controlled study in an acute porcine model. *Endoscopy*2007;39: 854-61.

[18] Meireles OR, Kantsevoy SV, Kalloo AN, al. e. Comparison of intraabdominal pressures using the gastroscope and laparoscope for transgastric surgery. *Surg. Endosc.*2007;21: 998-1001.

[19] Autorino R, Caddeddu JA, Desai MM, Gettman M, Gill IS, Kavoussi LR, Lima E, Montorsi F, Richstone L, Stolzenburg JU, Kaouk JH. Is LESS/NOTES really more? *Eur. Urol.*2011;59: 48-50.

[20] Varas Lorenzo MJ, Espinos Perez JC, Bardaji Bofill M. Natural orifice transluminal endoscopic surgery (NOTES). *Rev. Esp. Enferm. Dig.*2009;101: 275-282.

[21] Casa A, Sesti F, Marziali M, Gulemi L, Piccione E. Transvaginal hydrolaparoscopic ovarian drilling using bipolar electrosurgery to treat anovulatory women with polycystic ovary syndrome. *J. Am. Assoc. Gynecol. Laparosc.*2003;10: 219-222.

[22] Fernandez H, Alby JD, Gervaise A, de Tayrac R, Frydman R. Operative transvaginal hydrolaparoscopy for treatment of polycystic ovary syndrome: a new minimally invasive surgery. *Fertil. Steril.*2001;75: 607-611.

[23] Schulman JD, Dorfmann AD, Jones SL, Pitt CC, Joyce B, Patton LA. Outpatient in vitro fertilization using transvaginal ultrasound-guided oocyte retrieval. *Obstet. Gynecol.*1987;69: 665-668.

[24] Zhang XL, Yang YS, Sun G, Guo MZ. Natural orifice translumenal endoscopic surgery (NOTES): current status and challenges. *Chin. Med. J.* (Engl) 2010;123: 244-7.

[25] Thele F, Zygmunt M, Glitsch A, Heidecke CD, Schreiber A. How do gynecologists feel about transvaginal NOTES surgery? *Endoscopy*2008;40: 576-80.

[26] Peterson CY, Ramamoorthy S, Andrews B, Horgan S, Talamini M, Chock A. Women's positive perception of transvaginal NOTES surgery. *Surg. Endosc.*2009;23: 1770-4.

[27] Querleu D, Leblanc E, Ferron G, Narducci F, Rafii A, Martel P. Laparoscopic surgery and gynaecological cancers. *Bull Cancer*2007;94: 1063-1071.

[28] Narducci F, Occelli B, Lanvin D, Vinatier D, Leblanc E, Querleu D. Endoscopic aoritc dissection by the extraperitoneal approach: clinical study of 37 patients. *Gynecol. Obstet.Fertil.*2000;28: 108-114.

[29] Poulakis V. Quality of life after laparoscopic and open retroperitoneal lymph node dissection in clinical stage I nonseminomatous germ cell tumor: a comparison study. *Urology*2006;68: 154-160.

[30] Sonoda Y. Prospective evaluation of surgical staging of advanced cervical cancer via a laparoscopic extraperitoneal approach. *Gynecol. Oncol.*2003;91: 326-331.

[31] DiRe F, Baiocchi G. Value of lymph node assessment in ovarian cancer: status of the art at the end of the second millenium. *Int. J. Gynecol. Cancer*2000;10: 435-442.

[32] Zorron R, Soldan M, Filgueiras M, Maggioni LC, Pombo L, Oliveira AL. NOTES: transvaginal for cancer diagnostic staging: preliminary clinical application. *Surg. Innov.*2008;15: 161-5.

[33] Nassif J, Zacharopoulou C, Marescaux J, Wattiez A. Transvaginal extraperitoneal lymphadenectomy by Natural Orifices Transluminal Endoscopic Surgery (NOTES) technique in porcine model: feasibility and survival study. *Gynecol. Oncol.*2009;112: 405-8.

[34] Van der Zee AGJ, Oonk MH, De Hullu JA, Ansink AC, Vergote I, Verheijen RH, Maggioni A, Gaarenstroom KN, Baldwin PJ, Van Dorst EB, Van der Velden J, Hermans RH, van der Putten H, Drouin P, Schneider A, Sluiter WJ. Sentinel Node Dissection Is Safe in the Treatment of Early-Stage Vulvar Cancer. *J. Clin. Oncol.*2008;26: 884-889.

[35] Levenback C. Status of sentinel lymph node biopsy in gynaecological cancers. *Ann. Surg. Oncol.*2007;15: 18-20.

[36] Nassif J, Zacharopoulou C, Wattiez A. Staging of gynaecological malignancies by natural orifice transluminal endoscopic surgery (N.O.T.E.S.). *Surg. Oncol.*2009;18: 147-52.

[37] Frumovitz M, Ramirez PT, Levenback CF. Lymphatic mapping and sentinel lymph node detection in women with cervical cancer. *Gynecol. Oncol.*2008;110: S17-20.

[38] Selman T, Mann C, Zamora J, Appleyard TL, Khan K. Diagnostic accuracy of tests for lymph node status in primary cervical cancer: a systematic review and meta-analysis. *CMAJ*2008;178: 855-862.

[39] Bader AA. Where to look for the sentinel lymph node in cervical cancer. *Am. J. Obstet. Gynecol.*2007;197: 678. e1-7.

[40] Loar III PV, Reynolds RK. Sentinel node mapping in gynaecologic malignancies. *Int. J. Gynaecol. Obstet.*2007;99: 69-74.

[41] Ballester M, Dubernard G, Rouzier R, Barranger E, Darai E. Use of sentinel node procedure to stage endometrial cancer. *Ann. Surg. Oncol.*2008;15: 1523-1529.

[42] Ushijima K. Management of retroperitoneal lymph nodes in the treatment of ovarian cancer. *Int. J. Clin. Oncol.*2007;12: 181-186.

[43] Bourdel N, Kondo W, Botchorishvili R, Poincloux L, Niro J, Rabischong B, Jardon K, L. PJ, Mage G, Canis M. Assessment of sentinel nodes for gynecologic malignancies by natural orifices transluminal endoscopic surgery (NOTES): Preliminary report. *Gynecol. Oncol.*2009;115: 367-370.

[44] Cahill RA, Marescaux J. Natural orifice transluminal endoscopic surgery (N.O.T.E.S.) for oncologic disease. *Surg. Oncol.*2009;18: 91-3.

[45] Rolanda C, Lima E, Pego JM, al. e. Third-generation cholecystectomy by natural orifices: transgastric and transvesical combined approach. *Gastrointest. Endosc.*2007;65: 111-117.

[46] Gettman MT, Blute ML. Transvesical peritoneoscopy: initial clinical evaluation of the bladder as a portal for natural orifice translumenal endoscopic surgery. *Mayo Clin. Proc.*2007;82: 843-5.

[47] Canes D, Desai MM, Aron M, Haber GP, Goel RK, Stein RJ, Kaouk JH, Gill IS. Transumbilical single-port surgery: evolution and current status. *Eur. Urol.*2008;54: 1020-1029.

In: Laparoscopy: New Developments, Procedures and Risks   ISBN: 978-1-61470-747-9
Editor: Hana Terzic, pp. 243-251   © 2012 Nova Science Publishers, Inc.

Chapter XII

Retrieving Benign Specimens from the Peritoneal Cavity Following Laparoscopic Excision: A Review of the Literature

Andreas Stavroulis[1], Maria Memtsa[2] and Wai Yoong[3]*
[1] Minimal Access Surgery Clinical Fellow,
Department of Obstetrics and Gynaecology,
University College London Hospitals NHS Foundation Trust,
EGA Wing, 235 Euston Road, London, NW1 2BU
[2] Department of Obstetrics and Gynaecology,
University College London Hospitals NHS Foundation Trust,
EGA Wing, 235 Euston Road, London, NW1 2BU
[3] Department of Obstetrics and Gynaecology,
North Middlesex University Hospital NHS Trust,
Sterling Way, London, N18 1QX.

Abstract

The advantages of operative laparoscopy include small incisions, less postoperative pain, short hospital stay, earlier recovery and improved quality of life during the postoperative period. Different techniques have been described to facilitate the retrieval of excised masses without needing to enlarge the abdominal incision. Specimen extraction in laparoscopic surgery is more time consuming than open procedures and tissue removal must be performed in an expeditious manner if the cost-effectiveness of the technique is to be maintained. The authors review the various routes for the retrieval of benign specimens following laparoscopic excision and discuss associate risks and

[*] Corresponding author: Mr Wai Yoong, Department of Obstetrics and Gynaecology, North Middlesex University Hospital NHS Trust, Sterling Way, London, N18 1QX. Email: wai.yoong@nmh.nhs.uk

factors, which will influence the optimal choice of route. These routes include retrieval via the trocar using an endobag, morcellation, posterior colpotomy and mini-laparotomy. Natural Orifice Transluminal Endoscopy (NOTES) may be the operative and retrieval route of the future, is also briefly discussed.

Keywords: laparoscopy, excision, retrieval, benign mass.

Introduction

Laparoscopy has developed into an essential component of the operative gynaecological palette. The advantages of laparoscopic surgery include small incisions, less postoperative pain, short hospital stay, earlier recovery and improved quality of life during the postoperative period.

Major concerns about laparoscopic surgery for ovarian cysts include the risk of spillage of the cyst contents and subsequent complications such as pseudomyxoma peritonei (mucinous cystadenoma), chemical peritonitis (dermoid cyst or endometriomas) and the potential dissemination of malignancy. Because of the technical difficulty of the trocar insertion and specimen retrieval as well as poor visualization, conventional laparotomy is still the mode of treatment for most patients with large ovarian cysts.

A maximum tumour size beyond which endoscopic surgery is contraindicated has not been defined but some authors suggest that ovarian masses of greater than 10cm are best managed by laparotomy. [1] For specimens less than 10cm, retrieval through the transumbilical port following operative laparoscopy has been advocated on the basis that this site represents the thinnest and most distensible portion of the anterior abdominal wall. [2] However, while this technique may be possible for simple cysts, which can be decompressed, solid or semi-solid ovarian tumours (such as fibromas and dermoid cysts) may prove more challenging.

Different techniques have been described to facilitate the retrieval of excised masses without needing to enlarge the abdominal incision. Specimen extraction following laparoscopic surgery is more time consuming than open procedures and tissue removal must be performed in an expeditious manner if the cost-effectiveness of the technique is to be maintained. The route of retrieval must not compromise patient safety, either intra- or post-operatively.

The authors review the various routes of retrieval for large benign specimens following laparoscopic excision (as well as the pros and cons) and discuss associate risks and how these can be overcome.

Laparoscopy-Assisted Cystectomy for Large Adnexal Cysts

Large adnexal cysts exceeding 10cm on pre-operative imaging can be initially decompressed either through ultrasound guided [3] or laparoscopic aspiration followed by intracorporal ovarian cyst wall stripping performed endoscopically. [4] Limitations of laparoscopic treatment in these cases include spillage (chemical peritonitis eg dermoid or unsuspected malignancy), difficulty in introduction of Veress needle, limited visualisation of the ureters, and the technical challenge of retrieving the mass.

Göçmen et al [5] described the following technique for the removal of benign adnexal cysts of a diameter between 10 and 20cm:

Depending on the cyst size and location, either an umbilical or subcostal primary trocar is used. A 10mm suprapubic trocar is inserted in the cyst and its content aspirated using a cannula introduced through the suprapubic port. A grasping forceps inserted through a 5mm lateral port site is used to close the cyst puncture site and minimise spillage of cyst contents. After decompression, the suprapubic incision is enlarged to 20mm and a ring forceps is introduced through this. The cyst wall is then held by the ring forceps and the adnexal extracted onto the abdomen and an extracorporal cystectomy performed. Alternatively, a 5-mm trocar sleeve can be inserted in the close to the dome of the cyst, the trocar is then removed and suction-washing system is inserted into the mass through the sleeve. A purse suture or endoscopic loop can be placed around the cyst incision to avoid spillage. This method is thought to have a shorter operation time and less blood loss compared to the usual laparoscopic intracorporal ovarian cystectomy.

The risk of postoperative hernia is increased especially when enlarging laterally placed port sites[6] and most of these occur as Richter's hernias, without peritoneal lining, and contain small or large intestine or omentum. [7] This can be a serious complication requiring laparotomy in majority of the patients and intestinal resection in about 20%. [6] Even with 5-mm lateral port sites, the risk of hernia exists [8] as result of stretch and tear of the fascia secondary to the instrument manipulation or the passage of the tissue through the port site. It is true that the risk of a hernia at the umbilicus is less compared to ancillary ports, unless the umbilical wound is enlarged. [9] Currently, the closure of the fascia of port sites larger than 5mm is recommended, with the only exception being the umbilical port where practice is individualised.

Endopouches (Bag)

In order to avoid the possibility of cyst spillage, several authors have described the use of impermeable endoscopic specimen bags for the removal for laparoscopically excised mass. Apart from intraperitoneal spillage, the use of such a bag also has the advantage of avoiding contamination of the wound. The bags generally require a 10-12mm port, although the site can be enlarged for specimen removal. Once the cyst is securely in the bag, it can be decompressed to facilitate removal; if a solid (fibroma) or semi-solid (dermoid) mass is large, it can be "piecemealed" in the bag with scissors, harmonic scalpel or morcellator.

Commercial bags can be costly, difficult to manipulate and available only in standard sizes. Several enterprising authors have described 'easy-to-make' bags from surgical glove fingers (powder-free) [10], condoms [11] and zipper-type plastic bags. [12] While these are inexpensive, simple to make and available in a choice of sizes, "home made bags" are not subject to industry quality control and can tear when submitted to traction through the abdominal wall (although this can be reduced with the addition of a purse-ring suture, which allows easy closure and pulling as well as reopening) [10].

The endoscopic bag pouches are usually introduced and removed through a 10mm port site; this is primarily the umbilical port although other sites might be preferred. Many surgeons prefer to use a 5mm laparoscope for visualization through an ancillary port while retrieving the specimen in a bag through the umbilical 10mm one (likewise monitoring the morcellation of the mass). Exteriorising the endoscopic bag opening on the anterior abdominal wall before removal of the specimen avoids leakage or spillage into the peritoneal cavity which may lead to chemical peritonitis or malignant cell spread. Although there appeared to be little correlation between spillage and cyst size, specimens retrieved without endoscopic pouches were four times more likely to spill compared to specimens retrieved with endoscopic pouches [13].

In addition, a posterior colpotomy can also be used in conjunction with an endoscopic bag as described later.

Chatzipapas et al reported the "remote control" laparoscopic bag [14] which is made using a disposable suction connecting tubing and two long surgical sutures, which act as drawstrings. Its advantages include cost effectiveness, ease of use and safety and additional secondary ports are not required. Because the bag can be large, operating within the bag is a possibility, thus reducing the risk of spillage inside the peritoneal cavity.

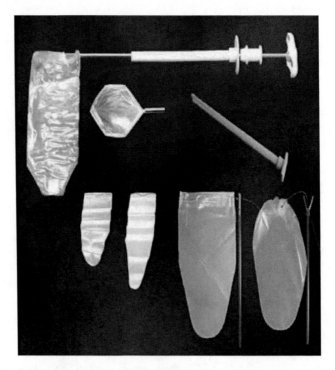

Figure 1. examples of endoscopic bags currently available.

An endoscopic bag extractor has also been reported [15] and this is an instrument that facilitates extraction of any type of endobag without the need of conventional minilaparotomy. After inserting it through the skin, its blades create an enlarged canal through which the bag can be removed without the risk of endobag rupture as the size of the canal can be adjusted.

Mini-Laparotomy

Randomized controlled trials have compared laparoscopy with mini-laparotomy in the management of ovarian cysts and concluded that operative laparoscopy is the best approach for the management of adnexal cysts but that mini-laparotomy can be considered an acceptable minimally invasive approach yielding similar results. [20-16] Clearly the major concern of the laparoscopic management of large adnexal masses is the probability of intraperitoneal spillage of an unexpected malignant cyst, in addition to the technical problem and longer operative time associated with larger masses. Although the above concerns are less with mini-laparotomy, as are with the conventional laparotomy, one could argue the anti-aesthetic result and the post-operative morbidity.

Usually the site for the mini-laparotomy is chosen at a suprapubic level. A diagnostic laparoscopy can be added to the traditional mini-laparotomy and this allows an inspection of the whole abdomen and therefore reducing the risk of unrecognised malignancy. It also aids the surgeon to plan where and how large the mini-laparotomy incision is to be made. The excised mass can then be removed through the incision. In addition, the cyst can be brought out through the incision and been excised the conventional way. When the size does not allow this, the cyst can be brought to the surface of the incision for the cyst contents to be aspirated, while controlling the spillage by either clump or a purse suture around the cyst incision site. Another example where this technique is preferred is during treatment of bowel endometriosis where the colorectal surgeons use a mini-laparotomy site to remove the excised bowel and when appropriate, re-anastomose it at the same time.

Randomised trials have shown that, while mini-laparotomy is associated with significant increase in minor postoperative discomfort and recovery time, more pain and need for analgesia as well as more aesthetic concerns, operative times are shorter and rates of intraperitoneal spillage are significantly reduced [16].

Morcellation

Electronic power morcellators excise large masses and enable the specimen to be brought out in strips through the sheath of the morcellator. They work by rotating a sharp cylindrical blade against the specimen and have an in-line valve to prevent loss of the pneumoperitoneum at time of tissue extraction and a blade protector (sheath) where the sharp blade can be brought back into to prevent inadvertent shearing of the tissue. Currently, many companies manufacture morcellators, each with its unique differences and cost. Larger diameter morcellators (which use larger incisions) remove tissue faster but is associated with a higher risk of subsequent hernia formation.

Morcellators do decrease the operative time [17] and the risk of port site herniation [18] as the fascia is not torn or stretched. There is a risk of inadvertent injury of adjacent organs and the operator must remember to bring the specimen towards the rotating morcellator tip rather than advance the morcellator towards the mass. It is important to try to remove all specimen fragments as accidental ovarian autograft has been reported. [19] Following initial laparoscopic myomectomy, fibroid remnants, which had been left behind, had to be removed through a second laparoscopic procedure as they were causing pain [20].

Colpotomy

Posterior colpotomy has been extensively documented in the past but has fallen out of favour because of the perceived technical difficulties, poor exposure, increased risk of pelvic sepsis, bowel perforation, haemorrhage, injury to the bladder and ureters, vaginal wall haematoma as well as vaginal scarring.

In more recent years, this attractive route has been reintroduced and successfully used to deliver solid and semi-solid tumours following operative laparoscopy (*figure 2*) [21]. Colpotomy is generally a safe and easily learnt technique as long basic surgical principles such as perioperative prophylactic antibiotics and good haemostasis, are followed.

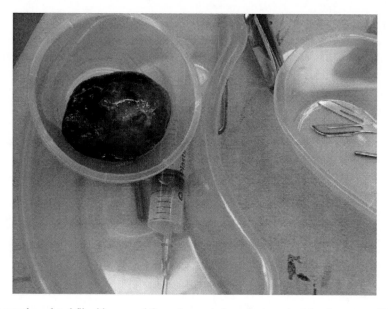

Figure 2. 7cm pedunculated fibroid removed through a posterior colpotomy incision (courtesy of Mr W Yoong, 2011).

To avoid spillage, which can occur with this technique, a laparoscopic assisted modification using an endoscopic bag has been described which allows large solid specimens to be removed safely and with minimal spillage [22]. With this technique, the excised specimen is placed in a bag, which is then placed into the Pouch of Douglas under direct laparoscopic view. When the vagina is incised, the sudden expulsion of CO_2 from the peritoneum delivers the "specimen in a bag" through the posterior colpotomy, after which the incision is sutured.

Pardi et al [23] used laparoscopy to assess adnexal mobility of dermoid cysts, which were then maneuvered into the Pouch of Douglas. A posterior colpotomy incision was made and the cyst exteriorised, after which a vaginal cystectomy was performed with or without cyst decompression. This technique combines the advantages of laparoscopy and open surgery, with laparoscopy being the first and last step of this procedure.

Natural Orifice Transluminal Endoscopic Surgery (NOTES)

NOTES represents the holy grail of minimally invasive intra-abdominal procedures, whereby access to the peritoneal cavity is achieved by incising and traversing the lumen of a natural orifice, in an attempt to avoid abdominal wall incisions [24]. Several natural orifices have been described as routes for access to the peritoneal cavity and these include oral, anal, vaginal, or urethral orifices, although the optimal access route is yet to be determined [25]. Ease of access and closure, potential for infection, security of closure, space limitations for instrument insertion and specimen retrieval, as well as relationship to the target anatomy are some of the factors considered in the debate of the best portal for performing NOTES. Because of its ease of access and capaciousness, the vagina is in fact the most commonly used NOTES portal of entry.

Historically, transvaginal access to the abdominal cavity or culdoscopy, was first performed by Albert Decker in 1928, and the technique was perfected by Palmer in 1942 using pneumoperitoneum. Since then, culdoscopy was widely used as a method to investigate subfertility, until the introduction of laparoscopy into clinical practice [24]. The first case of successful incidental vaginal appendicectomy at the time of vaginal hysterectomy was described by Bueno in 1949 [25], while, more recently, Tsin and colleagues [25] reported a modified laparoscopic technique of vaginal cholecystectomy after simultaneous hysterectomy ("culdolaparoscopy").

In early 2007, the first NOTES transvaginal cholecystectomy human cases were achieved by different groups. Access to the peritoneal cavity is obtained by simple dissection of the posterior fornix to enter the pouch of Douglas, while many groups favour a hybrid procedure during which laparoscopic umbilical visualisation after peritoneal insufflation is used before vaginal trocar placement [25]. Advantages of the transvaginal route include the ease of insertion of rigid instrumentation, suitability for specimen removal and proven safety record [24]. Closure of the vaginal wound is not a problematic issue, as it is performed under direct vision using absorbable sutures by conventional instruments and techniques. In addition, the potential for complications such as fistula and peritonitis is low [25]. On the other hand, bladder catheterisation and use of antibiotics is imperative, while more research into the potential development of dyspareunia and subfertility is needed in order to increase the procedure profile and, therefore patient acceptance. Contraindications to this approach include a fixed retroverted uterus and obliteration of the pouch of Douglas (due to adhesions either because of endometriosis, past pelvic infections or prior surgery), acute circumstances and male gender!

Discussion

Although laparoscopy has replaced open surgery for many gynaecological procedures, the retrieval of the excised specimen from the abdominal cavity following laparoscopic excision still represents a challenge and can be frustrating for the surgeon as the majority of procedures could be performed using ports of 5mm. Using ports of larger diameter or enlarging/stretching of the port sites has cosmetic drawbacks but can also increase the risk of vascular injuries, postoperative pain and hernia formation.

Specimens placed in impermeable endoscopic bags can be retrieved through 10mm ports, a mini laparotomy incision or posterior colpotomy. The route of retrieval should be specifically catered for individual patients who should be counseled about the advantages and disadvantages.

While it is still a relatively new technique, NOTES may be the operative and retrieval route of the future.

Conflict of interest: The authors declare no conflict of interest.

References

[1] Maiman M, Seltzer V, Boyce J. Laparoscopic excision of ovarian neoplasms subsequently found to be malignant. *Obstet. Gynecol.* 1991 Apr;77(4):563-5.

[2] Ghezzi F, Cromi A, Bergamini V, Uccella S, Siesto G, Franchi M, et al. Should adnexal mass size influence surgical approach? A series of 186 laparoscopically managed large adnexal masses. *BJOG.* 2008 Jul;115(8):1020-7.

[3] Nagele F, Magos AL. Combined ultrasonographically guided drainage and laparoscopic excision of a large ovarian cyst. *Am. J. Obstet. Gynecol.* 1996 Nov;175 (5):1377-8.

[4] Salem HA. Laparoscopic excision of large ovarian cysts. *J. Obstet. Gynaecol. Res.* 2002 Dec;28(6):290-4.

[5] Göçmen A, Atak T, Uçar M, Sanlikal F. Laparoscopy-assisted cystectomy for large adnexal cysts. *Arch. Gynecol. Obstet.* 2009 Jan;279(1):17-22.

[6] Boike GM, Miller CE, Spirtos NM, Mercer LJ, Fowler JM, Summitt R, et al. Incisional bowel herniations after operative laparoscopy: a series of nineteen cases and review of the literature. *Am. J. Obstet. Gynecol.* 1995 Jun;172(6):1726-31; discussion 1731-3.

[7] Lajer H, Widecrantz S, Heisterberg L. Hernias in trocar ports following abdominal laparoscopy. A review. *Acta Obstet. Gynecol. Scand.* 1997 May;76(5):389-93.

[8] Thapar A, Kianifard B, Pyper R, Woods W. 5 mm port site hernia causing small bowel obstruction. *Gynecol. Surg.* (2010) 7:71–73.

[9] Ghezzi F, Cromi A, Uccella S, Siesto G, Bergamini V, Bolis P. Transumbilical surgical specimen retrieval: a viable refinement of laparoscopic surgery for pelvic masses. *BJOG.* 2008 Sep;115(10):1316-20.

[10] Yao CC, Wong HH, Yang CC, Lin CS, Liu JC. Liberal use of a bag made from a surgical glove during laparoscopic surgery for specimens retrieval. *Surg. Laparosc. Endosc. Percutan Tech.* 2000 Aug;10(4):261-3.

[11] Chung SC, Li MK, Li AK. Lost stone during laparoscopic cholecystectomy: retrieval using a condom. *HPB Surg.* 1993 Aug;7(1):67-8.

[12] Weber A, Vázquez JA, Valencia S, Cueto J. Retrieval of specimens in laparoscopy using reclosable zipper-type plastic bags: a simple, cheap, and useful method. *Surg. Laparosc. Endosc.* 1998 Dec;8(6):457-9.

[13] Steiner RA, Wight E, Tadir Y, Haller U. Electrical cutting device for laparoscopic removal of tissue from the abdominal cavity. *Obstet. Gynecol.* 1993 Mar;81(3):471-4.

[14] Chatzipapas IK, Hart RJ, Magos A. The "remote control" laparoscopic bag: a simple technique to remove intra-abdominal specimens. *Obstet. Gynecol.* 1998 Oct;92(4 Pt 1):622-3.

[15] Köchli OR, Schnegg MP, Müller DJ, Surbek DV. Endobag extractor to remove masses during laparoscopy. *Obstet. Gynecol.* 2000 Feb;95(2):304-5.

[16] Panici PB, Palaia I, Bellati F, Pernice M, Angioli R, Muzii L. Laparoscopy compared with laparoscopically guided minilaparotomy for large adnexal masses: a randomized controlled trial. *Obstet. Gynecol.* 2007 Aug;110(2 Pt 1):241-8.

[17] Carter JE, McCarus SD. Laparoscopic myomectomy. Time and cost analysis of power vs. manual morcellation. *J. Reprod. Med.* 1997 Jul;42(7):383-8.

[18] Miller CE. Myomectomy. Comparison of open and laparoscopic techniques. *Obstet. Gynecol. Clin. North Am.* 2000 Jun;27(2):407-20.

[19] Marconi G, Quintana R, Rueda-Leverone NG, Vighi S. Accidental ovarian autograft after a laparoscopic surgery: case report. *Fertil. Steril.* 1997 Aug;68(2):364-6.

[20] Miller CE. Methods of tissue extraction in advance laparoscopy. *Current in Obstetrics and Gynecology* 2001,13:399-405.

[21] Teng FY, Muzsnai D, Perez R, Mazdisnian F, Ross A, Sayre JW. A comparative study of laparoscopy and colpotomy for the removal of ovarian dermoid cysts. *Obstet. Gynecol.* 1996 Jun;87(6):1009-13.

[22] Pillai R, Yoong W. Posterior colpotomy revisited: a forgotten route for retrieving larger benign ovarian lesions following laparoscopic excision. *Arch. Gynecol. Obstet.* 2010 Apr;281(4):609-11.

[23] Pardi G, Carminati R, Ferrari MM, Ferrazzi E, Bulfoni G, Marcozzi S. Laparoscopically assisted vaginal removal of ovarian dermoid cysts. *Obstet. Gynecol.* 1995 Jan;85(1):129-32.

[24] Box GN, Bessler M, Clayman R. Transvaginal Access: Current experience and Potential Implications for Urologic Applications. *J. Endourol.* 2009 May;23(5):753-757.

[25] Chukwumah C, Zorron R, Marks JM, Ponsky JL. Current Status of Natural Orifice Translumenal Endoscopic Surgery (NOTES). *Curr. Probl. Surg.* 2010 Aug;47:630-668.

In: Laparoscopy: New Developments, Procedures and Risks   ISBN: 978-1-61470-747-9
Editor: Hana Terzic, pp. 253-260   © 2012 Nova Science Publishers, Inc.

Chapter XIII

Against the Systematic Use of Laparoscopy in Infertility Assessment

Philippe Merviel[*], Emmanuelle Lourdel, Mélanie Brzakowski,
Stéphane Urrutiaguer, Odile Gagneur and Abdou Nasreddine
Department of Obstetrics and Gynecology, Reproductive Medicine
University of Picardie Jules Verne and CHU d'Amiens
124 rue Camille Desmoulins
F-80054 Amiens cedex 01, France.

Abstract

The aetiological assessment of an infertile couple includes several complementary biological and morphological examinations. Initial exploration of the female genital tract requires the performance of pelvic ultrasound and hysterosalpingography. Some medical teams perform hysteroscopy on an outpatient basis prior to the initiation of any therapeutic measures.

The value of systematic laparoscopy in infertility assessment is still subject to debate. After having been systematically employed in the 1970s and 1980s, laparoscopy was progressively abandoned as part of the initial infertility assessment over the following 20 years. However, systematic use of this technique has been suggested again in recent years - notably in view of the restriction of the number of in vitro fertilization (IVF) attempts to four per couple in France.

The aim of the present review is to evaluate arguments against the systematic use of laparoscopy and to try to draw up recommendations for practice.

In our opinion, laparoscopy is of course indicated in infertility assessments not only when anomalies are revealed by hysterosalpingography but also in the following circumstances:

---

[*] Corresponding author. *E-mail address:* Merviel.Philippe@chu-amiens.fr

- a history of infection (especially a positive Chlamydia antibody blood test) and/or pelvic surgery (a significant risk of adhesions).
- unexplained secondary infertility.
- unexplained infertility after the age of 37-38 (when choosing between artificial insemination and direct enrolment in an IVF programme).
- the failure of 3 or 4 cycles of good-quality intra-uterine inseminations (with ovarian stimulation and a sufficient number of spermatozoids).

Lastly, after the abandonment of microlaparoscopy, transvaginal hydrolaparoscopy (also known as fertiloscopy) now constitutes a surgical alternative to laparoscopy. Nevertheless, its value in initial infertility assessment remains to be defined.

Keywords: infertility – hysterosalpingography – *Chlamydia trachomatis* - laparoscopy - intrauterine insemination.

The aetiological assessment of an infertile couple includes several complementary biological and morphological examinations. Initial exploration of the female genital tract requires the performance of pelvic ultrasound and hysterosalpingography (HSG). Some medical teams perform hysteroscopy on an outpatient basis prior to the initiation of any therapeutic measures.

The value of systematic laparoscopy in infertility assessment is still subject to debate. After having been systematically employed in the 1970s and 1980s, laparoscopy was progressively abandoned as part of the initial infertility assessment over the following 20 years. However, systematic use of this technique has been suggested again in recent years - notably in view of the restriction (in France) of the number of *in vitro* fertilization (IVF) attempts to four per couple.

The aim of the present review is to evaluate arguments against the systematic use of laparoscopy and to try to draw up recommendations for practice.

1. Arguments against the Systematic Use of Laparoscopy

It is clear that laparoscopy is not appropriate for a patient with normal pelvic ultrasound and HSG results and a partner presenting moderate to severe sperm abnormalities. In fact, the indication is then IVF and (in some cases) intracytoplasmic sperm injection (ICSI) - an increasingly common situation in routine professional practice.

The systematic use of laparoscopy in infertility assessment is primarily restricted by the technique's inherent risks. Indeed, in a French study by Chapron [1], the risk of complications was 1.84 per 1000 diagnostic laparoscopies (11 per 5983 procedures), with seven haemorrhagic complications, three intestinal complications and one urological complication. The rate was higher still for surgical acts performed during laparoscopy (up to 11% for minor complications and 2.3% for major complications) [2]. A Finnish registry reported a complication rate of 0.6 per 1000 procedures [3].

In order to avoid surgery, some authors have combined HSG with other examinations. Hence, Ubaldi [4] concluded that laparoscopy can be deferred in young women having undergone vaginal pelvic ultrasound and who have a normal hysterosalpingogram (although the latter is not sensitive enough to detect adhesions). Likewise, Ayida [5] showed that a combination of hysterosalpingo-contrast sonography (HyCoSy: injection of ultrasound contrast and performance of pelvic ultrasound for imaging potential fallopian and peritoneal obstructions) and magnetic resonance imaging (MRI) enabled the diagnosis of a normal pelvis and thus the postponement of laparoscopy. Concerning HyCoSy alone, Boudghene [6] has shown a good HyCoSy–laparoscopy correlation (20 out of 23 cases), with no false positives. The technique's limitations include the inability to evaluate proximal lesions (endometriosis, salpingitis isthmica nodosa, etc.) or the condition of the ampullary mucosal folds. Lastly, Hauge [7] confirmed these HyCoSy results relative to laparoscopy, with a sensitivity of 92.8%, a specificity of 96.2%, a positive predictive value of 92.8% and a negative predictive value of 98.1%.

Once the uterine cavity has been filled, hysterosalpingography enables visualisation of the proximal fallopian tubes, the distal fallopian tubes and then the peritoneal mixing of the contrast agent. It is important to study the final images, which provide information on any infundibular obstructions and infertility-causing distal phymosis or peritubal adhesions. Identification of these adhesions with HSG is probably the most difficult aspect. The risk of post-operative adhesion depends on the surgical history: 1.6% after laparoscopy for ovarian cystectomy, drilling or myomectomy; 20% after a Pfannenstiel incision, 50% after median sub-umbilical laparotomy and 5% after a MacBurney incision and appendectomy - by far the most common previous surgical act in our patients. It is noteworthy that the risk of adhesions is 0.5% in women with no history of surgery. The pregnancy rate in the year after laparoscopic adhesiolysis has been estimated at 50%; however, the exact impact of adhesions on infertility has not been clearly established, since they rare occur in the absence of other problems. After adhesiolysis, the risk of extra-uterine pregnancy is still 5%.

Hysterosalpingographic analysis of the distal mucosal folds is also essential for estimating the likelihood of pregnancy. Thus, the outcome of the neosalpingostomy depends on the fallopian operability score. Salpingoscopy enables the physician to look at the fallopian mucosa, which are indirectly evaluated in terms of the aspect of the fallopian folds on the HSG. According to the Boer-Meisel score [8], the likelihood of pregnancy is 40-50% for grade I or II mucosae but is below 5% for grade III mucosae. The latter aspect of the fallopian mucosa is usually clearly visible on the hysterosalpingogram and thus does not necessitate laparoscopy - the couple can be directly enrolled in an IVF programme.

The problem of proximal fallopian obstruction remains. Mucous plugs or spasms can occur in the proximal fallopian tubes (i.e. in the interstitial region) and may prevent the injection of contrast agent into the distal tubes. Mol [9] has shown that when a proximal obstruction is seen on the hysterosalpingogram, 40% of the subsequent laparoscopic examinations were normal (i.e. the absence of spasm during laparoscopy or removal of the mucous plug by the greater pressure of methylene blue injection during laparoscopy, relative to contrast agent injection in HSG). Conversely, the same author found that 7% of women with normal HSG results displayed proximal fallopian obstruction (due to spasm) during laparoscopy. Overall, he concluded that when HSG had been performed within the previous ten months and had given normal results, laparoscopy only revealed 4.5% of fallopian lesions (36 out of 794 procedures); this percentage is very different from the values given above and may not justify the performance of useless, systematic laparoscopy in 95.5% of women. Observation of a proximal obstruction on the hysterosalpingogram justifies the performance of selective salpingography [10].

2. The Case of Endometriosis

Pelvic endometriosis is the pathology at the heart of the debate on systematic use of laparoscopy. Endometriosis can already be suggested by a clinical examination (pain), pelvic ultrasound (endometrioma) and/or HSG (rigidity of the cornua, tuba erecta, signs of salpingitis isthmica nodosa in the proximal fallopian tubes, etc.) but can only be truly confirmed by laparoscopy (black nodules, ligament retraction, adhesions, etc.). However, endometriosis presents a heterogeneous set of clinical symptoms and is even asymptomatic in many women [11]. It has not been established whether moderately severe endometriosis has a negative impact on fertility in the absence of other lesions; it is considered that endometriosis is associated with infertility in 10 to 50% of cases. Whereas Strathy [12] showed that the risk of infertility was multiplied 20-fold if endometriosis was present and Hughes [13] reported a monthly fertility rate of 2-10% for women with endometriosis versus 15-20% in the general population, Dugli and Saleh [14] did not find any relationship between endometriosis and the occurrence of pregnancy. Likewise, Marana [15] found that the pregnancy rate did not vary according to the endometriosis stage (except when fallopian lesions were present).

The main justification of use of laparoscopy in cases of endometriosis has been the Canadian study by Marcoux and Maheux [16] on 341 infertile women. It showed that destruction of the lesions in stage I or II endometriosis could improve the pregnancy rate. After 36 weeks of follow-up, cumulative pregnancy rates were significantly higher in the laparoscopy plus treatment group (i.e. destruction or exeresis of the lesions) (n=172) than in the laparoscopy-only group (n=169): 30.7 versus 17.7%, respectively (odds ratio (OR): 1.7; 95% confidence interval (CI): 1.2-2.6). In Marcoux and Maheux's study, 12 treatments of stage I-II endometriosis were need to obtain one additional pregnancy; if one considers that the prevalence of endometriosis is 30%, almost 40 women would have to be operated on to obtain that additional pregnancy. Donnez [17] subsequently confirmed this approach but combined drug treatment with the surgical procedure. Above all, laparoscopy appears to be essential prior to initiation of treatment with a gonadotropin releasing hormone (GnRH) agonist. However, the value of drug-based treatment of endometriosis in cases of infertility has not been demonstrated and only the surgical treatment of stage IV fallopian lesions (which are usually suspected after HSG) improves the pregnancy rate. Conversely, an Italian study [18] using a similar methodology (n=101) did not find any significant difference in the successful pregnancy rate one year after laparoscopy (19.6% in the destruction group versus 22.2% in the abstention group). These two studies [16, 18] were not free of bias. In the Canadian study, the women were informed of the result of the randomisation and the pregnancy rate observed in the control group was lower than expected. In the Italian study, histological confirmation of the endometriosis was not required, the duration of infertility was significantly longer and a large proportion of the women had taken GnRH agonists after laparoscopy. Of course, a meta-analysis [19] of the two studies concluded that treatment of stage I-II endometriosis lesions was beneficial (OR: 1.7; 95%CI: 1.1-2.5), essentially due to the difference in population size between these two studies, as is also recommended by the European Society of Human Reproduction and Embryology (ESHRE) [11] and the French National College of Gynaecologists and Obstetricians (CNGOF) [20]. Hence, the CNGOF states that "when laparoscopy is performed, surgical treatment of the lesions is recommended whenever possible, in order to improve fertility (grade B)".

There is still great debate as to whether it is necessity to perform laparoscopy with the sole objective of detecting stage I or II endometriosis (which does not clearly appear to be responsible for infertility, although treatment of the condition appears to be beneficial). Some authors are in favour of systematic laparoscopy for endometriosis screening [21-24], whereas others oppose use of this technique [25-28]. Even the ESHRE guidelines only recommend laparoscopy when endometriosis is symptomatic [11]. In a randomized, prospective series, Tanahatoe [29] showed that laparoscopy performed in the aftermath of six cycles of intra-uterine insemination (IUI) did not reveal further infertility-causing anomalies when compared with immediate, pre-IUI laparoscopy and thus does not have value in terms of improving the chances of pregnancy. Likewise, Werbrouck [30] studied the cumulative pregnancy rates after stimulation and IUI in women having undergone surgical treatment of mild or moderate endometriosis (n=58; 137 cycles), relative to women with unexplained infertility (n=49; 122 cycles). The pregnancy rates per cycle were identical (about 20%), as were the cumulative rates after four IUI cycles (about 70%). Hence, we believe that there is no value in using laparoscopy in the treatment of endometrial lesions because it will not improve the pregnancy rate.

Conclusions

This article is not a condemnation of the diagnostic and therapeutic value of laparoscopy but seeks to question the systematic use of this technique in infertility assessments.

In our opinion, laparoscopy is of course indicated in infertility assessments not only when anomalies are revealed by hysterosalpingography (or HyCoSy) but also in the following circumstances:

- a history of infection (especially a positive *Chlamydia* antibody blood test) and/or pelvic surgery (a significant risk of adhesions).
- unexplained secondary infertility.
- unexplained infertility after the age of 37-38 (when choosing between artificial insemination and direct enrolment in an IVF programme).
- the failure of 3 or 4 cycles of good-quality intra-uterine inseminations (with ovarian stimulation and a sufficient number of spermatozoids).

Lastly, after the abandonment of microlaparoscopy [31], transvaginal hydrolaparoscopy (also known as fertiloscopy) now constitutes a surgical alternative to laparoscopy [32-34]. Nevertheless, its value in initial infertility assessment remains to be defined.

Conflicts of interests

The authors have no conflicts of interest to declare.

References

[1]   Chapron C, Pierre F, Querleu D, Dubuisson JB. Complications of laparoscopy in gynecology. *Gynecol. Obstet. Fertil.* 2001;29:605-12.

[2]   Kontorvdis A, Chryssikipoulos A, Hassiakos D, Liapis A, Zourlas PA. The diagnostic value of laparoscopy in 2365 patients with acute and chronic pelvic pain. *Int. J. Gynecol. Obstet.* 1996;52:243-8.

[3]   Härkki-Siren P, Sjöberg J, Kurki T. Major complications of laparoscopy: a follow-up Finnish study. *Obstet. Gynecol.* 1999;94:94-8.

[4]   Ubaldi F, Wissanto A, Camus M, Tournaye H, Clasen K, Devroey P. The role of transvaginal ultrasonography in the detection of pelvic pathologies in the infertility workup. *Hum. Reprod.* 1998;13:330-3.

[5]   Ayida G, Chamberlain P, Barlow D, Koninckx P, Golding S, Kennedy S. Is routine diagnostic laparoscopy for infertility still justified ? A pilot study assessing the use of hysterosalpingo-contrast sonography and magnetic resonance imaging. *Hum. Reprod.* 1997;12:1436-9.

[6]   Boudghene FP, Bazot M, Robert Y, Perrot N, Rocourt N, Antoine JM, *et al.* Assessment of Fallopian tube patency by HyCoSy : comparison of a positive contrast agent with saline solution. *Ultrasound Obstet. Gynecol.* 2001;18:525-30.

[7]   Hauge K, Flo K, Riedhart M, Granberg S. Can ultrasound-based investigations replace laparoscopy and hysteroscopy in infertility ? *Eur. J. Obstet. Gynecol. Reprod. Biol.* 2000;92:167-70.

[8]   Boer-Meisel ME, te Velde ER, Habbema JD, Kardaun JW. Predicting the pregnancy outcome in patients treated for hydrosalpinx: a prospective study. *Fertil. Steril.* 1986;45:23-9.

[9]   Mol BMJ, Collins JA, Burrows EA, van der Veen F, Bossuyt PMM. Comparison of hysterosalpingography and laparoscopy in predicting fertility outcome. *Hum. Reprod.* 1999;14:1237-42.

[10] Woolcott R, Fisher S, Thomas J, Kable W. A randomized, prospective, controlled study of laparoscopic dye studies and selective salpingography as diagnostic tests of fallopian tube patency. *Fertil. Steril.* 1999;72:879-84.

[11] Kennedy S, Bergqvist A, Chapron C, D'Hooghe T, Dunselman G, Greb R, *et al.* ESHRE guideline for the diagnosis and treatment of endometriosis. *Hum. Reprod.* 2005;20:2698-704.

[12] Strathy JH, Molgaard CA, Coulam CB, Melton 3rd LJ. Endometriosis and infertility: a laparoscopy study of endometriosis among fertile and infertile women. *Fertil. Steril.* 1982;38:667-72.

[13] Hughes EG, Fedorkow DM, Collins JA. A quantitative overview of controlled trials in endometriosis-associated infertility. *Fertil. Steril.* 1993;59:963-70.

[14] Dlugi AM, Saleh WA, Jacobsen G. KTP/532 laser laparoscopy in the treatment of endometriosis-associated infertility. *Fertil. Steril.* 1992;57:1186-93.

[15] Marana R, Paielli FV, Muzzi L, Dell'Acqua S, Mancuso S. GnRH analogs versus expectant management in minimal and mild endometriosis-associated infertility. *Acta Eur. Fertil.* 1994;25:37-41.

[16] Marcoux S, Maheux R, Berube S. Laparoscopic surgery in infertile women with minimal or mild endometriosis. Canadian Collaborative Group on Endometriosis. *N. Engl. J. Med.* 1997;337:217-22.

[17] Donnez J, Squifflet J, Pirard C, Jadoul P, Wyns C, Smets M. The efficacy of medical and surgical treatment of endometriosis-associated infertility and pelvic pain. *Gynecol. Obstet. Invest.* 2002;54:2-7.

[18] Parazzini F. Ablation of lesions or no treatment in minimal-mild endometriosis in infertile women: a randomized trial. Gruppo Italiano per lo Studio dell'Endometriosi. *Hum. Reprod.* 1999;14:1332-4.

[19] Jacobson TZ, Barlow DH, Konninckx PR, Olive D, Farquhar C. Laparoscopic surgery for subfertility associated with endometriosis (cochrane review). *Cochrane Database Syst Rev* 2002;4:CD001398.

[20] Pouly JL, . Endometriosis related infertility. *J. Gynecol. Obstet. Biol. Reprod.* 2007;36:151-61.

[21] Corson SL, Cheng A, Gutmann JN. Laparoscopy in the "normal" infertile patient: a question revisited. *J. Am. Assoc. Gynecol. Laparosc.* 2000;7:317-24.

[22] Elsheikh A, Milingos S, Loutradis D, Kallipolitis G, Michalas S. Endometriosis and reproductive disorders. *Ann. N. Y. Acad Sci.* 2003;997:247-54.

[23] Akande VA, Hunt LP, Cahill DJ, Jenkins JM. Difference in time to natural conception between women with unexplained infertility and infertile women with minor endometriosis. *Hum. Reprod.* 2004;19:96-103.

[24] Hoshiai H. Current guidelines for treatment of endometriosis. The present status in Japan. *Drugs Today* 2005;41:17-21.

[25] Balasch J. Investigation of the infertile couple in the era of assisted reproductive technology: a time for reappraisal. *Hum. Reprod.* 2000;15:2251-7.

[26] Fatum M, Laufer N, Simon A. Should diagnostic laparoscopy be performed after normal hysterosalpingography in treating infertility suspected to be of unknown origin? *Hum. Reprod.* 2002;17:1-3.

[27] Lavy Y, Lev-Sagie A, Holtzer H, Revel A, Hurwitz A. Should laparoscopy be a mandatory component of the infertility evaluation in infertile women with normal hysterosalpingogram or suspected unilateral distal tubal pathology? *Eur. J. Obstet Gynecol. Reprod. Biol.* 2004;114:64-8.

[28] Erel CT, Senturk LM. Is laparoscopy necessary before assisted reproductive technology? *Curr. Opin. Obstet. Gynecol.* 2005;17:243-8.

[29] Tanahatoe SJ, Lambalk CB, Hompes PG. The role of laparoscopy in intrauterine insemination: a prospective randomized reallocation study. *Hum. Reprod.* 2005;20:3225-30.

[30] Werbrouck E, Spiessens C, Meulemen C, D'Hooghe T. No difference in cycle pregnancy rate and in cumulative live-birth rate between women with surgically treated minimal to mild endometriosis and women with unexplained infertility after controlled ovarian hyperstimulation and intrauterine insemination. *Fertil. Steril.* 2006;86:566-71.

[31] Benifla JL, Madelenat P. Microlaparoscopy under local anesthesia using a laparoscope under local anesthesia with sedation – arguments for ! *Gynecol. Obstet. Fertil.* 2000;28:78-83.

[32] Gordts S, Campo R, Rombauts L, Brosens I. Transvaginal hydrolaparoscopy as an outpatient procedure for infertility investigation. *Hum. Reprod.* 1998;13:99-103.

[33] Darai E, Dessolle L, Lecuru F, Soriano D. Transvaginal hydrolaparoscopy compared with laparoscopy for the evaluation of infertile women: a prospective comparative blind study. *Hum. Reprod.* 2000;15:2379-82.

[34] Nohuz E, Pouly JL, Bolandard F, Rabischong B, Jardon K, Cotte B, *et al.* Fertiloscopy: Clermont-Ferrand's experiment. *Gynecol. Obstet. Fertil.* 2006;34:894-9.

In: Laparoscopy: New Developments, Procedures and Risks   ISBN: 978-1-61470-747-9
Editor: Hana Terzić, pp. 261-278   ©2012 Nova Science Publishers, Inc.

Chapter XIV

Laparoscopic Approach of Failed Antireflux Surgery. Indications for Surgery and Technical Details

Elia Pérez-Aguirre, Andrés Sánchez-Pernaute[*],
Inmaculada Domínguez and Antonio Torres
Department of Surgery, Hospital Clínico San Carlos, Madrid, Spain.

Abstract

Introduction. A second operation after an unsuccessful antireflux surgery is a challenge for the esophago-gastric surgeon. A second laparoscopic access to the hiatus is usually technically demanding, as adherences of the previous operation generally complicate the identification of the anatomic structures. Inadvertent damage to abdominal or thoracic viscera is easier to perform. Besides, a functional satisfactory result is more difficult to achieve. In this setting, a thorough anatomic and functional study should be carried out for every patient to calibrate the possible benefits of a potential second operation with the risk of a revisional surgery, given that medical therapy is also available even for resistant cases. In the present work we report our last 10-year experience in the diagnostic workup and treatment of antireflux surgery failure, and we discuss the most convenient way to approach a revisional operation.

Patients and method. From January 2001 to December 2010, 39 consecutive patients have been evaluated in our department for a failure of a previous antireflux operation. Patients were usually referred for a maintenance or recurrence of preoperative symptoms, and occasionally for the appearance of new symptoms after the operation. A diagnostic workup was carried out comprising a personal interview, functional tests including pHmetry and manometry, and recently high resolution manometry and impedanciometry,

[*] Correspondence should be submitted to: Andrés Sánchez-Pernaute, MD, PhD, Department of Surgery, 3ª planta, ala Sur, Hospital Clínico San Carlos, c/Martín Lago s/n, Madrid 28040, Spain, Telephone: +34 1 330 3184, Fax:+34 1 330 3183, e-mail:asanchezp.hcsc@salud.madrid.org, pernaute@yahoo.com

endoscopy, a barium swallow X-ray study and in the past two years a computed tomography (CT) with 3d reconstruction. Patients were classified according to the different mechanisms of failure into: a) fundoplication disruption, b) fundoplication slippage, c) fundoplication migration to the thorax or type I hiatal hernia, d) paraesophageal herniation, d) twisted fundoplication, e) misdiagnosis, f) mixed failure and e) another non-previously classified failure including a finally unidentified cause of failure.

Results. Thirty-nine patients with failure of a first fundoplication were evaluated, 24 women and 15 men, with a mean age of 49 years at the first operation. Gastroesophageal reflux was the indication for surgery in 82% of the patients, and hiatal hernia with no evidence of reflux in the other 5. Globally, some kind of hiatal hernia was present in 22 patients, 80% of them a type I hernia; a giant hernia with an intrathoracic stomach was present in 7 patients. Seventeen patients had a histologically proven Barrett's esophagus, in 4 cases submitted previously to argon or radiofrequency ablation. Most first operations consisted on a standard calibrated Nissen laparoscopic fundoplication. The mean time for symptoms recurrence was 31 months. The first symptom of recurrence was mostly heartburn, followed by dysphagia. Thirty-four patients have been submitted to a second operation. The most frequent diagnosis was fundoplication disruption (10 cases), followed by migration of the fundoplication to the thorax (9 cases) and paraesophageal hernia (8 patients). Reoperations consisted mostly on fundoplication "redo" (21 patients) and mesh hiatoplasty (17 cases). Ten patients have documented recurrence after the second operation (29%), with 6 patients being submitted to a third operation (17.6%).

Conclusions. Revisional surgery of the hiatus is indicated mainly for failure to control gastroesophageal reflux or for thoracic ascension either of a part of the stomach or of the first fundoplication. Recurrence after a revisional surgery presents in one-quarter of the re-operated patients. A complete diagnostic workup and a meticulous operation are mandatory to reduce the recurrence rate, given that a third operation carries out a high risk of esophagectomy.

Introduction

Laparoscopic surgery of the esophageal hiatus has undoubtedly become the gold standard treatment for gastroesophageal reflux disease (GERD) and hiatal hernia (HH) (1, 2, 3). The most frequently operation performed today is the laparoscopic "floppy Nissen" fundoplication, a modification from the original Nissen procedure, in which a complete mobilization of the gastric fundus by means of division of the short gastric vessels, mobilization of the distal esophagus, closure of the diaphragmatic crura over a large esophageal bougie (usually 60 French) and a 2 – 3 cm total posterior fundoplication performed also over a calibrating intraluminal bougie, are the essential steps (4). Variations are frequent worldwide; many surgeons do not find necessary to calibrate the procedure, and many others do not routinely perform short gastric vessels division (5). The results of the operation are good in the control GERD, generally better than those obtained with proton-pump inhibitors (PPI), and as the procedure is performed through a minimally invasive access, it should be considered nowadays as the ideal treatment for complicated GERD or for patients who wish not to be lifetime dependents on PPI treatment.

However laparoscopic fundoplication is not 100% effective in the control of GERD, and a 3 to 5% failure rate is expected even in the most experienced hands (6, 7). When the procedure has been performed to treat a giant type III hiatal hernia, the problem is higher, as the rate of anatomic failures may be around 30% (8).

In specialized centers, surgeons are frequently confronted to treat patients with failure of a previous antireflux operation. This is a real surgical challenge, both from a technical and from a functional point of view. A second operation on the gastroesophageal junction is difficult to perform, as the anatomy of this delicate region has been changed and it is usually difficult to correctly identify the different structures. Lesions on the upper part of the stomach or on the esophagus are not infrequent, and if they pass unadverted or they are not appropriately treated, consequences for the patient could be dramatic. Even if the operation courses uneventful, a perfect functional result after a previous failure is difficult to get.

In this work we present our experience in the laparoscopic approach of revisional antireflux operations over the last ten years. Based on our results, we conclude some technical advices to follow when performing this kind of reoperations.

Patients And Methods

From the year 2000 to 2010, 39 patients have been evaluated in our department for a failure of a first antireflux operation. Six patients had been operated in another hospital, and the other 33 had been operated in our department. Twenty-four were female and 15 male, and their mean age was 49 years (23 – 73). The indication for the first operation had been GERD in 82% of the cases, and 7 patients had been submitted to surgery because of a symptomatic HH; however, some kind of hernia was present in 60% of the patients, mostly type I sliding hernia.

All our patients had been submitted to a complete workup consisting on pH-metry, manometry, barium swallow and endoscopy, to objectively document the presence of GERD, measure esophageal motility, find out the presence of esophagitis or other complications of GERD and correctly delineate the anatomy of the esophagus and gastroesophageal junction.

After these, patients were submitted to surgery. Laparoscopy in our department is performed with five portals, three of 5 mm diameter, and two of 10 – 12 mm diameter. The pars membranosa of the lesser omentum is opened, with care to preserve the hepatic branch of the vagus nerve. Occasionally a left hepatic artery is found coming from the left gastric artery; it may be preserved, but it is usually divided to facilitate the operation. The right crus of the diaphragm is dissected, and the posterior esophagus completely dissected free from right to left. A tape is passed to encircle the distal esophagus. With a gentle downwards traction, the phrenoesophageal membrane is opened. Then the left part of the gastric fundus is dissected by division of the short gastric vessels, which is performed with the harmonic scalpel. At least 4 cm of tubular esophagus should be obtained after a proper mediastinal dissection. Care should be taken to preserve both vagus nerves. The diaphragmatic crura are closed with number "0" non-absorbable sutures over a large bore endoluminal bougie, 54 to 60 French. Then a 2 cm long, loose, 360° posterior wrap is build over the same Maloney bougie with three "00" non-absorbable stitches. The wrap is anchored to the esophagus and to the right crus of the diaphragm. This is an actualization of Donahue's floppy Nissen fundoplication, which was introduced to decrease the side-effects of the original techinque (4) (Figure 1).

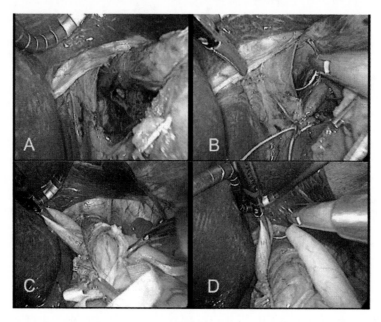

Figure 1. Four moments of a "floppy" Nissen fundoplication. A: Complete mobilization of the distal esophagus. B. Closure of the diaphragmatic hiatus with interrupted non-absorbable sutures. C: Passage of the fundic wrap behind the esophagus. D. First suture of the fundoplication performed over a large bore intraluminal bougie.

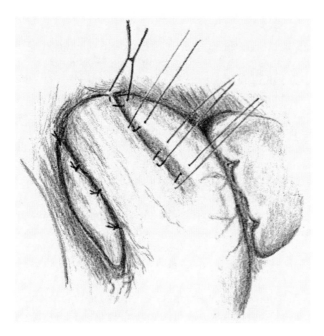

Figure 2. The partial posterior fundoplication described by André Toupet. Modified from reference "10".

When the patient has a severe motor disturbance of the esophageal body, a partial wrap is recommended. In these cases we prefer the posterior fundoplication described by André Toupet (9, 10) (Figure 2), instead of the anterior one described by Jacques Dor (11). The primer consists on a 270° posterior wrap anchored with two rows of interrupted sutures to both sides of the esophagus and the diaphragm; the latter is an anterior 180° fundoplication in which the anterior wall of the gastric fundus is sutured to both sides of the esophagus and to the diaphragm. Though it is not necessary, we routinely divide the short gastric vessels for both procedures, in the same way that it is performed for the total fundoplication.

When a large HH is found, and more than 4 stitches are necessary to close the hiatal defect, a prosthetic reparation of the diaphragm is performed. The mesh is placed around the esophagus and fixed with four non-absorbable stitches at the four cardinal points to the diaphragm (Figure 3).

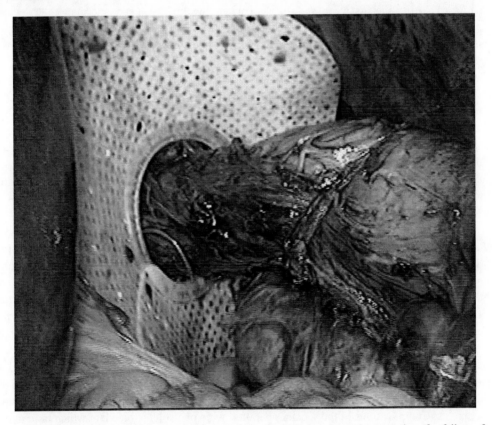

Figure 3. Circular mesh employed to reinforce the hiatus in large hernias and reoperations for failure of antireflux surgery.

In this series, 31 patients had been submitted to a floppy Nissen procedure, 4 to a Rossetti modification, 3 to a Toupet partial fundoplication and 1 to an anterior Dor's technique. The Rossetti modification of the original Nissen fundoplication consists on the performance of the wrap with the anterior fundic wall; only occasionally the author considered necessary to open the bursa omentalis and divide the short gastric vessels (12).

All the procedures were completed laparoscopically except for one: it was a patient who suffered from a refractory hypotension secondary to a low cardiac output after the pneumoperitoneum introduction and the forced anti-Trendelemburg position.

A mesh reinforcement of the diaphragm was employed in one patient.

Only 2 patients had some kind of postoperative complications: one had aspiration pneumonia and one had an upper digestive tract hemorrhage.

Results

GERD symptoms were resolved in all cases, but 3 patients experimented persistent dysphagia after the operation. Patients were visited at the first, sixth and twelve months, and then yearly. After the first year, endoscopy, barium swallow, pHmetry and manometry were routinely performed. Failure of the procedure was defined as the persistence of preoperative symptoms, recurrence of the symptomatology, the appearance of new unbearable symptoms secondary to the fundoplication, or misdiagnosis. The mean time from the operation to diagnosis of failure of the procedure was 31 months, with 35% of the patients diagnosed in the first postoperative year, 48.7% before the first 2 years and 74% within the first 3 years. The most frequent symptom of recurrence was gastroesophageal reflux (51%), followed by dysphagia (23%). After a complete preoperative study, which usually included all anatomic and functional tests as performed before the first operation, the suspected diagnosis was fundoplication disruption in 10 cases, disruption plus hiatal hernia (type I) in 2, fundoplication slippage in 4 cases, slippage with type I herniation in 3, migration to the thorax in 9 patients, paraesophageal hernia in 8, too-tight plication in 1 case, gastric stenosis in 1 case, and one patient was reoperated with no clear diagnosis of the cause of failure.

Thirty-four patients have been submitted to revisional surgery. A fundoplication disruption was found in 7 patients, and in 2 more there was an associated type I hiatal hernia; 5 fundoplications were found slipped or twisted (Figure 4), 2 of them with associated hernia; in 6 patients a paraesophageal hernia was found, and in 11 cases fundoplication migration to the thorax was the diagnosis, in 2 of them with partial fundoplication disruption. The other patients had a tight Nissen fundoplication, a gastric cancer and in one case no clear diagnosis was obtained after the exploration. The second operative technique consisted on the performance of a new Nissen fundoplication in 21 patients, change into a Toupet fundoplication in 5, a Collis gastroplasty in 1, a gastrectomy for a gastric cancer in 1 and a simple reduction of the herniation in 6 cases. Reinforcement of the diaphragm with a prosthetic mesh was performed in 17 cases, all of them with a circular mesh around the esophagus. Complications of the second operation were one splenic bleeding which motivated conversion to open surgery and splenectomy, and 2 gastric wall lesions (Figure 5), which were both intraoperatively diagnosed and treated with mechanical suture. All patients but one experimented improvement of their symptoms after the operation.

In the follow up, 10 patients have suffered a second failure (29%), though only 6 of them required a third operation (17.6%). The second failure was more frequent among patients with a first re-operation for recurrent reflux (usually disruption) than when it had been performed for some kind of thoracic ascension (migration, paraesophageal or sliding hernia). Four of the patients had a new herniation, one had severe gastroesophageal reflux with Barrett's esophagus and the other one a persistent dysphagia after reduction of a previous Nissen to a partial fundoplication which was still a severe barrier for an aperistaltic esophagus. Two thoracic approaches were performed (Belsey Mark IV procedures), one patient was submitted to a laparoscopic HH reduction and hiatal closure, one to a laparoscopic duodenal diversion, one to a new Nissen fundoplication and one to a Toupet dismantling for persistent dysphagia.

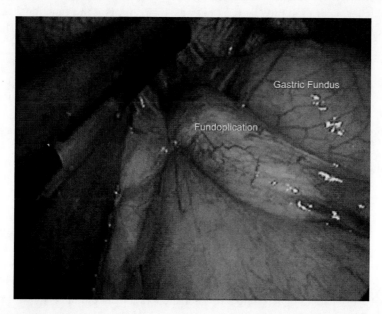

Figure 4. A "twisted" Nissen. Note the fundoplication is wrongly placed on the gastric body, making the effect of a gastric hernia.

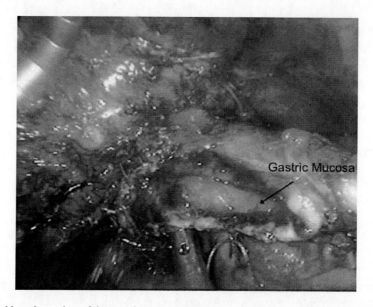

Figure 5. Accidental opening of the gastric mucosa during the dismantling of a partial fundoplication.

Discussion

Revisional surgery after a failed antireflux operation is a difficult task for the esophago-gastric surgeon. The first reports about reoperations in the esophageal hiatus published in the 1980's reflected how revisional surgery differed from primary operations in that morbidity was much higher, with mortality rates as high as 18%, and that the functional results were much worse, with control of reflux esophagitis in only 65% of the patients (13). The presence of adherences from the previous operation increased the risk of esophageal or gastric perforation, which happened in one third of the patients. Maher et al (14) published in 1985 a series of 55 reoperated patients on which a varied surgical approach could get a mean 80% success rate, with low morbidity and mortality; the authors defended a thoracic approach for reoperation, to avoid the "footprints" of the previous operator. David Skinner presented in 1992 a large series of re-operated patients with long follow up (15). The author reported a 72% success rate for the second operation, with a 1.7% mortality rate and 21% morbidity rate; a third operation was followed by a 66% success rate, which fell down to 50% after the fourth one. The second operation was a resective surgery for more than 20% of the patients. Some advices from Skinner had been effective for many years, and some of them are still in the "Decalogue" of the reoperative surgery: 1) it is of the greatest importance to carry out a thorough preoperative workup to perfectly know which is the real problem of the patient, what has happened and why; 2) though the surgeon should have a decision made on which technique to perform, the final decision should rely on the operative findings; 3) a transthoracic approach is advisable, even more when the first operation was made through the abdomen; 4) every patient undergoing a revisional operation should have a bowel preparation for the possibility of an esophageal resection and colonic interposition; 5) of course, reoperations on the hiatus should be always performed in highly specialized centers.

But the surgical scenario changed from head to toe with the beginning of the 1990's. Laparoscopy was the responsible for this change, and it was motivated by two facts: in first place, the minimal aggression of the "new" procedures induced a shift towards surgical treatment instead of medical therapy for uncomplicated GERD; in second place, many surgeons, not specialized in antireflux operations, and probably with "business orientation", began performing a good number of procedures, mostly in the private setting and with few, if any, preoperative studies to document the presence of GERD and to analyze the esophageal function. This situation led to an increase in the number of surgical failures, many of them secondary to a wrong technique. The minimally invasive access made the postoperative anatomy more suitable for a new intervention, and so the number of revisional operations also increased.

At the turn of the century some authors began reporting good experiences in the laparoscopic approach to revisional surgery of the hiatus. Hunter et al (16) published a comparative study between the results of open and laparoscopic revision, with rates of success around 90% for both approaches, minimal morbidity and anecdotic mortality. Laparoscopy was feasible for a reoperation after antireflux failure, and morbidity was low. However, 10 to 20% of the patients submitted to a second operation had to be operated again. The experience of the Emory University was probable one of the bests in the world, but even experienced centers could not repeat such a good results. Swanström et al (17), from Portland, Oregon, with an ample experience in laparoscopic surgery of the esophagus, reported a low rate of complications after revisional surgery, but a lower success rate than the group of Emory, with only 74% of excellent or good results after the second surgery. Gooszen et al (18), from Utrecht in The Nederlands reported a 73% rate of improvement or resolution in patients reoperated for recurrent reflux.

It seems clear that after the introduction of laparoscopic surgery, and after surgeons gained enough experience and skills to perform primary and secondary operations, morbidity of revisional surgery has decreased to acceptable rates, but functional results of reoperations are yet significantly worse than those obtained after primary procedures.

The first problem to face is to select the appropriate candidate for reintervention, i.e., the most suitable patient to obtain a clear benefit from a second surgery. The initial workup should focus on the addressing of the responsible cause of the surgical failure. The moment of presentation of the failure informs if there has been a real failure or the case is a persistence of the disease. In case of persistence, the first operation has been either wrongly indicated (misdiagnosis) or deficiently performed. In case of misdiagnosis, the real diseases should be searched for, but no time should be wasted and fundoplication should be promptly dismantled. If there is not a misdiagnosis, the diagnostic work-up is the same for persistence of the disease than for recurrence of the symptomatology. A complete functional study of the esophagus is compulsory, to diagnose the presence of gastroesophageal reflux (pHmetry), and to analyze esophageal motility and emptying (manometry and impedanciometry). Sometimes it is advisable to perform a Bilitec 2000 test to rule out the presence of alkaline reflux. Occasionally an esophageal emptying study by means of scintigraphy is also performed. The data obtained with these tests have to be compared with the first preoperative studies, to know how the operation has altered, improved or deteriorated, the esophageal function. An endoscopy has also to be performed to rule out esophagitis, and to study the endoluminal anatomy of the gastroesophageal junction (herniation or not) and stomach (correct fundoplication – centered –, hourglass stomach, twisted fundoplication...). A barium swallow is crucial to study migration to the thorax, paraesophageal herniation or sliding herniation, and it helps in the diagnosis gastroesophageal reflux and in the study of esophageal emptying. Recently we have added to our armamentarium the routine study with multi-slice computed tomography. Both the axial and coronal images (Figure 6), and the 3D reconstruction (Figure 7) seem to be of great utility for the surgeon before performing the revisional surgery. With all these studies an approximate diagnosis of the cause of the failure should have been obtained.

Now the question is, which are the patients who will respond better to a reoperation in the esophageal hiatus after a previous failure? The answer to this question is not easily found in the surgical literature. Gooszen et al (18) found that patients with a severe motor disturbance in the distal third of the esophagus, those who had suffered from a thoracic migration of the first wrap, and those being re-operated through the abdomen, were the ones who had a worse prognosis after the second operation. In Emory, John Hunter only found as a predictive negative factor for the second operation the presence of a HH in the first surgery (19).

In our experience, almost 20% of the patients submitted to revisional surgery of the hiatus need a third operation. Though our numbers are small and do not permit to get statistical differences, we can extract some conclusions from them. We observed 3 second-failures among 7 patients submitted to reoperation for a recurrent reflux, 42.8%, and 3 second-failures among 15 patients reoperated for a thoracic ascension of the stomach of the first fundoplication, 20%, $p = 0.5$. In 17 out of 34 patients, a mesh was left in the second operation. The second recurrence rate was 17% for patients with a hiatal mesh and 34% for those without hiatal prosthetic reinforcement (p = 0.43). These numbers do not reach statistical significance, but it seems that a thorough tension-free closure of the esophageal hiatus is associated to a lower rate of surgical failure. The mesh repair probably explains the differences found between literature series and ours, as the previously cited ones do not use any kind of hiatal reinforcement in reoperations (16, 18, 19).

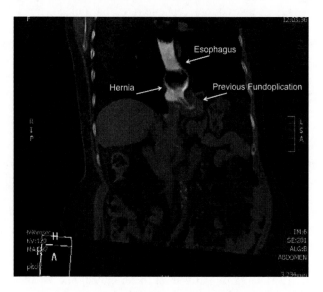

Figure 6. Computed tomography of a patient with a fundoplication failure. There is a slippage of the stomach through the fundoplication and through the diaphragmatic hiatus, making the effect of a type I hiatal hernia. The fundoplication is "anchored" to the diaphragm. Courtesy of Dr. Ricardo Rodríguez, Dept. Radiology, Hospital Clínico San Carlos.

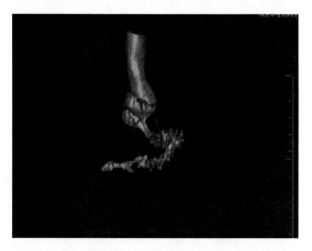

Figure 7. 3D reconstruction of the CT showed in Figure 6. The mesh ring is visible marking the diaphragm. In this image, it seems that the herniation is paraesophageal, with the gastroesophageal junction almost in its original place. Courtesy of Dr. Ricardo Rodríguez, Dept. Radiology, Hospital Clínico San Carlos.

The second question is to select the adequate technique for each problem. In the past, many surgeons considered that the second approach should always be performed through the thorax, as this was the way to avoid the adherences generated by the first operation (15, 20, 21) (Figure 8). Nowadays most of the experienced groups perform the second operation through the abdomen, and usually laparoscopically (16, 22).

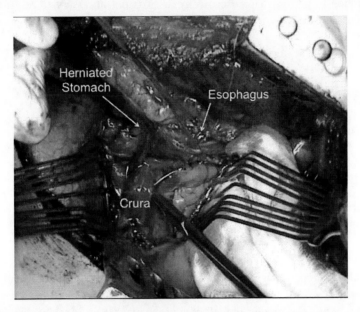

Figure 8. Migration into the thorax. Repair through a Belsey Mark IV operation.

Focusing on the precise technique, little is found apart from personal likings. It is clear that when severe dysphagia is the problem, and there is no other pathology to justify it, as a twisted Nissen, migration to the thorax or paraesophageal herniation, or a tight diaphragmatic closure, the second technique should not be a total fundoplication; but even this could be argued nowadays, as many surgeons consider that a short and floppy Nissen should not be a tight barrier even for a diseased esophagus (4). We think that if there is a severe motility disorder, a Toupet fundoplication is enough (10), and it is better to need some PPI any time than to be submitted to pneumatic dilations for a severe dysphagia and to repeat endoscopies for food impaction.

In cases of migration to the thorax or in the presence of a paraesophageal hernia, most of the groups consider performing some kind of reinforcement of the hiatal closure (23, 24). We place systematically a circular mesh, a PTFE plus Prolene dual mesh with a silicon ring protecting the inner part in touch with the esophagus (Figure 3). Other authors, however, defend the enlarging of the esophagus to perform a non-tension closure (25, 26, 27). This is achieved by means of a fundic wedge resection easily performed with a linear stapler over a gastric bougie, as it is performed when building up a sleeve gastrectomy for morbid obesity. In this way the rate of postoperative hernia is reduced, but pathologic reflux may persist, as the tubulized stomach serving as a new esophagus secretes acid, with no barrier against its rise into the unprotected proximal esophagus.

It is useful to remember that there are interesting alternatives for very special patients, as it is a duodenal diversion. When there is an unbearable reflux with severely altered esophageal motility, it is of no use trying to perform a new partial fundoplication. The best position is to totally eliminate the acid and alkaline reflux by means of a high gastric division with a Roux-en-Y gastrojejunostomy, as defended by Attila Csendes from Chile (28). This is an easy operation to perform laparoscopically, as it is not necessary to resect the excluded distal stomach, and there is no need to dissect the previously operated gastroesophageal junction.

How to Perform a Safe Operation?
Tips and Clues to Approach
the Operated Hiatus

We systematically approach the patient laparoscopically. Even patients submitted to a previous laparotomy can benefit from a second laparoscopic approach. Only for multioperated patients or for those with HH recurrence after a prosthetic transabdominal repair of the diaphragm, the thorax should be the choice.

The first steps of the operation should be directed in a very safe way. We almost systematically commence the reoperation through the great curvature of the stomach. It is frequent that the first operation had not a complete mobilization of the stomach by division of all the short gastric vessels, so this is usually – at least partially – a "virgin territory". After a complete dissection of the fundus, the left crus of the diaphragm is easily approached (Figure 9), and from here, we rapidly go into the mediastinum, which is also a "safe territory" (Figure 10). Then dissection turns to the right crus, usually occult behind the right part of the fundic wrap, which is found adherent to the undersurface of the left lobe of the liver. Here a great care is taken not to enter into the stomach. Once the mediastinum has been accessed from the left hand-side, the upper part of the phrenoesophageal membrane is dissected, and the upper aspect of the esophagus is identified. If there is any problem in a safe identification of the esophagus, dissection must be continued upwards, where there should be little, if any, footprints from the previous operation. The anterior vagus nerve is systematically searched for in this part of the operation. The tubular esophagus is encircled with a surgical tape, and our steps are directed to the right crus of the diaphragm. Here, the posterior vagus will be completely dissected (Figure 11) to avoid its damage and in some occasions to place the new wrap between the nerve and the esophagus, warranting a correct posterior fundoplication. If there is still any stitch closing the hiatus, it should be removed. Dissection continues up to the plane of the pulmonary veins, to get at least 3 to 4 centimeters of abdominal esophagus. It is frequent to open accidentally the right or left pleura, what is should not be a problem if the anesthesist is aware of it; in case of necessity, a pleural drainage should be inserted.

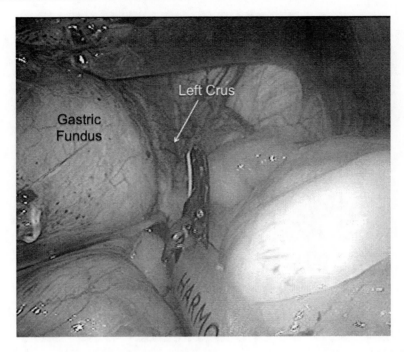

Figure 9. Revisional surgery. Dissection is commenced in the short gastric vessels up to the left crus of the diaphragm.

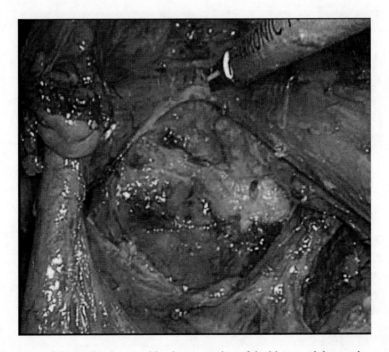

Figure 10. A vision of the mediastinum, with a huge opening of the hiatus and the esophagus dissected in the upper part of the image.

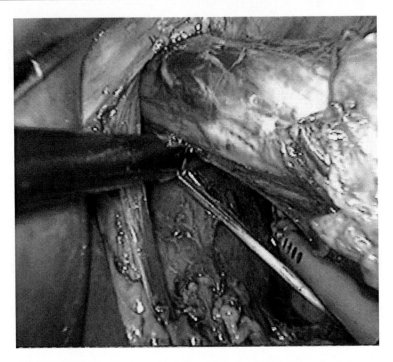

Figure 11. Dissection of the posterior branch of the vagus nerve.

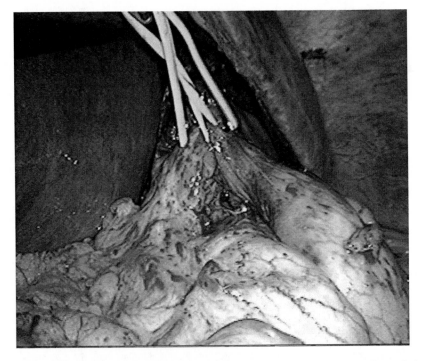

Figure 12. Redo-Nissen. The previous fundoplication has been totally dissected from the underlying esophagus.

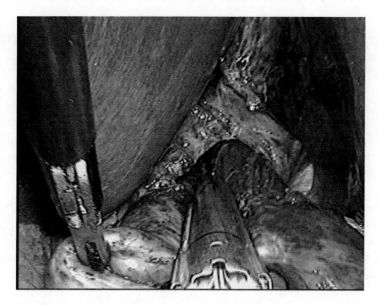

Figure 13. A stapler has been introduced to divide the fundoplication.

Although a correct fundoplication may be left untouched, if there is any doubt, the previous wrap should be dismantled (Figures 12, 13 & 14). We employ for this two parallel shots of a linear stapler, to completely remove the previous sutures. If the aim is to convert into a Toupet's procedure, a simple attach of the staple lines to both sides of the esophagus is enough to complete the operation. If the aim is to redo the Nissen, a new calibration is mandatory, to elude a tight plication.

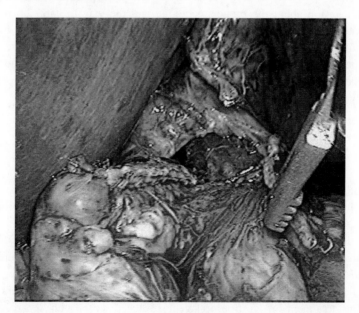

Figure 14. After firing the stapler, the previous Nissen fundoplication is converted into a partial posterior wrap.

A systematic gastroplasty is not our policy. Only in case there is insufficient esophagus in the abdomen, and there is no real possibility of getting a longer segment, a pseudo-Collis should be performed as described previously (27).

Finally, we defend the use of prostheses to reinforce the diaphragm. We have found that when there is any kind of migration to the thorax, or if a paraesophageal hernia has developed, there is a lower rate of recurrences when a mesh is interposed. We currently employ the circular mesh already described, which has a silicon ring protecting the esophagus. We have placed more than forty meshes in the last 5 years, including primary operations and revisions for failure, and we have only recorded one case of erosion into the esophagus detected in an endoscopy. The patient has a mild dysphagia, and tolerates a soft diet.

In our series there was only one case in which we could not affirm what was the real cause of the failure. In these occasions, there are two possibilities: a) to completely dismantle the previous fundoplication and repeat it trying to perform it correctly, or b) to try another kind of plication. Probably it is wiser to follow Skinner's commentary, and consider that if a properly build up fundoplication did not work, another type of wrap should be performed (15).

Finally, there is another point to consider: the esophageal function and the esophageal anatomy. It is absurd to try to perform a new barrier when there is a severe motor disturbance of the esophageal body, and when there is dysplasia it is a high risk to leave insufficiently treated a Barrett's esophagus. In these cases, a much better quality of life and overall, a safer policy from an oncological point of view, is to remove the diseased esophagus and to interpose a colonic segment (29). The operation should be performed with a vagal preservation, as defended by DeMeester (30).

In conclusion, operations over a previously operated esophageal hiatus are difficult to perform. The decision about the proper technique and the way to carry out the revisional surgery are both a challenge for the esophageal surgeon. These cases should be treated only in highly specialized departments, with experience in all the reviewed procedures, thoracic or abdominal, open or minimally invasive, resective or not. Recurrent reflux is not a malignant condition – though it could behave worse than that –, and morbidity of a second operation should be in the lowest rate, as mortality should be zero.

References

[1]   Hinder RA, Filipi CJ, Wetscher G, Neary P, DeMeester TR, Perdikis G. Laparoscopic Nissen fundoplication is an effective treatment for gastroesophageal reflux. *Ann Surg* 1994; 220:472-481.

[2]   Peters JH, Heimbucher J, Kauer WK, Incarbone R, Bremner CG, DeMeester TR. Clinical and physiologic comparison of laparoscopic and open Nissen fundoplication. *J Am Coll Surg* 1995; 180:385-393.

[3]   Peters JH, DeMeester TR, Crookes P, Oberg S, de Vos Shoop M, Hagen JA, Bremner CG. The treatment of gastroesophageal reflux disease with laparoscopic Nissen fundoplication: prospective evaluation of 100 patients with "typical" symptoms. *Ann Surg* 1998; 228:40-50.

[4]   Donahue PE, Samelson S, Nyhus LM, Bombeck CT. The floppy Nissen fundoplication. Effective long-term control of pathologic reflux. *Arch Surg* 1985; 120:663-668.

[5]   Yang H, Watson DI, Lally CJ, Devitt PG, Game PA, Jamieson GG. Randomized trial of division versus nondivision of the short gastric vessels during laparoscopic Nissen fundoplication: 10-year outcomes. *Ann Surg* 2008; 247:38-42.

[6]   Soper NJ, Dunnegan D. Anatomic fundoplication failure after laparoscopic antireflux surgery. *Ann Surg* 1999; 229:669-677.

[7]   Campos GM, Peters JH, DeMeester TR, Oberg S, Crookes PF, Tan S, DeMeester SR, Hagen JA, Bremner CG. Multivariate analysis of factors predicting outcome after laparoscopic Nissen fundoplication. *J Gastrointest Surg* 1999; 3:292-300.

[8]   Hashemi M, Peters JH, DeMeester TR, Huprich JE, Quek M, Hagen JA, Crookes PF, Theisen J, DeMeester SR, Sillin LF, Bremner CG. Laparoscopic repair of large type III hiatal hernia: objective follow up reveals a high recurrence rate. *J Am Coll Surg* 2000; 190:553-560.

[9]   Toupet A. Technique d'oesophago-gastroplastie avec phreno-gastropexie dans le cure radicales des hernies hiatales et comme complement de l'operation de Heller dans les cardiospasmes. *Mem Acad Chir* 1963; 89:394-399.

[10] Katkhouda N, Khalil MR, Manhas S, Grant S, Velmahos GC, Umbach TW, Kaiser AM. André Toupet: surgeon technicial par excelence. *Ann Surg* 2002; 235:591-599.

[11] Dor J, Humbert P, Paoli JM, Miorclerc M, Aubert J. Treatment of reflux by the so-called modified Heller-Nissen technique. *Presse Med* 1967; 75:2563-2565.

[12] Krupp S, Rossetti M. Surgical treatment of hiatal hernias by fundoplication and gastropexy (Nissen repair). *Ann Surg* 1966; 164:927-934.

[13] Zucker K, Peskin GW, Saik RP. Recurrent hiatal hernia repair. *Arch Surg* 1982; 117:413-414

[14] Maher JW, Hocking MP, Woodward ER. Reoperations for esophagitis following failed antireflux procedures. *Ann Surg* 1985; 201:723-725.

[15] Skinner DB. Surgical management after failed antireflux operations. *World J Surg* 1992; 16:359-363.

[16] Hunter JG, Smith CD, Branum GD, Waring JP, Trus TL, Cornwell M, Galloway K. Laparoscopic fundoplication failures. Patterns of failure and response to fundoplication revisión. *Ann Surg* 1999; 230:595-606.

[17] Khajanchee YS, O'Rourke R, Cassera MA, Gatta P, Hansen PD, Swanström LL. Laparoscopic reintervention for failed antireflux surgery. Subjective and objective outcomes in 176 consecutive patients. *Arch Surg* 2007; 142:785-792

[18] Furnée EJB, Draaisma WA, Broeders IAMJ, Smout AJPM, Vlek ALM, Gooszen HG. Predictors of symptomatic and objective outcomes after surgical reintervention for failed antireflux surgery. *Brit J Surg* 2008; 95:1369-1374

[19] Smith CD, McClusky DA, Rajad MA, Lederman AB, Hunter JG. When fundoplication fails. Redo? *Ann Surg* 2005; 241:861-871.

[20] Belsey RHR. Mark IV repairs of hiatal hernia by the transthoracic approach. *World J Surg* 1977; 1:475-483.

[21] Maher JW, Hocking MP, Woodward ER. Reoperations for esophagitis following failed antireflux procedures. *Ann Surg* 1985; 201:723-725.

[22] Pennathur A, Awais O, Luketich JD. Minimally invasive redo antireflux surgery: lessons learned. *Ann Thorac Surg* 2010; 89:S2174-S2179.

[23] Zehetner J, DeMeester SR, Ayazi S, Kilday P, Augustin F, Hagen JA, Lipman JC, Sohn HJ, DeMeeser TR. Laparoscopic versus open repair of paraesophageal hernia: the second decade. *J Am Coll Surg* 2011; 212:813-820.

[24] Targarona EM, Bendahan G, Balague C, Garriga J, Trias M. Mesh in the hiatus: a controversial issue. *Arch Surg* 2004; 139:1286-1296.

[25] Pera M, Deschamps C, Taillefer R, Duranceau A. Uncut Collis-Nissen gastroplasty: early functional results. *Ann Thorac Surg* 1995; 60:915-921.

[26] Swanstrom LL, Marcus DR, Galloway GQ. Laparoscopic Collis gastroplasty is the treatment of choice for the shortened esophagus. *Am J Surg* 1996; 171:477-481.

[27] Lin E, Swafford V, Chadalavada R, Ramshaw BJ, Smith CD. Disparity between symptomatic and physiologic outcomes following esophageal lengthening procedures for antireflux surgery. *J Gastrointest Surg* 2004; 8:31-39.

[28] Braghetto I, Csendes A, Burdiles P, Botero F, Korn O. Results of surgical treatment for recurrent postoperative gastroesophageal reflux. *Dis Esophagus* 2002; 15:315-322.

[29] Gadenstätter M, Hagen JA, DeMeester TR, Ritter MP, Peters JH, Mason RJ, Crookes PF. Esophagectomy for unsuccessful antireflux operations. *J Thorac Cardiovasc Surg* 1998; 115:296-302.

[30] DeMeester SR. Vagal-sparing esophagectomy: Is it a useful addition? *Ann Thorac Surg* 2010; 89:S2156-S2158.

In: Laparoscopy: New Developments, Procedures and Risks   ISBN: 978-1-61470-747-9
Editor: Hana Terzić, pp. 279-283   ©2012 Nova Science Publishers, Inc.

Chapter XV

Laparoscopy and Modern Management of Abdominal Trauma

A. Yakubu,[*a,b, c,] **V. N. Sitnikov**[d] **and V. Sarkisyan**[e]

[a] Rostov State Medical University, Rostov – On – Don, Russian Federation
[b] Jahun General Hospital, Jahun, Jigawa State, Nigeria.
[b] Kazaure General Hospital, Kazaure, Jigawa State, Nigeria.
[d] Rostov Emergency Specialist Hospital No: 2,
Rostov – On – Don, Russian Federation
[e] Thoracoabdominal Trauma, Rostov State Emergency,
Rostov – On – Don, Russian Federation.

Summary

The incidence of abdominal injury in all traumas is 1.5 to 18% and follows a pattern of continuous increase globally. Blunt abdominal injuries are usually associated with serious complications and a high mortality of 25 to 65% as a result of difficulty in prompt diagnosis and management, and are frequently associated with other types of injuries.

Diagnostic peritoneal lavage, ultrasonography, abdominal radiographs, and computed tomography are commonly used for triage of patients with abdominal trauma. The listed diagnostic modalities are commonly used in hemodynamically stable patients with abdominal trauma as a means of diagnostic procedure and decision making for conservative or operative management. Some of the investigations are found to be unnecessary as the victims are hemodynamically unstable and require immediate operation. The time taken for triage using these methods sometime causes delay and leads to serious complications and even death due to inappropriate management in 17% of cases.

---
[*] Rostov State Medical University, Surgery No. 4, Hachishevasky 29, Rostov – On – Don, 344022, Russian Federation, E-mail: drakyakubu@yahoo.com

Hemodynamically unstable patients with abdominal trauma usually undergo exploratory laparotomies which are sometime negative, and expose the patients to additional needless surgical trauma.

Patients with small bowel, diaphragmatic and retroperitoneal involvement resulting from blunt abdominal trauma show no clear clinical or radiological signs on initial examination. In such cases missed diagnosis occurs in 47%.

Laparoscopy has been used for selected hemodynamically stable patients as a diagnostic procedure and to aid decisions for nonoperative or operative management. However, it is not commonly used as either diagnostic or therapeutic tool in unstable patients. Therefore, it is imperative to develop a technique and algorithm for management of patients with acceptable outcome at this era of modern surgical technology. For this purpose we chose this topic in this book to disseminate our vast experience in management of more than 3000 patients with abdominal trauma.

Trauma is a global public health problem of growing proportions, and is the main cause of death during the first half of human life span and the fifth leading cause of death in all age groups. Considering the high morbidity, mortality, disability, and age group involved in trauma, it is an important social factor that affects the working class worldwide today. Generally, the extremities of the patients' age range are less involved [1], as demonstrated by [2].

The causes were mainly road traffic accidents and falls for blunt injuries and interpersonal violence for stab and gunshot injuries.

Polytrauma is associated with multiple injuries occurs at war fields, where modern techniques have almost no role to play. Here the convectional laparotomy still remains the cornerstone for management of abdominal trauma; management of such cases requires special experts. In connection with this it is not included in this chapter of the book.

The incidence of abdominal injury in all traumas is 1.5 to 18% and follows a pattern of continuous increase globally. Blunt abdominal injuries are usually associated with serious complications and a high mortality of 25 to 65% as a result of difficulty in prompt diagnosis and management, and are frequently associated with other types of injuries as shown by [2].

Isolated trauma of the abdomen is seen in 5.1 to 20.4% of cases, but combined injuries are seen in 18.3–64% of cases [3]. Noncompliant organs such as liver, spleen, and kidneys are at high risk of injury due to parenchymal fracture 24– 60%). Urinary bladder and bowel are susceptible to injury too [4, 5,1]. Solid and hollow organ injury is observed in 4–31% [6].

The position, shape, and surface area of the diaphragm place it at high risk in all types of thoracoabdominal trauma and difficult to reveal during the initial evaluation [7, 1, 8]. Missed diagnosis, which occurs in 47% of cases, is still a problem in AT patients, and leads to inappropriate management in 17% of cases, which results in needless laparotomies, complications, and death [9].

Patients with AI are hemodynamically unstable and require immediate operation. They should be taken immediately to the operation room without further unnecessary investigations or interventions; most victims are hemodynamically unstable [1].

Clinical findings are essential in the management of all patients with AT but considering the fact that most patients (25–69.3%) are in profound shock or coma [1]), diagnostic techniques such as computer tomography and ultrasonography are more important in triage and management of AT [10, 4, 1].

It is imperative to develop a technique and algorithm for management of patients with acceptable outcome at this era of modern surgical technology. For this purpose we chose this topic in this book to disseminate our vast experience in management of more than 3000 patients with abdominal trauma.

Criteria for selecting patients for both VAL include penetrating injuries to abdominal or lumbar area, significant lacerations of the anterior abdominal wall and lumbar regions, signs and symptoms of internal-organ involvement, fractures of the lower ribs and pelvic bones, hemodynamic instability, and clinical or radiological findings that indicated an urgent surgical intervention.

Use of VAL as approach in unstable patients with abdominal trauma developed gradually than in hemodynamically stable patients. However, today its role in management of both stable and non-stable is well established and indications are increasing daily. VAL in the past was limited for and mainly in diagnostic purposes in stable victims. As the technology and experience have improved indications have also become more of therapeutic.

We have shown that there are no absolute contraindications observed for laparoscopy in abdominal trauma [6]. However co – morbid conditions, such as respiratory, cardiovascular and renal insufficiency, and excessive anterior abdominal wall scarring are relative indications for conversion.

VAL is performed in an operating room under general anesthesia. Arterial blood pressure, arterial oxygen saturation (SaO2), end-tidal carbon-dioxide capnography, and electrical cardiac activity are monitored closely. Once airway control is obtained and proper monitoring equipment attached, the patient and the video monitors are placed in the appropriate position for VAL. The patient's position is equally important for proper placement of instruments, good visualization of the involved part of the abdominal cavity, and performing any of the indicated interventions. Therapeutic laparoscopy is successfully used for splenectomy, small-bowel repair, liver repair, large-bowel repair, duodenum repair, gastric wall repair, diaph ragm repair, ligation of bleeders in the mesentery and omentum and distal pancreatectomy.

Pneumoperitoneum, which is necessary in VAL, leads to reduction of lung volume and cardiac index, systemic hypercapnia, and an increase in cardiac filling pressures and systemic vascular resistance. Because of this effect the technique is commonly used in hemodynamically stable patients with AI [9, 3, 8].

To avoid this disastrous effect of pneumoperitonium carbon dioxide is insufflated into the peritoneal cavity at low rate of 0.5mL per minute to a maximum intra-abdominal pressure of 9–12 mmHg. Trocar access incisions are placed in such that they could easily be used for opened laparotomy or thoracotomy in the case the VAL is aborted for conversion. Following the completion of procedures gas (CO2) is released from the abdominal cavity at a rate of 2.0 mL per minute, following the completion of the laparoscopy. Blood and clots are evacuated with suction instruments, abdominal cavities are drained, and damaged organs are repaired.

In cases where therapeutic VAL is not feasible the procedures are aborted and laparotomy/thoracotomy is performed for further management.

This technique makes it possible to use VAL in hemodynamically unstable patients with abdominal injuries. To easy the patients' management a simple algorithm is designed (Fig.1).

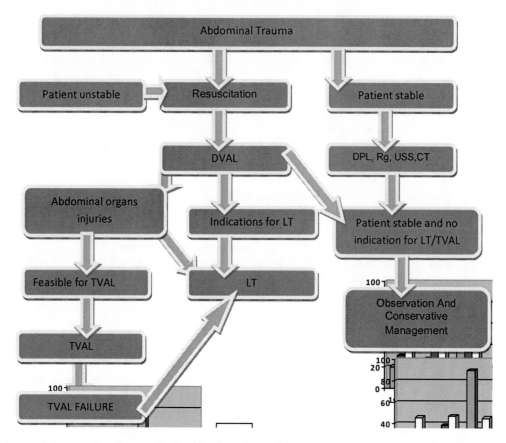

Figure 1. Diagnostic – therapeutic algorithm in patients with abdominal trauma. DVAL,Diagnostic video – assisted laparoscopy; DPL,Diagnostic peritoneal lavage; Rg, Radiography; USS, Untrasonography; CT, Computed tomography; LT, Laparotomy; TVAL, Therapeutic video – assisted laparoscopy.

VAL technique has shown 100% sensitivity, 88% specificity, and 91% accuracy, in evaluation and treatment of patients with AI [6, 9, 7]. Fifty percent of cases that usually undergo exploratory laparotomy can be successfully managed by the technique. In some these cases laparotomy turns to be a needless surgical trauma which even worsened the patients' postoperative condition and significantly affected their management outcome. VAL in expert hand protects 73% of cases from needless laparotomies and related postoperative complications [1]. There is a conversion rate of 10% from VAL to laparotomy.

Prognosis highly defends on duration of injury before surgery, involved organ, blood loss and associated injuries. Pneumonia, wound site infection, wound infiltration, evisceration, and bands intestinal obstruction are less common postoperative complications. Mortality and postoperative complications can be decreased to 4.7 and 7.9%, respectively [6].

Use of video-assisted laparoscopy in abdominal trauma has the following impacts:

1. VAL surgery is increasingly used in the abdominal trauma victims.
2. Diagnostic VAL has a significant role to play when conventional imaging is inadequate.

3. It provides a magnified view of blood vessels and organs, enabling clear sight of the injury, its location, and characteristics, and early determination of further definitive lines of management, especially when diagnosis is difficult and a hollow viscus injury is suspected.
4. It is less traumatic, and entails less postoperative pain, shorter hospital stay, minimal surgical scarring, and rapid return to full activities.
5. It is a safe, feasible, and effective procedure for the evaluation and treatment of hemodynamically stable and unstable patients with abdominal trauma.
6. It reduces the number of nontherapeutic laparotomies performed, postoperative complications and mortality rate.

References

[1] Lawrence W, Gerard M (2003) Management of injured patients. In: James R, William C, Frank R (eds) *Current surgical diagnosis and treatment.* Lange, New York, pp. 230–255

[2] M. Cherkasov, V. Sitnikov, B. Sarkisyan, O.Degtirev, M.Turbin, A. Yakub (2008) Laparoscopy versus laparotomy in management of abdominal Trauma. *Surg Endosc* 22:228–231

[3] Lujan A, Parrilla P, Robles R, Torralba J, Sanchez F, Arenas J (1995) Laparoscopic surgery in the management of traumatic hemoperitoneum in stable patients. *Surg Endosc* 9:879–881

[4] Jason S, Erica C, Scott D, Bin J, Michael S (2005) Abdominal trauma: a disease in evolution. *ANZ J Surg* 75:790–810

[5] Juan A, Hector A, William V, Walter W, Esteban G, Gustavo A, James M, George V, Demetrios D (2002) Penetrating thoracoabdominal injuries: ongoing dilemma-which cavity and when? *World J Surg* 26:539–543

[6] V. Sitnikov, A. Yakubu, V.Sarkisyan, M.Turbin (2009) The role of video-assisted laparoscopy in management of patients with small bowel injuries in abdominal trauma. *Surg Endosc* 23:125–129

[7] Friese R, Coln C, Gentilello L (2005) Laparoscopy is sufficient to exclude occult diaphragm injury after penetrating abdominal trauma. *J Trauma* 58:789–792

[8] Martinez M, Briz J, Carillo1 E (2001) Video thoracoscopy expedites the diagnosis and treatment of penetrating diaphragmatic injuries. Surg Endosc 15:28–32 *Surg Endosc* (2008) 22:228–231

[9] Carey JE, Koo R, Miller R, Stein M (1995) Laparoscopy and thoracoscopy in evaluation abdominal trauma. *Am Surg* 61:92–95

[10] Demetriades D, Velmahos G (2003) Technology-driven triage of abdominal trauma. The emerging era of nonoperative management. *Annu Rev Med* 54:1–15

Index

F

G

H

I

M

N

O

P

Q

R

T

U

V

W

Y